# Women's Health in IBD

## The Spectrum of Care From Birth to Adulthood

# Women's Health in IBD

## The Spectrum of Care From Birth to Adulthood

## Editors

### Bincy P. Abraham, MD, MS

Lynda K. and David M. Underwood Center for Digestive Disorders Houston
Methodist Hospital and Weill Cornell Medical College
Houston, Texas

### Sunanda V. Kane, MD, MSPH

Division of Gastroenterology and Hepatology
Mayo Clinic Rochester
Rochester, Minnesota

### Kerri L. Glassner, DO

Lynda K. and David M. Underwood Center for Digestive Disorders Houston
Methodist Hospital and Weill Cornell Medical College
Houston, Texas

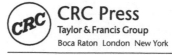

## CRC Press

Taylor & Francis Group
Boca Raton London New York

CRC Press is an imprint of the
Taylor & Francis Group, an **informa** business

First published 2022 by SLACK Incorporated

Published 2024 by CRC Press
2385 NW Executive Center Drive, Suite 320, Boca Raton FL 33431

and by CRC Press
4 Park Square, Milton Park, Abingdon, Oxon, OX14 4RN

*CRC Press is an imprint of Taylor & Francis Group, LLC*

Library of Congress Control Number: 2021951314

Cover Artist: Lori Shields

ISBN: 9781630918286 (pbk)
ISBN: 9781003526957 (ebk)

DOI: 10.1201/9781003526957

# Contents

# Contents

# About the Editors

*Bincy P. Abraham, MD, MS* earned her medical degree from University of Texas Medical Branch, Galveston, Texas, where she continued with residency training in internal medicine and fellowship in gastroenterology. During fellowship, she earned her degree in Master of Clinical Investigation and received specialized training in inflammatory bowel disease (IBD) through the Crohn's and Colitis Foundation in Cedars Sinai Hospital in Los Angeles. She is currently the Distinguished Professor and Director of the Fondren Inflammatory Bowel Disease Program at the Underwood Digestive Diseases Center of Houston Methodist Hospital. She is also the Program Director for the Gastroenterology Fellowship program. Her particular interest in IBD includes the transition of adolescent patients with IBD from pediatric to adult care as well as women's issues and pregnancy in IBD. She has chaired the Southern Regional chapter of the CCFA Medical Advisory Committee, has served as president of the Texas Gulf Coast Gastroenterology Society, and is involved in national committees for and is a Fellow of the American College of Gastroenterology, and American Gastroenterology Association, and Crohn's and Colitis Foundation.

*Sunanda V. Kane, MD, MSPH* received her MD from Rush Medical College in Chicago and did her residency there as well. Her Fellowship was at the University of Chicago where after training she joined the faculty until 2007, when she moved to Mayo Clinic in Rochester, Minnesota. Dr. Kane also holds a Master in Public Health from the University of Illinois Chicago; her Master's thesis was on the relationship between oral contraceptives and the development of IBD. Her career has been spent studying and championing gender related issues in IBD in the areas of menstrual related issues, fertility, pregnancy, and menopause. She has edited several textbooks within both gastroenterology and IBD specifically. She has written a book for patients on the management of IBD which is now in its second and soon third edition. Along with patient care, Dr. Kane continues to engage in teaching activities, research and serves as the Chair of Quality for her Division. She has been active as well in national societies and is Past President of the American College of Gastroenterology.

*Kerri L. Glassner, DO* earned her medical degree from Rocky Vista University College of Osteopathic Medicine, Parker, Colorado. She completed her residency in internal medicine and fellowship in gastroenterology at Houston Methodist Hospital, Houston, Texas. During fellowship, she received specialized training in IBD through the Crohn's and Colitis Foundation at Mayo Clinic, Rochester, Minnesota. She is currently an assistant professor of clinical medicine at the Fondren Inflammatory Bowel Disease Program at the Underwood Digestive Diseases Center of Houston Methodist Hospital. Her specific interests include pregnancy in IBD and liver disease in IBD. She is a member of the American College of Gastroenterology, American Gastroenterology Association, and Crohn's and Colitis Foundation.

# About the Editors

# Contributing Authors

*Anita Afzali, MD, MPH (Chapter 7)*
Associate Professor of Medicine
Director of Clinical Operations
Medical Director
OSU Inflammatory Bowel Disease Center
Abercrombie & Fitch Endowed Chair in
  Inflammatory Bowel Disease
Division of Gastroenterology, Hepatology
  and Nutrition
The Ohio State University Wexner Medical
  Center
Columbus, Ohio

*Jessica Barry (Chapter 2)*
Department of Pediatric Gastroenterology,
  Hepatology, Nutrition
Cleveland Clinic Children's Outpatient Center
Cleveland, Ohio

*Nirupama Bonthala, MD (Chapter 3)*
Cedars-Sinai Medical Center
Los Angeles, California

*Madalina Butnariu, MD (Chapter 7)*
Assistant Professor of Clinical Medicine
Division of Gastroenterology, Hepatology
  and Nutrition
The Ohio State University Wexner Medical
  Center
Women's Health in IBD Director
OSU Inflammatory Bowel Disease Center
Capsule Endoscopy Director
Columbus, Ohio

*Kindra Clark-Snustad, DNP, ARNP
  (Chapter 7)*
Inflammatory Bowel Disease Program
Division of Gastroenterology
University of Washington
Seattle, Washington

*Jordyn Feingold, MD (Chapter 4)*
Resident Physician
Department of Psychiatry
Icahn School of Medicine at Mount Sinai
New York, New York

*Sonia Friedman, MD (Foreword)*
Associate Professor of Medicine
Harvard Medical School
Associate Physician
Brigham and Women's Hospital
Boston, Massachusetts

*Jill K. J. Gaidos, MD (Chapter 8)*
Associate Professor
Department of Gastroenterology, Hepatology,
  and Nutrition
Virginia Commonwealth University and
  McGuire VA Medical Center
Richmond, Virginia

*Kelly Issokson, MS, RD, CNSC (Chapter 3)*
Cedars-Sinai Medical Center
Los Angeles, California

*Shelly Joseph, MD (Chapter 1)*
Postdoctoral Clinical Fellow
Division of Pediatric Gastroenterology,
  Hepatology, & Nutrition
Johns Hopkins University School of Medicine
Baltimore, Maryland

*Laurie Keefer, PhD (Chapter 4)*
Professor of Medicine and Psychiatry
Icahn School of Medicine at Mount Sinai
New York, New York

*Emilie S. Kim, MD (Chapter 5)*
Jill Roberts Center for IBD
Division of Gastroenterology and Hepatology
Weill Cornell Medicine
New York, New York
New Jersey Medical School
Rutgers University
Newark, New Jersey

*Dana J. Lukin, MD, PhD (Chapter 5)*
Jill Roberts Center for IBD
Weill Cornell Medicine
New York, New York

*Rebecca Matro, MD (Chapter 9)*
Division of Gastroenterology and Hepatology
Scripps Clinic
La Jolla, California

*Katrina H. Naik, MD (Chapter 8)*
Department of Internal Medicine
George Washington University
Washington, DC

*Maria Oliva-Hemker, MD (Chapter 1)*
Stermer Family Professor and Director of
   Pediatric Inflammatory Bowel Disease
Division of Pediatric Gastroenterology,
   Hepatology & Nutrition
Johns Hopkins University School of Medicine
Baltimore, Maryland

*Jessica Philpott, MD (Chapter 2)*
Staff Gastroenterologist
Assistant IBD Fellowship Director
Cleveland Clinic Digestive Disease Institute
Center for Inflammatory Bowel Disease
Cleveland, Ohio

*Eamonn M. M. Quigley, MD (Chapter 11)*
Lynda K. and David M. Underwood Center
   for Digestive Disorders
Houston Methodist Hospital and Weill
   Cornell Medical College
Houston, Texas

*Akriti P. Saxena, MD (Chapter 6)*
Pennsylvania Hospital
University of Pennsylvania
Philadelphia, Pennsylvania

*Ellen J. Scherl, MD (Chapter 5)*
Jill Roberts Center for IBD
Division of Gastroenterology and Hepatology
Weill Cornell Medicine
New York, New York

*Anil Sharma, MD (Chapter 9)*
Division of Gastroenterology and Hepatology
Oregon Health and Science University
Portland, Oregon

*Daniela Guerrero Vinsard, MD (Chapter 10)*
Department of Internal Medicine
University of Connecticut Health Center
Farmington, Connecticut

*Ryan Warren, RD (Chapter 5)*
Weill Cornell Medicine
New York, New York

*Sharmeel K. Wasan, MD (Chapter 6)*
Clinical Associate Professor of Medicine
Boston University School of Medicine
Gastroenterology Fellowship Program
   Director
Boston Medical Center
Boston, Massachusetts

# Foreword

The most common age of onset of inflammatory bowel disease (IBD) is between 15 and 35 years and most adult studies describe a female predominance with a female to male ratio of 1.1 to 1.8:1. In the past 20 years, there has been a revolution in IBD treatment with many biologics that are safe in pregnancy, burgeoning research in the areas of fertility and sexual function, and increasing knowledge in the areas of growth, nutrition, menstrual disorders, bone health, and menopause. Yet women, who constitute more than 50% of the adult IBD population, and who undergo complex hormonal, psychological and physical changes throughout their lifetimes, are often reduced to a "special population" in IBD curriculums. Women with IBD face challenges in multiple areas of life. They have increased sexual dysfunction, in particular dyspareunia and increased difficulty achieving orgasm, impaired body image, and increased depression and anxiety. Women with Crohn's disease, especially those who have had surgery, have an increased waiting time to pregnancy and women with active IBD and those who have had pelvic surgery have decreased fertility. Women with IBD who wish to become pregnant worry about the risks of passing IBD to their child and/or an IBD flare or IBD medication harming their child. Health care providers must be aware of and sensitive to these issues and know how to manage them. Sexual dysfunction, infertility and pregnancy, and the many nutritional, endocrine, and mental health issues specific to women cannot be relegated to a "special populations" section but need to be at the center of what every trainee is learning.

In that regard, *Women's Health in IBD: The Spectrum of Care From Birth to Adulthood*, edited by Bincy P. Abraham, Sunanda V. Kane, and Kerri L. Glassner is a perfect companion for all health care providers wishing to learn about women's health and IBD. It is an extremely comprehensive, well-written, and up-to-date text with the most current information regarding pediatrics, nutrition, and mental, endocrine, and reproductive health. All of the authors are experts in the field. The tables are informative yet concise and perfectly summarize the main points of the book. The chapters contain all of the information needed to care for female IBD patients from birth to childhood, adolescence, and adulthood. This book is truly a gem and should be an indispensable part of fellowship training as well as an integral part of patient-centered care. The editors' and authors' take-home message is that women's health is relevant to all areas of IBD and should be at the forefront of gastroenterology education, clinical research, and clinical practice.

—*Sonia Friedman, MD*

# Introduction

This book was written for anyone providing care to women with inflammatory bowel disease. There are many issues unique to women and understanding those issues will help optimize their care. The book is divided into chapters starting with pre-pubescent topics and progressing chronologically through the different stages of life. It is meant to be a guide with information that is current and evidence based. We realize that all patients should receive care that is individualized to their needs; this book helps provide some background as to what those issues may be and how to manage them.

# 1

# Birth to Puberty in Women With IBD

Shelly Joseph, MD | Maria Oliva-Hemker, MD

## Introduction

Inflammatory bowel disease (IBD), the umbrella term for the chronic gastrointestinal inflammatory conditions known as Crohn's disease (CD) and ulcerative colitis (UC), presents unique diagnostic and treatment difficulties in children. The incidence of pediatric IBD (onset at ≤ 17 years) continues to rise, with an annual incidence of approximately 10 cases per 100,000 and an estimated prevalence of 34 to 58 per 100,000 in North America.[1] Similar to what has been noted in adults with IBD, the reach of pediatric IBD now extends internationally, including in those regions where it was thought to be rare such as Asia and Africa.[2] Given that up to 25% of individuals with IBD are diagnosed by 20 years of age, it is not difficult to surmise that they will carry a notable lifelong disease burden.[3] This chapter will focus on particular challenges associated with IBD in children and the impact of disease on linear growth and pubertal development. Although pediatric IBD is typically diagnosed and managed similarly in both sexes, specific issues pertaining to girls and adolescent females will be highlighted when appropriate.

## Diagnostic Challenges in Pediatric IBD

The precise etiology of IBD is unknown, however it is thought to result from the interplay of genetic susceptibility in combination with a dysregulated immune response to the intestinal microbial environment in the setting of one or more environmental triggers.[4] Unlike in adults, where the prevalence of CD approximates that of UC, CD is about twice as common in children.[5] While most

Abraham BP, Kane SV, Glassner KL, eds.
*Women's Health in IBD: The Spectrum of Care
From Birth to Adulthood* (pp 1-19).
© 2022 Taylor & Francis Group.

reports indicate no difference in the adult male to female ratios for UC, epidemiologic studies of sex differences have historically demonstrated a female predominance of CD with ratios ranging from 1.1 up to 1.8.[6] This is in contrast to pediatric data where the sex distribution is reversed in CD with a male to female ratio of approximately 1.5 to 1.[5] At diagnosis, children tend to have more severe disease activity, greater disease extension into the small intestine for CD, and more colonic involvement in UC.[7,8] The more than 240 genetic loci implicated in IBD pathogenesis, the earlier disease onset in children, as well as the greater disease severity, underscore a possible increased genetic burden of disease in younger populations compared to adults.[9,10]

IBD diagnosis in children relies on clinical data obtained from the collective integration of a patient's physical exam, history, laboratory data, imaging studies, and endoscopic findings. There are challenges in obtaining the history at varying stages of development—in young children the caregiver typically provides the entire history and makes assumptions about the child's symptoms. The older child or adolescent may be hesitant to tell their caregivers or clinical providers about the symptoms that they might be experiencing due to embarrassment or fear of medical testing. Deciding whether a child should be evaluated for IBD can be problematic because the presenting signs and symptoms are often non-specific and can be associated with a number of other more common illnesses of childhood. Chronic abdominal pain, for example, is the most common gastrointestinal symptom in children presenting with CD, and it is also the most common gastrointestinal symptom in general among all children, effecting as many as 75%.[11] Diarrhea is another frequently encountered symptom in childhood that can be associated with infectious gastroenteritis. Oral aphthae, low grade fevers, rashes, and fatigue can occur with viral illnesses in childhood. Arthralgia, the most frequent extraintestinal manifestation of pediatric IBD effecting up to 25% to 35% of children, can be confused with growing pains or sports injuries.[5] Perianal disease including skin tags, anal fissures, and perianal abscesses have been noted to occur in up to 18% of children with CD, and these children are often misdiagnosed with constipation.[5] Weight loss can serve as a hallmark of malnutrition and chronic disease and can certainly be seen in children with IBD; however, it is important to highlight that the worldwide obesity epidemic has expanded the clinical picture and it can no longer be assumed that an overweight or obese child does not have IBD. In fact, approximately 10% of children with CD and 20% to 34% of children with UC have a body mass index (BMI) percentile that falls in the overweight or obese categories for age (BMI $\geq$ 85th percentile for age).[12,13] Normal results of routine blood tests such as a complete blood count, comprehensive panel, erythrocyte sedimentation rate, or C-reactive protein are insufficient to rule out an IBD diagnosis as they can be normal especially in mild, emerging disease in 21% of children with CD and 54% with UC.[14]

Ultimately, if the clinical provider does not recognize the signs of IBD in a child, diagnostic delays can occur. Although hematochezia from colitis typically does lead to a shorter time of diagnosis—from 0.75 to 4 months—CD of the small intestine, which often presents with intermittent abdominal pain in children, may have a diagnostic delay of more than 12 months.[11] Particular to children is the presentation of delayed linear growth and pubertal development which will be discussed in more detail later in this chapter. Growth failure by itself, which in some cases may be the only presenting sign of CD, can carry a diagnostic lag time of up to 18 months.[5,11]

Once there is a high enough degree of suspicion for IBD in a child, endoscopic confirmation of the diagnosis is recommended with both upper endoscopy and colonoscopy with ileal intubation. The endoscopic findings of IBD are similar in adults and children, although in some cases—especially in younger children, the histologic changes may be more consistent with acute inflammation rather than the typical chronic architectural changes such as intestinal crypt distortion and branching. Children generally tend to have more small bowel disease in CD with the ileocolonic phenotype occurring in as many as 63% of cases. Extensive colitis occurs in approximately 82% of children with UC compared to 48% of adults who have more proctitis or left sided colitis.[7,8] Unlike adults, where UC typically starts in the rectum and extends proximally in a diffuse manner, pediatric UC can be associated with rectal sparing in 5% to 15% of cases, histologic patchy gastritis in up to 22% of cases, and can have isolated cecal-appendiceal inflammation producing patterns that can be easily confused with CD.[15-17] Treatment goals remain the same whether children are diagnosed with CD, UC, or indeterminant colitis. Induction and maintenance of remission with corticosteroid sparing treatment regimens are preferred for the preservation of optimal growth potential and bone health, to prevent complicating disease behaviors, and to ensure an optimal quality of life.

## Very-Early-Onset IBD

Although the majority of children with IBD will be diagnosed in their elementary, middle, or high school years (median age 12.4 years) over the last decade the most rapidly increasing age group being diagnosed with IBD is children ≤ 5 years of age, who are referred to as having very-early-onset (VEO)-IBD.[1,18,19] Their presentation frequently involves diarrhea with or without blood and the initial disease phenotype is almost uniformly one of colitis, although over time the disease extent may progress to include increased small bowel involvement once children are 6 years and older.[19-21] Most of these very young children will be diagnosed with the typical polygenic or "classic" IBD, but initially it may be difficult to distinguish between CD vs UC and so they are often classified as having indeterminate colitis or IBD-type unclassified. Children with this type of VEO-IBD initially have milder disease activity compared to older children, but their disease may develop a more aggressive phenotype in the first 5 years post diagnosis as evidenced by the findings that they are more likely to be administered corticosteroids and immunomodulators.[19] It is uncertain as to why there has been an increased incidence of VEO-IBD within the last decade. Leading theories attribute the pathogenesis to the complex relationship between an infant's developing immune system and the intestinal microbiome, both of which are shaped in the first few years of life and are influenced by a variety of environmental exposures including antibiotic exposures, infant feeding habits, and maternal diet.[18]

Interestingly, as many as 15% to 20% of children with VEO-IBD are diagnosed with monogenic disorders that are being increasingly identified.[22] They commonly present in early infancy or within the first 2 years of life with more severe intestinal inflammation or perianal disease, although the endoscopic and histologic findings can be very similar to those seen in CD or UC. Their clinical course can be refractory to multiple immunosuppressive medications with associated high morbidity.[22] Monogenic IBD-phenotypes, which require genetic testing to distinguish them from "classical" IBD, have been grouped broadly into 5 categories—epithelial barrier defects, phagocyte defects, hyper/autoinflammatory conditions, B cell and T cell defects, and immune-regulation defects (Table 1-1).[18,22] In children who present with recurrent infections, persistent diarrhea, weight loss, and malabsorption, the more familiar primary immunodeficiency syndromes (also in Table 1-1) should also be considered.[21,22] Conditions such as common variable immunodeficiency, chronic granulomatous disease (CGD), Wiskott-Aldrich syndrome (WAS), immune dysregulation polyendocrinopathy and enteropathy (IPEX), CTLA4 deficiency, and XIAP deficiency are typically nonresponsive to routinely used IBD therapies. Indeed, immunomodulating therapies used in IBD such as anti–tumor necrosis factor (TNF) medications are contraindicated in the treatments of immunodeficiencies since they can further alter an abnormally functioning immune system.[22] Although some of these conditions, such as CGD, have a primarily x-linked mode of inheritance and therefore are more often diagnosed in males, family history might reveal that female relatives who are x-linked carriers of disease have a predilection for developing discoid lupus which is seen in 3% of the patients diagnosed with CGD and in 6% of the female relatives.[23] Genetic counseling is important for young women with family histories of immunodeficiency conditions as it can inform genetic counseling for future reproductive planning.[24]

The North American Society for Pediatric Gastroenterology, Hepatology, and Nutrition has provided recommendations for the evaluation of children ≤ 5 years of age in order to ensure that those with monogenic or immunodeficiency diseases are appropriately identified.[18] Even if children are older, but have a history of recurrent bacterial, viral, or fungal infections or have a course that has been refractory to multiple medications, these conditions should be suspected. Recommendations

## Table 1-1. Monogenic and Immune-Mediated Conditions Associated With Very-Early-Onset IBD

| CATEGORY | DISEASE | GENE | PHENOTYPE |
|---|---|---|---|
| Epithelial barrier defect | ADAM17 deficiency | ADAM17<br>Autosomal recessive | UC-like, inflammatory skin lesions |
| | X-linked ectodermal dysplasia | IKBKG<br>X-linked | CD-like, skin lesions, immunodeficiency |
| | Dystrophic bullosa | COL7A1<br>Autosomal recessive | Epidermolysis bullosa, strictures |
| | Kindler syndrome | FERMT1<br>Autosomal recessive | UC-like, strictures, epidermolysis bullosa |
| | TTC7A deficiency | TTC7A<br>Autosomal recessive | Intestinal atresia, immunodeficiency |
| | Familial diarrhea | GUCY2<br>Autosomal dominant | CD-like, strictures, diarrhea |
| | Neonatal inflammatory skin and bowel disease | EGFR<br>Autosomal recessive | CD-like, skin and hair lesions |
| Phagocyte defects | CGD | Multiple: CYBB (X-linked), CYBA, NCF1, NCF2, NCF4<br>Autosomal recessive | Granulomatous, CD-like, skin lesions, immunodeficiency |
| | LADI | ITGB2<br>Autosomal recessive | CD-like, immunodeficiency |
| | LADII | SLC35C1<br>Autosomal recessive | CD-like, immunodeficiency |
| | Glycogen storage disease type Ib | SLC37A4<br>Autosomal recessive | Granulomatous, CD-like, immunodeficiency |

*(continued)*

are directed at early identification of genetic disorders to identify the subset who will benefit from targeted therapies or from hematopoietic stem cell transplantation. Family history of early onset of IBD or IBD-like illnesses with perianal and fistulizing manifestations and a history of recurrent infections should raise the index of suspicion for these conditions. Basic immune function testing can begin with immunoglobulin levels (IgA, IgE, IgM, IgG), vaccine titers to assess humoral immunity if there is a positive history of receiving routine childhood vaccines, and a neutrophil respiratory burst assay to assess for CGD such as the dihydrorhodamine test.[18] Referral to an immunologist or geneticist should be strongly considered to enable more sophisticated immunologic evaluation and genetic testing.[18] Genetic panels can be obtained that can analyze hundreds of genes associated with inherited disorders of the immune system but ultimately whole exome sequencing or whole genome sequencing are increasingly being employed when targeted panels are uninformative.[18,22]

## Table 1-1 (continued). Monogenic and Immune-Mediated Conditions Associated With Very-Early-Onset IBD

| CATEGORY | DISEASE | GENE | PHENOTYPE |
|---|---|---|---|
| Hyper/ autoinflammatory | Mevalonate kinase deficiency | MVK<br>Autosomal recessive | CD-like, fevers |
| | FMF | MEFV<br>Autosomal recessive | CD/UC-like, fevers |
| | XLP-1 | SH2D1A<br>X-linked | CD-like, HLH |
| | XLP-2 | XIAP<br>X-linked | CD-like, penetrating disease, granulomatous, HLH |
| | Granulomatous colitis | TRIMM22<br>Autosomal recessive | CD-like, granulomatous, VEO IBD |
| | Hermansky–Pudlak 1,4,6 | HSP 1/4/6<br>Autosomal recessive | CD-like, fistulizing |
| Immune regulation defects | IL-10 signaling defects | Multiple: IL10RA, IL10RB, IL10<br>Autosomal recessive | CD-like, perianal disease, fistulizing, infantile onset, malignancy |
| | IPEX-like | IL2RA<br>Autosomal recessive | CD-like, skin lesions |
| | IPEX-like | STAT1<br>Autosomal dominant | CD-like, skin lesions |

*(continued)*

# IBD Effects on Growth

Growth failure and pubertal delay have been demonstrated in children with both UC and CD; however, overall there is a stronger association of growth derangement in CD.[25,26] Some of the earliest research in pediatric IBD involved analysis of its effects on growth. One such single-center study evaluated detailed growth charts for 48 children with IBD using 3 separate validated methods to estimate adult height and compared those results to their achieved adult height.[27] During the study period, 37% of the children with CD and 10% of those with UC had evidence of growth failure by at least 2 out of the 3 height estimation methods used. Although most were able to achieve the adolescent growth spurt, 31% of all children with IBD had permanent growth failure which translated to a 6 to 8 cm height deficit in girls and a 7 to 9 cm in boys on analysis of height-for-age growth curves. These results are supported by other early studies including one that prospectively followed 69 children diagnosed with IBD at 3-month intervals for 1 to 3 years, obtaining height velocity measurements and height-for-age z-scores.[28] In children, z-scores are reported as they represent a calculated number of standard deviations from the mean by age, thus accounting for dynamic changes in average growth measurements over time. This study found that 25% of the children

## Table 1-1 (continued). Monogenic and Immune-Mediated Conditions Associated With Very-Early-Onset IBD

| CATEGORY | DISEASE | GENE | PHENOTYPE |
|---|---|---|---|
| B/T cell defects | SCID | Multiple: ADA, LIG4, ZAP70, CD3γ<br>Autosomal recessive | CD-like, skin lesions, immunodeficiency |
| | CVID | Multiple: ICOS, LRBA | CD-like, skin lesions, immunodeficiency |
| | Agammaglobulinemia | BTK<br>X-linked<br>PIK3R1<br>Autosomal recessive | CD-like, immunodeficiency |
| | WAS | WAS<br>X-linked | UC-like, skin lesions, immunodeficiency |
| | Omenn syndrome | DCLRE1C<br>Autosomal recessive | CD-like, immunodeficiency |
| | Hyper Ig-E syndrome | DOCK8<br>Autosomal recessive | Granulomatous, CD-like, skin lesions |
| | IPEX syndrome | FOXP3<br>X-linked | Autoimmune enteropathy, skin lesions |
| | CTLA4 deficiency | CTLA4<br>Autosomal dominant | Lymphocytic colitis, immunodeficiency |

CD, Crohn's disease; CGD, chronic granulomatous disease; CVID, common variable immunodeficiency; FMF, familial Mediterranean fever; HLH, hemophagocytic lymphohistiocytosis; IBD, inflammatory bowel disease; IPEX, immune dysregulation, polyendocrinopathy and enteropathy, X-linked; LADI/II, leukocyte adhesion deficiency I/II; SCID, severe combined immunodeficiency; UC, ulcerative colitis; WAS, Wiskott–Aldrich syndrome; XLP I/2, X- linked lymphoproliferative syndrome 1/2.

observed had below-average height velocity z-scores and 40% had reduced height-for-age values, with patients with CD being 2 times more likely to have growth delays than patients with UC.[28] Growth delays are often thought of as a manifestation of active IBD symptoms, however, it can be the only presenting symptom as illustrated by a sentinel pediatric study that evaluated the growth of 50 pre-pubertal children with CD and found that 21 of those children demonstrated a reduction in height velocity prior to onset of any gastrointestinal symptoms.[29] This points to growth failure serving as an independent, early manifestation of disease.[10,34]

A child's height potential, which is largely determined by genetics, can be estimated clinically by calculating the mid-parental height. For girls, this is calculated by subtracting 13 cm from the father's height, adding this value to the mother's height and obtaining the average of those 2 numbers as per the following calculation:

$$girl's\ midparental\ height = \frac{[father's\ height\ (cm) - 13cm] + mother's\ height\ (cm)}{2}$$

For boys, the mother's height plus 13 cm plus the father's height is averaged.[30,31] Most children's final height will fall within approximately 8.5 cm of the calculated midparental height. This value is often utilized in conjunction with trends in age-based growth charts developed by the World Health Organization for children aged 0 to 2 years and by the Centers for Disease Control and Prevention (CDC) for children aged 2 to 18 years to monitor disease severity and response to therapies in pediatric IBD.[32] Likewise, bone age can estimate growth potential by measuring closure of a child's growth plates, typically by evaluating a radiograph of the left hand; with some recent evidence suggesting that children with IBD have the potential to continue to grow beyond projected closure of their growth plates, indicating possible delayed skeletal maturation.[33]

Growth impairment is the result of multiple factors, including decreased consumption of calories, malabsorption, and excess nutrient losses. Poor caloric intake is influenced by ongoing disease symptoms such as abdominal pain, nausea, and anorexia. Small bowel inflammation can result in malabsorption of macro- and micronutrients thereby contributing to growth impairment, osteopenia, and nutrient deficiencies. Colitis can lead to fecal protein loss and protein malnutrition.[5,34] Given the median age of onset of IBD of approximately age 12 years, the malnutrition that can be associated with CD or UC unfortunately occurs during a critical period of growth in childhood and adolescence when there are increased nutritional requirements at baseline to sustain the needs of rapid growth and development.[19,35]

A state of heightened systemic inflammation also results in increased metabolic demand and a higher overall catabolic state that improves only with improved disease control.[34] In fact it has been suggested that the inflammatory process itself effects the release of inflammatory cytokines linked to the inhibition of growth factors. Specifically, the inflammatory cytokine interleukin 6 (IL-6) has been shown to inhibit secretion of insulin like growth factor-1 (IGF-1) by hepatocytes and cartilage.[35] IL-6 acts by activating inflammatory cytokine pathways which in turn activate a signal transducer and activator 3 transcription factor that functions to regulate cellular response to cytokines and growth factors. This complex signaling pathway results in up-regulation of acute phase reactants and tissue inflammation but also down regulates tissue response to growth hormone and IGF-1.[36] Other pro-inflammatory mediators known to be increased in IBD such as interleukin-1 beta and TNF alpha (TNF-α) have also been shown to down regulate expression of growth hormone receptors and intermediate signaling molecules that result in diminished expression of growth hormone and IGF-1.[36,37]

Prepubertal girls after the age of 3 years typically grow at a rate of 5 to 6 cm/year.[31] Then with puberty a linear growth spurt occurs in female adolescents that produces an average height velocity increase of 8.25 cm/year. This increased height velocity slows after onset of menses (menarche) resulting in approximately 2 more years of increased growth velocity.[38] Onset of puberty and the associated attainment of peak growth velocity occurs in girls, approximately 2 years earlier than boys.[38] Hypotheses regarding the regulation and timing of pubertal onset are derived from research on primates and in observations of pathologic conditions of puberty such as hypogonadism. They suggest that various neurotransmitters including leptin, gamma-amino butyric acid, glutamate, norepinephrine, and dopamine may act on hypothalamic glial cells to signal the changes in gonadotropin-releasing hormone (GnRH) secretion that herald the initiation puberty. Furthermore, the findings that monogenic mutations can result in syndromes of abnormal pubertal development including Kallmann's syndrome and hypogonadotropic hypogonadism suggest that genetic factors likely also contribute to the sexual dimorphisms seen in male vs female timing of puberty.[39]

There has been extensive investigation evaluating the impact that IBD may have on achievement of adult height. Reported deficits in attainment of adult height vary from 3 to 9 cm in boys and girls with boys being more significantly negatively affected than girls in terms of their IBD associated growth impairment.[27-29] It has been speculated that girls might be somewhat protected from loss of growth potential experienced by boys due to the relationship between onset of puberty and timing of the growth spurt and the average age of onset of IBD in childhood. There is an increased incidence of IBD prior to puberty in boys compared with girls, which points to the earlier impact that inflammation might have on growth hormones prior to puberty thereby exacerbating the deleterious effects IBD has on growth potential in boys.[27]

Other studies have investigated sex-based differences in tissue responsiveness to growth hormones (GH), growth hormone levels, and sex hormones. Sex differences in tissue responsiveness to GH and IGF-1 have been attributed to cell signaling pathways mediated by the signal transducers and activators of transcription (STAT) proteins. Differences in STAT protein expression in males compared with females observed in mice indicate that these proteins are implicated in the differences between the way tissues respond to regulate transcription of GH and IGF-1 in males. In murine studies of growth, males were shown to have a less consistent response to the pulsatile release of GnRH in the STAT-GH cell signaling pathway.[40] Pediatric clinical data has shown that IGF-1 levels are reduced in boys compared to girls even prior to puberty. The rationale as to why this occurs remains unclear but given the known influence that inflammatory cytokines can have on growth as described previously, inferences can be made that inflammation has a stronger negative effect on expression of GH and IGF-1 in boys compared to girls.[41]

Although human GH has been used to treat GH deficiency and growth failure seen in conditions such as Turner's syndrome, renal failure, and idiopathic short stature; insufficient evidence exists to suggest that GH modifies the disease course in pediatric IBD. As such, injection of human GH is not routinely recommended and if considered should be used only in consultation with a pediatric endocrinologist.[42] Management of growth failure in IBD is aimed at supporting appropriate nutritional status and significantly limiting the use of corticosteroids due to their deleterious effects on growth and bone development.[43] Additionally, pediatric studies have shown that clinical response to corticosteroids does not translate to histologic mucosal healing or sustained remission.[43] If corticosteroids are required, typical daily doses of 1 mg/kg to a maximum dose of 40 mg (rarely up to 60 mg) are prescribed and tapered as quickly as possible approximately over 6 to 10 weeks. For ileocolonic CD, pediatric clinical trials comparing oral prednisone to budesonide, which has reduced steroid systemic availability, have shown equivalent remission rates of 47% and 50% ($P < .05$) based on disease activity indices, but more significantly reported side effects in the prednisone group compared to the budesonide group (71% vs 32%, $P < .05$).[44]

Head-to-head randomized therapeutic clinical trials are not available in children; however,[45] a clinical effectiveness study using a large prospective cohort of children stratified to either early (within 3 months) anti-TNF therapy (infliximab or adalimumab) vs early immunomodulators (methotrexate, azathioprine, or 6-mercaptopurine), demonstrated statistically significant improvement in average height z-scores only in the anti-TNF group. Similarly, the patients receiving anti-TNF therapy had statistically significantly higher rates of corticosteroid-free clinical remission at 1 year, 85.3% vs 60.3% ($P = .0017$), compared with the immunomodulatory group.[45] In light of this type of evidence, clinical guidelines issued by the European Society of Pediatric Gastroenterology, Hepatology and Nutrition (ESPGHAN) stipulate that when a child has increased risk factors for poor CD outcomes such asextensive disease, severe endoscopic ulceration, osteoporosis, or severe growth impairment defined as z-score greater than -2.5; then anti-TNF medications should be considered as first line treatment options to induce and maintain remission and preserve growth potential.[43] Recommendations such as these have led to decreased use of azathioprine, 6-mercaptopurine, and methotrexate as monotherapy in pediatric IBD.[43,45] Additionally, the combination of azathioprine and 6-mercaptopurine with anti-TNF agents is used sparingly in children with IBD due to the non-trivial risk of developing fatal hepatosplenic T-cell lymphoma, especially in young males under 35 years.[46] If combination therapy is required to reduce drug immunogenicity, methotrexate has become the preferred option although its use in children can be limited due to nausea and vomiting. Use of methotrexate in girls of child-bearing potential requires an open discussion regarding teratogenicity, sexual activity, and preventative contraception use.

Finally, in the pediatric literature there are robust data with CD showing that exclusive enteral nutrition (EEN) using formulas of all types from polymeric to amino-acid based are equivalent to corticosteroids for induction of clinical remission while at the same time improving nutritional status and helping to reverse growth impairment. In fact, studies report EEN significantly improving mucosal healing in 74% to 80% of children compared to 33% to 40% ($P < .05$) for oral corticosteroids.[47,48] EEN can be consumed orally or administered via nasogastric tube if not tolerated orally, typically for a period of 6 to 12 weeks. During this time whole foods in the diet are significantly reduced to between 0% to 20% of daily calories.[43,49] If induction of remission is achieved, the diet is then gradually liberalized to include reintroduction of solid table foods over a period of days to weeks with no specific guidelines regarding the food reintroduction schedule established. EEN is more widely used in Canada and Europe when compared with the United States. To improve palatability, other exclusion diets that do incorporate whole foods have shown some initial promise and are undergoing further investigation.[49] However, except for milder cases of CD, maintenance of remission with dietary therapy alone is difficult to achieve without additional medical therapy given frequent disease resurgence once the restrictive diet is terminated.

# IBD Effects on Puberty

Along with growth impairment, delay in pubertal development is also a common finding, particularly with CD. The hypothalamic-pituitary-gonadal axis (HPG axis) begins to form in the developing fetus as early as the first trimester of pregnancy and produces hormones at the pubertal level shortly after birth once maternal hormones are withdrawn. This is termed the "mini puberty" of infancy and results in such phenomena as neonatal acne. In girls, the HPG axis then becomes mostly quiescent until puberty when GnRH begins to be secreted by the hypothalamus in a pulsatile fashion.[50] This transition from quiescent to pulsatile secretion of GnRH serves as the driving force behind the development of sexual maturity and secondary sex characteristics that we recognize and understand to define puberty.

In the United States, puberty in girls typically occurs between the ages of 8 and 13 years with an average age of onset of 10.2 years.[38] For Black and Hispanic girls, puberty begins approximately 1 year earlier than in non-Hispanic White females. Consequently, it is not abnormal to see thelarche starting as early as age 7 years in these racial and ethnic groups. The average age of menarche, which occurs approximately 2.5 years after the onset of puberty, also occurs at a slightly earlier age in Black and Hispanic girls; however, the average age of menarche overall in the United States across all races is approximately 12 years.[38] It takes girls in the United States approximately 4 years to complete puberty and to reach sexual maturity; however, there is much variability in this process which can be as short as 2 years and rarely as long as 8 years in extreme circumstances. Although the onset of puberty has demonstrated an overall global trend toward a younger median age in the past decade, a recent meta-analysis of worldwide data shows that US findings surrounding puberty are consistent with those seen in Europe, Asia, and the Middle East with regards to median age onset of thelarche generally falling between age 8 to 11 years with the exception of Africa showing a slightly later median age range of 10 to 13 years.[42]

Puberty in females can be divided into separate processes (Table 1-2) that occur largely in a concerted temporal relation to one another and include thelarche, or breast development; adrenarche/pubarche, which results in the development of pubic and axillary hair; a linear growth spurt characterized by increase in height velocity; and menarche, or the onset of menstruation.[31,38,50] Clinically, Tanner staging is used to help identify pubertal development on physical exam in girls which is heralded by Tanner stage II.[51] With the onset of puberty, the hypothalamus both becomes more sensitive to, and increases its production of, GnRH in a pulsatile fashion that then signals the anterior pituitary gland to secrete the gonadotropins luteinizing hormone (LH) and follicle stimulating hormone (FSH) also in a cyclic and pulsatile fashion.[31,50] These gonadotropins then facilitate production of hormones by female gonads, the ovaries. LH first stimulates production of androgens by the ovarian theca cells, which are then converted to estrogens by aromatase enzymes in the ovarian

## Table 1-2. Normal Stages of Female Pubertal Development

| THELARCHE | Breast development<br>Mean age onset: 8 to 9 years (~1 year earlier in Black and Hispanic groups) |
| --- | --- |
| PUBARCHE | Associated with adrenarche, development of axillary and pubic hair<br>Mean age onset: 8 to 10 years |
| LINEAR GROWTH | Increased height velocity, average increase of 8.25 cm/year<br>Mean age of onset: 9 years |
| MENARCHE | Start of menstruation<br>Mean age of onset: 12 years |

granulosa cells. FSH acts on the ovarian granulosa cells to facilitate the conversion of androgen to estradiol in the ovary.[50] Estrogen plays an essential role in the reproductive development and formation of secondary sexual characteristic of girls during puberty such as its role in thelarche; this process is termed *feminization*. Menarche results from cyclic secretion of the sex hormones estrogen and progesterone in response to cyclic changes in levels of gonadotropins LH and FSH.[50]

Like the HPG axis in stimulation of the gonads to secrete sex hormones, the hypothalamic-pituitary-adrenal (HPA) axis functions by stimulating the adrenals to produce androgens which play an important role in adrenarche and subsequent development of pubic and axillary hair. The activity of the adrenal gland is largely regulated by adrenocorticotropic hormone that is secreted by the pituitary gland along the HPA axis. The adrenal glands are responsible for the production of approximately 50% of female androgens, which is in contrast to male development in which the majority of androgens are secreted by the testes and a minority are produced by the adrenals.[50] The adrenal glands' role in female androgen production becomes significant when we consider the strong effect that repetitive and sustained use of exogenous corticosteroids have in suppressing adrenocorticotropic hormone and thus suppressing the endogenous secretion of hormones by the adrenal glands. The role that corticosteroids can play in suppression of the HPA axis further supports the need to limit corticosteroid use in young girls with IBD who are often at a pivotal stage of sexual development. Adrenal gland function is also known to be influenced by other mediators that have been implicated in the pathogenesis of growth impairment in children with IBD including insulin, IGF-1, and GH as discussed previously.[52] Poor nutrition and inflammatory states can suppress these metabolic growth factors which can in turn negatively impact the function of the adrenal glands, and thereby hinder female sexual development.

Delayed puberty is defined as a lack of achievement of Tanner stage II, typically starting with thelarche in girls, by age 13 years.[38] However, knowing that pubertal onset, and specifically thelarche can occur as early as age 7 years in Black and Hispanic girls should elicit a higher index of suspicion for delays sooner in those populations especially in the presence of other vague complaints such as chronic abdominal pain. Primary amenorrhea is considered when there is lack of initiation of menses by age 15 or 3 years after the start of thelarche. Menstrual irregularity, however, is not uncommon in young women during puberty given that up to 50% of menstrual cycles in the 2 years following menarche can be anovulatory and thus irregular.[38] Regardless of consideration of anovulatory cycles, if any of the following occur, referral to an endocrinologist and/or gynecologist should be considered:

- Persistent menstrual irregularity beyond 2 years following menarche
- Greater than 90 days between menses
- Lack of menses by age 15
- Lack of breast development by 13 years
- Significant growth arrest

The decision regarding timing of referra for further evaluation; however, is a clinical one that is individualized by patient with lower thresholds in young women with chronic disease such as IBD in order that appropriate therapeutic interventions can be initiated in a timely manner.

There are many possible causes of pubertal delay. Most commonly it is due to benign constitutional delay which results in a delay of the pubertal growth spurt that occurs when there is a delay in the GnRH surge. This is a phenomenon that typically affects boys, and runs in families, however, it can also affect girls. The ultimate outcome for constitutional delay is eventual growth velocity "catch up" without any impairment of the other pubertal phases or final adult height. Conversely, pubertal delay can be the result of primary or secondary gonadal failure. Primary gonadal failure can be due to an underlying syndrome or genetic mutation that specifically affects sexual development such as Turner syndrome, 46-XY gonadal dysgenesis, or androgen insensitivity syndrome. Secondary gonadal failure can be due to malnutrition and chronic illness, as seen in IBD, which can result in a functional delay in sexual development due to diminished production of gonadotropins in this already increased catabolic state of pubertal growth.[31,38,53]

The delay in onset of puberty and the prolongation of duration of puberty overall noted with IBD—and more specifically CD—is often associated with delays in growth velocity.[31,53-55] A study that followed 106 children with pediatric-onset IBD through adulthood and collected data on their growth and attainment of peak height velocity as a proxy for overall pubertal development found no pubertal delays identified in the children with UC. However, 23% of the girls and boys with CD had delays in their peak height velocity attainment that was greater than 2 standard deviations below their national average.[56] Similar pubertal delays have applied to age of menarche in girls with CD. A study of 34 girls with CD compared to over 500 girls without CD obtained from a national US sample found that median age of menarche in the girls with CD was delayed to 13.9 years compared to the national average age of 12 ($P < .00005$).[57] The actual delay in menarche was at least 2 years with just over half of the girls with CD experiencing menarche by age 14 years.[57]

Delay in onset of menses is important to consider in the context of the relationship between age of menarche and linear growth. Although some might presume that a delay in onset of menses and progression of puberty could theoretically prolong puberty and growth potential, this has not been the case for observed outcomes. Delays in menarche have been linked to diminished overall growth potential. A study examining racial differences in pubertal development followed > 2500 girls longitudinally for an average of 6 years during their development and found that those girls who had menarche after age 13 years were on average 4 cm shorter than those girls with earlier menarche.[58] This finding suggests that an alteration of normal age of menarche can result in linear growth impairment and has been postulated to contribute to some of the observed growth derangements seen in young women with IBD.[31,42]

The cause of pubertal delay in girls with IBD is likely influenced by a number of factors including nutritional status, degree of intestinal inflammation, physical stress, and growth hormones. Chronic undernutrition due to overall diminished caloric intake and utilization can reduce the minimal body fat percentage necessary to support pubertal processes such as menarche. Primary or secondary cessation of menses, for example, can be seen in some high-performance athletes and can be reversed in the setting of increased caloric intake and limitations to exercise regimens.[59] This phenomenon, termed *functional hypothalamic amenorrhea*, results in suppression of the HPG axis and disruption in the pulsatile secretion of GnRH, FSH, and LH without a clear organic cause. Studies have suggested a threshold of 30 kcal/kg/day required to sustain HPG axis functions in adolescence.[59]

Chronic undernutrition can also result in diminished levels of IGF-1 even in the presence of elevated GH, a finding described as GH resistance. Low IGF-1 levels will in turn disrupt the HPG axis and result in pubertal derangements. Similar to what occurs with delayed linear growth, inflammatory cytokines such as TNF-α and IL-6 result in reduced sex steroid production with resultant adverse effect on pubertal development.[31,59] Most of this information has been derived from mouse studies demonstrating that pro-inflammatory mediators including TNF-α suppress androgen production and activation. However, similar to the suppression of growth, the inherent inflammatory process in IBD also contributes to observed pubertal delay. For example, diminished peak height velocity as low as 1 to 2 cm/year was observed more often in children with frequently relapsing IBD.[54] Conversely, reviews of patterns of growth and pubertal development among a population of children in the UK found that resumption of normal pubertal development was strongly associated with attainment of clinical remission of disease as demonstrated in children with CD and pubertal delay who started puberty within 1 year of undergoing resection of diseased bowel.[55] In addition to judicious timing of surgical intervention for IBD, efforts at reversing growth and pubertal delays now include medical therapies such as anti-TNF, anti–IL-12/IL-23, and anti-integrin therapies in combination with attention to appropriate nutrition.

## Amenorrhea, Dysmenorrhea, and Menstrual Irregularities

Complete pubertal suppression due to ovarian failure has been described rarely in adult case reports and in association with autoimmune ovarian dysfunction, but has not clearly been associated with IBD.[60,61] A study following 52 women with premature ovarian failure found that approximately 40% carried a diagnosis of an autoimmune disease but of those only about 2% had CD.[62] Studies of ovarian insufficiency and amenorrhea are lacking in pediatric IBD; however, if a girl with CD or UC demonstrates evidence of primary or secondary amenorrhea, an interdisciplinary evaluation should be considered by her pediatrician or gastroenterologist with consultations from a dietitian, endocrinologist, or gynecologist as needed. Given the known effects of the inflammatory process on puberty, assessment of disease clinical activity should be undertaken with history, physical examination, imaging, laboratory studies, and endoscopic evaluations as indicated.

If active intestinal inflammation and malnutrition are determined to not be the cause of amenorrhea, the history and physical exam typically informs the next steps in the evaluation. For example, a complete lack of pubertal development by age 13 years might suggest HPG axis dysfunction; hirsutism and acne might point to polycystic ovarian syndrome; and abdominal pain with imperforate hymen could reveal hematometrocolpos/outflow tract obstruction. Pregnancy must certainly be excluded, especially for the adolescent patient. There is little data available to suggest a relationship between IBD and conditions that might predispose to menstrual irregularities in the adolescent such as endometriosis or polycystic ovarian syndrome.[63] Although healthy young women can experience menstrual irregularities for the first 1 to 2 years following onset of menarche due to anovulatory cycles, if irregular cycles are still being experienced beyond 2 years post menarche there is a 67% likelihood that oligomenorrhea could be the sustained result of an underlying pathology and prompts additional evaluation.[38]

Independent of IBD, young women can experience dysmenorrhea and associated changes in bowel habits such as decreased appetite, nausea, abdominal pain, and changes in stool consistency during different phases of the menstrual cycle.[64] Largely adult survey-based studies looking at gastrointestinal symptoms during menstruation have shown that 34% of women who did not have bowel complaints at baseline reported changes in bowel habits at the time of menstruation and that up to 50% of women with functional gastrointestinal disorders reported worsening of their symptoms with menstruation.[65] Animal models have suggested that the etiology of bowel symptoms experienced during menstruation can be attributed to direct effects that sex hormones have on gut permeability, smooth muscle receptors, the enteric nervous system, and motility of the gastrointestinal tract; however, human studies evaluating the effects of ovarian hormones on intestinal motility have been conflicting.[63] Proposed mechanisms of action have included increased uterine prostaglandin secretion during the luteal phase of the menstrual cycle with resultant increased inflammation and cramping abdominal pain.[66] Additionally, decreased progesterone during menses has been associated with increased gastrointestinal motility and a possible etiology of looser stools.[63] Estrogen has been linked to increased pain perception and increased visceral pain sensitivity through its action on both central and enteric nervous system pain receptors, which might contribute to the experience of abdominal pain in girls with and without IBD.[63]

Women with IBD might describe a cyclic pattern of symptoms, such as looser stools and worsening abdominal cramping during the week prior to and during menstruation in a predictable pattern.[63,67] This has been demonstrated in several adult survey studies, one of which evaluated menstrual symptoms in 238 women with IBD (151 with CD) aged 18 to 65 years vs a healthy control group. Fifty-nine percent of women with CD and 42.5% with UC ($P = .01$), vs 28% of controls ($P < .0001$) were likely to experience worsening of diarrhea leading up to and during menstruation. Similar findings of worsening abdominal pain prior to and during menses were also noted.[68] Another study of women 18 to 48 years of age surveyed 49 women with UC, 49 with CD, 46 with irritable bowel syndrome, and 90 healthy controls. Eighty percent of all women surveyed reported gastrointestinal symptoms during menses, most commonly diarrhea. This study notably showed that the incidence of any symptoms were higher among women with CD vs controls and that those women with CD and irritable bowel syndrome were more likely to report diarrhea than controls.[67] Another prospective questionnaire based study of 91 adult women with a mean age of 35 years noted similar catamenial exacerbation of diarrhea and abdominal pain in women with IBD compared to healthy controls, but went further in highlighting that despite these worsening bowel symptoms, 80% of the women with IBD remained in clinical remission during the course of the study.[69] Clinicians need to be aware of this phenomenon and inquire about menstrual cycle patterns with respect to stools in order to avoid confusing this cyclic pattern of transient change in bowel habits with a disease flare.

In treating dysmenorrhea and oligomenorrhea, consideration may be given to prescribing oral contraceptives (OCPs) or nonsteroidal anti-inflammatory medications (NSAIDs). Robust pediatric data addressing OCP use and possible increased risk of developing IBD is absent. Extrapolation to pediatrics from adult cohort and case-control studies has been controversial due to conflicting evidence lacking strong statistical significance.[70] A notable adult meta-analysis that pooled data from 2 cohort and 7 case-control studies collectively evaluating more than 30,000 women with IBD revealed a non-significant, mildly increased pooled relative risk of OCPs use and the subsequent development of IBD of 1.44 (95% confidence interval [CI] 1.12 to 1.86).[71] One of the larger case-control studies that looked at 581 patients compared to 433 healthy controls found that young women with CD were likely to start taking OCPs at an earlier age vs healthy controls noting an average age of starting use of 18 ± 3 years.[72] Given the lack of clinically significant data to suggest a strong causative relationship between OCPs and IBD development or exacerbation, their use is neither widely avoided, nor contraindicated in pediatric patients with IBD.

NSAIDs are often used to treat dysmenorrhea in women and are another class of medication that has been implicated in exacerbation and development of IBD. Like the research done on OCPs, data primarily comes from adult cohort and case-control studies and mouse models. In the interleukin-10 knockout murine model of colitis, administration of selective cyclooxygenase 1 and 2 inhibitors resulted in a reduction of protective intestinal prostaglandin levels by 75% with associated rapid progression to colitis.[73] Clinical studies supporting the mouse model findings include an increased odds ratio of 2.9 (95% CI 1.32 to 6.64) for developing colitis following current or recent NSAID exposure in 785 hospitalized adults.[74] However, a meta-analysis evaluating NSAID use in the ambulatory setting pooled data from 5 cohort and 8 case-control studies from 1983 to 2016 and concluded that there was no consistent, statistically significant association between NSAID and cyclooxygenase-2 inhibitor use and exacerbation of IBD with the concession that in sub-analysis of studies with the lowest bias there did seem to be some increased risk of NSAID use and CD flare that did not translate to UC.[75] Based on the data derived from adult studies, ESPGHAN has issued guidelines suggesting that NSAID use in pediatric IBD be limited to low doses and short courses.[76,77]

# Immunizations

Preventative health maintenance plays an essential role in the management of pediatric IBD. Given that the bulk of an individual's lifetime vaccines are administered in childhood, this aspect of preventative health maintenance is essential to consider. Immunosuppressive therapies remain the mainstay of IBD treatment, and a chronic state of undernutrition and inflammation puts children at increased risk for infection; therefore, protection against vaccine preventable illness of childhood and those that have further reach into the adult years such as hepatitis B, varicella (VZV), pneumococcal pneumonia, and human papillomavirus (HPV) is strongly recommended.[78] Pediatric guidelines issued jointly by North American Society of Pediatric Gastroenterology Hepatology and Nutrition and ESPGHAN stipulate that children with IBD should follow the routine vaccination guideline and schedule as determined by the CDC and supported by American Academy of Pediatrics, with the caveat that live vaccines should be avoided when a child is on immunosuppressive treatment; and, if needed, live vaccines should be given prior to initiation of immunosuppressive therapy.[79-81] Immunosuppressive treatments are defined as the equivalent of 20 mg/day or 2 mg/kg/day or more of corticosteroids for 14 days or longer, and other medications such as 6-mercaptopurine, azathioprine, methotrexate, and anti-TNF therapies. With respect to these types of medications, it is suggested to wait 1 to 3 months prior to live vaccine administration for safety and to allow for appropriate immune response.[80,82]

To help decide whether additional vaccination should be contemplated in a pediatric patient with IBD, screening for immunity to hepatitis B and VZV is often considered by assessment with serologic titers. In the setting of lack of immunity, there may be time to allow for re-vaccination or booster shot administration prior to starting immunosuppressive medications, but this will depend on the severity of the patient's symptoms. It has been noted that even if VZV titers suggest a nonimmune status, confirming that 2 VZV vaccinations have been given may be sufficient. A notable survey-based study administered to patients aged 13 to 75 years at routine IBD visits showed that of the 169 patients who had a positive history of VZV vaccination, all had detectable antibodies with 96% of those demonstrating adequate seropositivity to confer immunity against disease.[83]

Acute influenza infection can present with fevers and arthralgias mimicking an IBD flare but can also result in more severe symptoms among those with chronic illness or those on immunosuppressive medications. Thus, annual vaccination for seasonal influenza with the inactivate vaccine has been part of the routine health maintenance guidance for children and adults with IBD and all members of their household.[82] Routine HPV vaccination in adolescence should also be emphasized given the increased risk of HPV infection and subsequent cervical dysplasia in women with IBD. A study of 134 pap smears from 40 women with IBD reported that 42.5% had abnormal pap smears with higher grade dysplasia compared to only 7% in over 300 healthy controls ($P < .001$).[84] Some of these findings may be attributed to increased risk of developing HPV in the setting of immunosuppression as demonstrated by an increased odds ratio of 1.5 (95% CI 1.2 to 4.1, $P = .021$) in those women with a greater than 6-month exposure to immunomodulating thiopurines, corticosteroids, and anti-TNF medications.[84] For girls and boys, the CDC has recommended that HPV vaccination can begin as early as age 9 years and consists of a series of 2 vaccines if administered prior to age 15 in healthy children or 3 vaccines if administered after age 15 or within groups of patients who might have abnormal immune responses to vaccines such as individuals with IBD.[79,85]

Vaccines given in adolescence typically have lower completion rates than those given in early childhood. A review of vaccination records of 153 children with IBD revealed that 93.5% of children were up to date for age on their early childhood measles/mumps/rubella vaccine and 85.6% on diphtheria/tetanus/pertussis/haemophilus influenza combination vaccine vs 42% of those children being up to date for age on HPV vaccination which is given in adolescence.[85,86] Barriers to routine vaccination in children once they develop IBD include confusion surrounding the administration of vaccines in the context of receiving immunosuppressants, concern surrounding active disease flare, caregiver refusal due to lack of awareness and understanding of significance, and fear of side effects.[83] However, the good news for children with IBD is that most childhood vaccinations do occur before the age of 6 years, and guidance for delayed vaccination is provided through catch-up vaccination timelines issued by both the CDC with the support of the American Academy of Pediatrics.[79,81] Therefore improved vaccination rates can be achieved with increased emphasis on provider and caregiver education surrounding vaccination recommendations in children with IBD.

# Conclusion

Pediatric-onset and VEO-IBD are increasing in incidence and prevalence throughout the world. A high index of suspicion is required for making a timely diagnosis in children due to the non-specific and sometimes subtle presenting signs and symptoms. Early diagnosis and subsequent appropriate management are key to promoting optimal growth and pubertal development given how IBD can adversely impact these 2 important processes of childhood. Menstrual irregularities, dysmenorrhea, and oligomenorrhea are commonly seen in young women with IBD and can be mitigated by successful treatment and optimal nutritional support. IBD management in children and adolescents should avoid or minimize use of corticosteroids and focus on achievement of durable steroid-free remission and mucosal healing. Ensuring that children with IBD have successfully completed their childhood vaccination schedule is important to decreasing morbidity and mortality from vaccine preventable infections.

---

## KEY POINTS

1.  Pediatric-onset IBD presents a diagnostic challenge, given the non-specific presenting signs and symptoms in children; unlike adult-onset IBD, children are more likely to present with CD, and are more likely to be male.

2.  Very-early-onset IBD, in children 5 years or younger, is a rapidly expanding group and should raise suspicion for underlying genetic or immunologic conditions that require targeted treatments.

3.  Treatment of pediatric-onset IBD favors the use of steroid-sparing agents such as anti-TNF medications to minimize deficits in linear growth and pubertal delay.

4.  Young women with IBD are likely to experience predictable patterns of worsening bowel symptoms and dysmenorrhea in relation to their menstrual cycle. The reason for this is multifactorial and not completely understood.

# References

1.  Benchimol EI, Bernstein CN, Bitton A, et al. Trends in epidemiology of pediatric inflammatory bowel disease in Canada: distributed network analysis of multiple population-based provincial health administrative databases. *Am J Gastroenterol.* 2017;112(7):1120-1134.

2.  Benchimol EI, Fortinsky KJ, Gozdyra P, Van den Heuvel M, Van Limbergen J, Griffiths AM. Epidemiology of pediatric inflammatory bowel disease: a systematic review of international trends. *Inflamm Bowel Dis.* 2011;17(1):423-439.

3.  Kappelman M, Moore K, et al. Recent trends in the prevalence of Crohn's disease and ulcerative colitis in a commercially insured US population. *Dig Dis Sci.* 2013;58(2):519-525.

4.  Knights D, Lassen KG, Xavier RJ. Advances in inflammatory bowel disease pathogenesis: linking host genetics and the microbiome. *Gut.* 2013;62(10):1505-1510.

5.  Mamula P, Markowitz JE, Baldassano RN. Inflammatory bowel disease in early childhood and adolescence: special considerations. *Gastroenterol Clin North Am.* 2003;32(3):967-995.

6.  Andres PG, Friedman LS. Epidemiology and the natural course of inflammatory bowel disease. *Gastroenterol Clin North Am.* 1999;28(2):255-281.

7.  Van Limbergen J, Russell RK, Drummond HE, et al. Definition of phenotypic characteristics of childhood-onset inflammatory bowel disease. *Gastroenterology.* 2008;135(4):1114-1122.

8.  Vernier–Massouille G, Balde M, Salleron J, et al. Natural history of pediatric Crohn's disease: a population-based cohort study. *Gastroenterology.* 2008;135(4):1106-1113.

9.  Jostins L, Ripke S, Weersma RK, et al. Host–microbe interactions have shaped the genetic architecture of inflammatory bowel disease. *Nature.* 2012;491(7422):119-124.

10. Liu JZ, van Sommeren S, Huang H, et al. Association analyses identify 38 susceptibility loci for inflammatory bowel disease and highlight shared genetic risk across populations. *Nat Genet.* 2015;47(9):979-986.

11. Heikenen JB, Werlin SL, Brown CW, Balint JP. Presenting symptoms and diagnostic lag in children with inflammatory bowel disease. *Inflamm Bowel Dis.* 1999;5(3):158-160.

12. Long MD, Crandall WV, Leibowitz IH, et al. The prevalence and epidemiology of overweight and obesity in children with inflammatory bowel disease. *Inflamm Bowel Dis.* 2011;17(10):2162-2168.

13. Body mass index in children with newly diagnosed inflammatory bowel disease: observations from two multicenter North American inception cohorts. *J Pediatr.* 2007;151(5):523-527.

14. Mack DR, Langton C, Markowitz J, et al. Laboratory values for children with newly diagnosed inflammatory bowel disease. *Pediatrics.* 2007;119(6):1113-1119.

15. Sharif F, McDermott M, Dillon M, et al. Focally enhanced gastritis in children with Crohn's disease and ulcerative colitis. *Am J Gastroenterol.* 2002;97(6):1415-1420.

16. Levine A, de Bie CI, Turner D, et al. Atypical disease phenotypes in pediatric ulcerative colitis 5-year analyses of the EUROKIDS registry. *Inflamm Bowel Dis.* 2013;19(2):370-377.

17. Differentiating ulcerative colitis from Crohn disease in children and young adults: report of a working group of the North American society for Pediatric Gastroenterology, Hepatology, and Nutrition and the Crohn's and Colitis Foundation of America. *J Pediatr Gastroenterol Nutr.* 2007;44(5):653-674.

18. Kelsen JR, Sullivan KE, Rabizadeh S, et al. North American Society for Pediatric Gastroenterology, Hepatology, and Nutrition position paper on the evaluation and management for patients with very early-onset inflammatory bowel disease. *J Pediatr Gastroenterol Nutr.* 2020;70(3):389-403.

19. Oliva-Hemker M, Hutfless S, Al Kazzi ES, et al. Clinical presentation and five-year therapeutic management of very early-onset inflammatory bowel disease in a large North American cohort. *J Pediatr.* 2015;167(3):527-532.

20. Heyman MB, Kirschner BS, Gold BD, et al. Children with early-onset inflammatory bowel disease (IBD): analysis of a pediatric IBD consortium registry. *J Pediatr.* 2005;146(1):35-40.

21. Ouahed J, Spencer E, Kotlarz D, et al. Very early onset inflammatory bowel disease: a clinical approach with a focus on the role of genetics and underlying immune deficiencies. *Inflamm Bowel Dis.* 2020;26(6):820-842. doi:10.1093/ibd/izz259

22. Uhlig HH, Schwerd T, Koletzko S, et al. The diagnostic approach to monogenic very early onset inflammatory bowel disease. *Gastroenterology.* 2014;147(5):990-1007.

23. Guerrerio AL, Frischmeyer-Guerrerio PA, Lederman HM, Oliva-Hemker M. Recognizing gastrointestinal and hepatic manifestations of primary immunodeficiency diseases. *J Pediatr Gastroenterol Nutr.* 2010;51(5):548-555.

24. Speckmann C, Lehmberg K, Albert MH, et al. X-linked inhibitor of apoptosis (XIAP) deficiency: the spectrum of presenting manifestations beyond hemophagocytic lymphohistiocytosis. *Clin Immunol.* 2013;149(1):133-141.

25. Fumery M, Duricova D, Gower-Rousseau C, Annese V, Peyrin-Biroulet L, Lakatos PL. Review article: the natural history of paediatric-onset ulcerative colitis in population-based studies. *Aliment Pharmacol Ther.* 2016;43(3):346-355.

26. Malik S, Wong SC, Bishop J, et al. Improvement in growth of children with Crohn disease following anti-TNF-[alpha] therapy can be independent of pubertal progress and glucocorticoid reduction. *J Pediatr Gastroenterol Nutr.* 2011;52(1):31-37.

27. Markowitz, Jamies, Grancher K, Rosa J, Aiges H, Daum F. Growth failure in pediatric inflammatory bowel disease. *J Pediatr Gastroenterol Nutr.* 1993;16(4):373-389.

28. Motil KJ, Grand RJ, Davis-Kraft L, Ferlic LL, Smith EO. Growth failure in children with inflammatory bowel disease: a prospective study. *Gastroenterology.* 1993;105(3):681-691.

29. Kanof ME, Lake AM, Bayless TM. Decreased height velocity in children and adolescents before the diagnosis of Crohn's disease. *Gastroenterology.* 1988;95(6):1523-1527.

30. Tanner JM, Goldstein H, Whitehouse RH. Standards for children's height at ages 2-9 years allowing for heights of parents. *Arch Dis Child.* 1970;45(244):755-762.

31. Deplewski D, Gupta N, Kirschner BS. Puberty and pediatric-onset inflammatory bowel disease. In: Mamula P, Grossman AB, Baldassano RN, Kelsen JR, Markowitz JE, eds. *Pediatric inflammatory bowel disease.* Springer International Publishing; 2017:171-179.

32. Growth charts—WHO child growth standards. https://www.cdc.gov/growthcharts/who_charts.htm#The%20 WHO%20Growth%20Charts. Website. Updated 2019.

33. Gupta N, Liu C, King E, et al. Continued statural growth in older adolescents and young adults with Crohn's disease and ulcerative colitis beyond the time of expected growth plate closure. *Inflamm Bowel Dis.* 2020;26(12):1880-1889. doi:10.1093/ibd/izz334

34. Thomas AG, Miller V, Taylor F, Maycock P, Scrimgeour CM, Rennie MJ. Whole body protein turnover in childhood Crohn's disease. *Gut.* 1992;33(5):675-677.

35. Conklin, Laurie, Oliva-Hemker M. Nutritional considerations in pediatric inflammatory bowel disease. *Expert Rev Gastroent.* 2010;4(3):305-317.

36. Soendergaard C, Young AJ, Kopchick JJ. Growth hormone resistance—special focus on inflammatory bowel disease. *Int J Mol Sci.* 2017;18(5):1019.

37. Wolf M, Sebastian Böhm, Brand M, Kreymann G. Proinflammatory cytokines interleukin 1β and tumor necrosis factor α inhibit growth hormone stimulation of insulin-like growth factor I synthesis and growth hormone receptor mRNA levels in cultured rat liver cells. *Eur J Endocrinol.* 1996;135(6):729-737.

38. Bordini B, Rosenfield RL. Normal pubertal development: part II: clinical aspects of puberty. *Pediatr Rev.* 2011;32(7):281-292.

39. Nathan BM, Palmert MR. Regulation and disorders of pubertal timing. *Endocrin Metab Clin.* 2005;34(3):617-641.

40. Herrington J, Smit LS, Schwartz J, Carter-Su C. The role of STAT proteins in growth hormone signaling. *Oncogene.* 2000;19(21):2585-2597.

41. Gupta N, Lustig R, Kohn MA, McCracken M, Vittinghoff E. Sex differences in statural growth impairment in Crohn's disease: role of IGF-1. *Inflamm Bowel Dis.* 2012;17(11):2318-2325.

42. DeBoer MD, Denson LA. Delays in puberty, growth and accrual of bone mineral density in pediatric Crohn's disease: despite temporal changes in disease severity, the need for monitoring remains. *J Pediatr.* 2013;163(1):17-22.

43. Ruemmele FM, Veres G, Kolho KL, et al. Consensus guidelines of ECCO/ESPGHAN on the medical management of pediatric crohn's disease. *J Crohns Colitis.* 2014;8(10):1179-1207.

44. Levine A, Weizman Z, Broide E, et al. A comparison of budesonide and prednisone for the treatment of active pediatric Crohn disease. *J Pediatr Gastroenterol Nutr.* 2003;36(2).248-252

45. Walters TD, Kim M, Denson LA, et al. Increased effectiveness of early therapy with anti-tumor necrosis factor-α vs an immunomodulator in children with Crohn's disease. *Gastroenterology.* 2014;146(2):383-391.

46. Rosh JR, Gross T, Mamula P, Griffiths A, Hyams J. Hepatosplenic T-cell lymphoma in adolescents and young adults with Crohn's disease: a cautionary tale? *Inflamm Bowel Dis.* 2007;13(8):1024-1030.

47. Berni Canani R, Terrin G, Borrelli O, et al. Short- and long-term therapeutic efficacy of nutritional therapy and corticosteroids in paediatric Crohn's disease. *Digest Liver Dis.* 2006;38(6):381-387.

48. Borrelli O, Cordischi L, Cirulli M, et al. Polymeric diet alone versus corticosteroids in the treatment of active pediatric Crohn's disease: a randomized controlled open-label trial. *Clin Gastroenterol Hepatol.* 2006;4(6):744-753.

49. Levine A, Wine E, Assa A, et al. Crohn's disease exclusion diet plus partial enteral nutrition induces sustained remission in a randomized controlled trial. *Gastroenterology.* 2019;157(2):440-450

50. Bordini B, Rosenfield RL. Normal pubertal development: part I: the endocrine basis of puberty. *Pediatr Rev.* 2011;32(6):223-229.

51. Abbassi V. Growth and normal puberty. *Pediatrics.* 1998;102:507-511.

52. Guercio G, Rivarola MA, Chaler E, Maceiras M, Belgorosky A. Relationship between the growth hormone/insulin-like growth factor-I axis, insulin sensitivity, and adrenal androgens in normal prepubertal and pubertal girls. *J Clin Endocrinol Metab.* 2003;88(3):1389-1393.

53. Ballinger AB, Savage MO, Sanderson IR. Delayed puberty associated with inflammatory bowel disease. *Pediatr Res.* 2003;53(2):205-210.

54. Brain CE, Majrowski W, Leonard J, Camacho-Hubner C, Savage MO, Walker-Smith J. Characteristics of pubertal development in inflammatory bowel disease (IBD). *Pediatr Res.* 1993;33(5):S86.

55. Brain CE, Savage MO. Growth and puberty in chronic inflammatory bowel disease. *Baillière's Clin Gastroenterol.* 1994;8(1):83-100.

56. Hildebrand H, Karlberg J, Kristiansson B. Longitudinal growth in children and adolescents with inflammatory bowel disease. *J Pediatr Gastroenterol Nutr.* 1994;18(2):165-173.

57. Gupta N, Lustig RH, Kohn MA, Vittinghoff E. Menarche in pediatric patients with Crohn's disease. *Dig Dis Sci.* 2012;57(11):2975-2981.

58. Freedman DS, Khan LK, Serdula MK, Dietz WH, Srinivasan SR, Berenson GS. Relation of age at menarche to race, time period, and anthropometric dimensions: the Bogalusa heart study. *Pediatrics.* 2002;110(4):e43.

59. Ackerman KE, Misra M. Amenorrhoea in adolescent female athletes. *Lancet Child Adol Health.* 2018;2(9):677-688.

60. Caroppo E, D'Amato G. Resumption of ovarian function after 4 years of estro-progestin treatment in a young woman with Crohn's disease and premature ovarian insufficiency: a case report. *J Assist Reprod Genet.* 2012;29(9):973-977.

61. Forges T, Monnier-Barbarino P, Faure GC, Béné MC. Autoimmunity and antigenic targets in ovarian pathology. *Hum Reprod Update.* 2004;10(2):163-175.

62. Grossmann B, Saur S, Rall K, et al. Prevalence of autoimmune disease in women with premature ovarian failure. *Eur J Contracep Repr.* 2020;25(1):72-75.

63. Bharadwaj S, Kulkarni G, Shen B. Menstrual cycle, sex hormones in female inflammatory bowel disease patients with and without surgery. *J Dig Dis.* 2015;16(5):245-255.

64. Heitkemper M, Shaver JF, Mitchell ES. Gastrointestinal symptoms and bowel patterns across the menstrual cycle in dysmenorrhea. *Nurs Res.* 1988;37(2):108-113.

65. Moore J, Barlow D, Jewell D, Kennedy S. Do gastrointestinal symptoms vary with the menstrual cycle? *BJOG: Int J Obstet Gy.* 1998;105(12):1322-1325.

66. Saha S, Zhao Y, Shah SA, et al. Menstrual cycle changes in women with inflammatory bowel disease: a study from the ocean state Crohn's and colitis area registry. *Inflamm Bowel Dis.* 2014;20(3):534-540.

67. Kane SV, Sable K, Hanauer SB. The menstrual cycle and its effect on inflammatory bowel disease and irritable bowel syndrome: a prevalence study. *Am J Gastroenterol.* 1998;93(10):1867-1872.

68. Bernstein MT, Graff LA, Targownik LE, et al. Gastrointestinal symptoms before and during menses in women with IBD. *Aliment Pharmacol Ther.* 2012;36(2):135-144.

69. Lim SM, Nam CM, Kim YN, et al. The effect of the menstrual cycle on inflammatory bowel disease: a prospective study. *Gut Liver.* 2013;7(1):51-57.

70. Loftus, EV Jr. Clinical epidemiology of inflammatory bowel disease: incidence, prevalence, and environmental influences. *Gastroenterology.* 2004;126(6):1504-1517.

71. Godet PG, May GR, Sutherland LR. Meta-analysis of the role of oral contraceptive agents in inflammatory bowel disease. *Gut.* 1995;37(5):668-673.

72. Bernstein CN, Rawsthorne P, Cheang M, Blanchard JF. A population-based case control study of potential risk factors for IBD. *Am J Gastroenterol.* 2006;101(5):993-1002.

73. Berg DJ, Zhang J, Weinstock JV, et al. Rapid development of colitis in NSAID-treated IL-10–deficient mice. *Gastroenterology.* 2002;123(5):1527-1542.

74. Evans JM, McMahon AD, Murray FE, McDevitt DG, MacDonald TM. Non-steroidal anti-inflammatory drugs are associated with emergency admission to hospital for colitis due to inflammatory bowel disease. *Gut.* 1997;40(5):619-622.

75. Moninuola OO, Milligan W, Lochhead P, Khalili H. Systematic review with meta-analysis: association between acetaminophen and nonsteroidal anti-inflammatory drugs (NSAIDs) and risk of Crohn's disease and ulcerative colitis exacerbation. *Aliment Pharmacol Ther.* 2018;47(11):1428-1439.

76. Turner D, Ruemmele FM, Orlanski-Meyer E, et al. Management of paediatric ulcerative colitis, part 2: acute severe colitis—an evidence-based consensus guideline from the European Crohn's and Colitis Organization and the European Society of Paediatric Gastroenterology, Hepatology and Nutrition. *J Pediatr Gastroenterol Nutr.* 2018;67(2):292-310.

77. Turner D, Ruemmele FM, Orlanski-Meyer E, et al. Management of paediatric ulcerative colitis, part 1: ambulatory care—an evidence-based guideline from European Crohn's and Colitis Organization and European Society of Paediatric Gastroenterology, Hepatology and Nutrition. *J Pediatr Gastroenterol Nutr.* 2018;67(2):257-291.

78. Lu Y, Jacobson D, Bousvaros A. Immunizations in patients with inflammatory bowel disease. *Inflamm Bowel Dis.* 2009;15(9):1417-1423.

79. Birth-18 years immunization schedule. CDC. https://www.cdc.gov/vaccines/schedules/hcp/imz/child-adolescent.html.

80. Rufo PA, Denson LA, Sylvester FA, et al. Health supervision in the management of children and adolescents with IBD: NASPGHAN recommendations. *J Pediatr Gastroenterol Nutr.* 2012;55(1):93-108.

81. Immunization schedule. https://www.aap.org/en-us/advocacy-and-policy/aap-health-initiatives/immunizations/Pages/Immunization-Schedule.aspx.

82.  Sands BE, Cuffari C, Katz J, et al. Guidelines for immunizations in patients with inflammatory bowel disease. *Inflamm Bowel Dis.* 2004;10(5):677-692.

83.  Melmed G, Ippoliti A, Papadakis K, et al. Patients with inflammatory bowel disease are at risk for vaccine-preventable illnesses. *Am J Gastroenterol.* 2006;101(8):1834-1840.

84.  Kane S, Khatibi B, Reddy D. Higher incidence of abnormal pap smears in women with inflammatory bowel disease. *Am J Gastroenterol.* 2008;103(3):631-636.

85.  Farshidpour M, Charabaty A, Mattar MC. Improving immunization strategies in patients with inflammatory bowel disease. *Ann Gastroenterol.* 2019;32(3):247-256.

86.  deBruyn JCC, Soon IS, Fonseca K, et al. Serologic status of routine childhood vaccines, cytomegalovirus, and epstein-barr virus in children with inflammatory bowel disease. *Inflamm Bowel Dis.* 2019;25(7):1218-1226.

# 2

# Transitional Care for Women With IBD

Jessica Philpott, MD | Jessica Barry

## Introduction

Transitional care for inflammatory bowel disease (IBD) involves both the discernible transfer of a patient from child-centered to adult-centered care and the transition of the primary responsibility of management of the disease from the family to the patient. As approximately 25% of patients with IBD are diagnosed by pediatric providers, and IBD is largely a chronic, incurable disease, a notable portion of IBD patients will undergo this process. Roughly half of these patients are female. Health care transition often happens at a time for women with IBD when body image, reproductive health care, and the socioeconomic challenges accompanying "adulting" in the 21st century are forefront in the life of an IBD patient. This is a time when negative body image, psychiatric comorbidities, inadequate reproductive health care, and developmental delays due to chronic illness, if present, are particularly destructive to the life course of an individual. It is important to note that for women with IBD pregnancy may in fact be the event that provokes the transition from pediatric to adult medicine and this creates a different timeline than other transition scenarios. Health care providers in both the child-centered care world and adult side who understand the educational, social, and health needs of women with IBD and structured transition interventions and resources are important to provide comprehensive care to these patients.

Abraham BP, Kane SV, Glassner KL, eds.
*Women's Health in IBD: The Spectrum of Care
From Birth to Adulthood* (pp 21-37).
© 2022 Taylor & Francis Group.

# Definitions

Several terms are necessary to define in order to have an effective conversation about transitional care for IBD (Table 2-1). For the purposes of this chapter, transition will be used to refer to the comprehensive process of both acquisition of skills and the process of disease self-management and transfer to adult providers. Transition readiness in general is referred to as having acquired sufficient skills to transition successfully to adult providers, suggesting that one has attained ability to independently manage one's disease with the assistance of the health care world. Carlsen et al have suggested that this includes the domains of 1) proper medical management, 2) management of emotions, and 3) living a meaningful life with IBD.[1] Self-efficacy is commonly equated with transition readiness, but the 2 terms are not synonymous. Perceived self-efficacy in general is defined as an individual's perception of their ability to plan and effect actions necessary to manage certain situations.[1] Self-efficacy as it applies to IBD means disease self-management. Health care independence can be defined as the ability to achieve, make decisions, and initiate actions by oneself in regards to one's health care.[2] Adherence to medication and other health care recommendations is identified as an important aspect of self-efficacy as a health care consumer. Adherence is linked to better outcomes for IBD, and published rates range from 7% to 72% and can be even lower for adolescents.[3,4] Understanding the reasons for lower adherence are important. Studies suggest that not having time, feeling medication interfered with "normal life," lack of belief that the medication is helping, and fear of side effects contribute to non-adherence.[4] In addition, in the experience of the authors, socioeconomic factors have great impact. Particularly in the United States, navigating the health care system in regard to the affordability of therapies often requires hours on the phone to make sure prior authorizations are achieved. If a parent is no longer accomplishing this task for a transitioned patient, this may not get done. Interestingly, employment, an event often accompanying transfer to adult medicine, is associated with lower adherence.[5] As non-adherence is a major obstacle to self-efficacy and disease control, understanding the reasons and providing support and education is essential in management of these patients.

# The Needs of Patients and Their Families

The needs of a patient who transfers from pediatric to adult care and their family are 1) medical, 2) psychosocial, 3) economic, and 4) educational. If these needs are not addressed, the transition and transfer might be challenging. The medical needs of individuals who are diagnosed with IBD as children can be quite complex. Children with IBD are more likely to have extensive disease and more rapid progression.[6] Pediatric patients with Crohn's disease are more likely to have ileocolonic disease compared with isolated ileal disease, and proximal disease (esophagus, stomach, duodenum) is also more common. Often, more aggressive medical therapy is required to control disease, and thus monitoring for side effects and long-term risk. Individuals presenting with ulcerative colitis under the age of 18 years are also more likely to have pancolonic disease and proctitis is uncommon.[7] Of note, delay in puberty and delay or loss of growth, in particular pubertal growth is reported.[8] Not only are there medical challenges, but these individuals experience psychological diseases and social challenges. Studies suggest that up to 25% of youth with IBD experience depression, which is higher than that reported for other chronic diseases of childhood,[9,10] with high rates of anxiety. IBD patients with depression may have more difficulty with adherence. They have higher rates of absenteeism, but in general meet comparable educational success.[11]

Understanding if young women with IBD experience different challenges, needs, or outcomes than males is important, but there are not adequate data to report. In regards to health-related quality of life (QOL), one study reports global, but not statistically significant, lower measures in girls with IBD than boys,[12] while a separate study reported that adolescent boys had lower QOL.[13] For educational outcomes, a case-control study of Swedish school children with IBD identified male sex

## Table 2-1. Definitions

| TERM | DEFINITION | ASSESSMENT EXAMPLES |
|---|---|---|
| Transition | Comprehensive process of both acquisition of skills and process of disease self-management and transfer to adult providers. | |
| Transition readiness | Acquisition of sufficient skills to transition successfully to adult providers. Possessing the knowledge set, the skills required for self-efficacy, and the social support to successfully transfer to adult medicine and transition to health care independence. | • Proper medical management<br>• Management of emotions<br>• Living a meaningful life with IBD |
| Self-efficacy | An individual's perception of their ability to plan and effect actions necessary to manage certain situations. | Self-efficacy at it applies to IBD:<br>• Disease self-management (scheduling appointments, monitoring symptoms, communicating with health care providers, and taking medicines) |
| Health care independence | The ability to achieve, make decisions, and initiate actions by oneself regarding one's health care. | |
| Adherence | The extent to which a person's behavior (including taking medication, dietary choices, and lifestyles) intersects with recommendations from a health care provider. | |

as associated with lower educational achievement in both the study and the control group. Certainly, further study to understand the different needs and challenges faced by young women in this age group compared to men are needed.

There is growing evidence that structured transition programs result in improved psychosocial outcomes.[14] Developing a comprehensive program to address these needs requires a multidisciplinary approach. Addressing the concerns and needs of parents and other caregivers is important and should be included in transition programs. Parents note concern with losing relationships with pediatric providers and perception of lower quality care from adult providers. A survey study of providers, patients, and parents found that each group had different views on what was most important for the patients to achieve in order to transition care,[15] with lack of agreement as to when transition readiness occurred.[16] In order to fully address the challenges of young women diagnosed with IBD as children, successful transition programs should comprehensively address the needs of patients and their families.

# Impact of Gender on Transition Readiness

Whether or not gender does or should have impact on transition readiness is unclear. Yerushalmy-Feler et al noted significantly better transition readiness in female patients from a cohort of 17 to 18-year-old patients with IBD.[17] Reporting the results of the 2009-10 National Survey of Children with Special Health Care Needs in the United States, McManus et al did find that male sex was associated with less successful transition,[18] and Gray et al also found that female patients were at a significantly higher rate of meeting the institutional benchmark for transition readiness.[19] In a recent survey of patients by the Crohn's and Colitis Foundation, female gender was again associated with greater transition readiness.[20] In regard to transgender patients, we are aware of no data as to the impact that transition from pediatric to adult medicine has on these patients. While these data suggest that gender may have some impact on successful transfer and transition, further data will be helpful in verifying this association and developing programs that more specifically meet the needs of young women.

# Young Women With Chronic Diseases

Acceptance of the diagnosis of a chronic disease at a young age is challenging for both young males and females. Even at a young age the need for education and support among women with chronic diseases is paramount when considering that the rates of physical disability are higher in women than in men and chronic diseases increase this risk.[21]

The psychosocial impact on young women with chronic illness can affect their beliefs about treatment adherence, leading to difficulties with medication compliance, self-care, and stress management related to living with their chronic disease.[22] The negative consequences of failure to achieve timely and consistent medical care are often brought on by the refusal to accept the diagnosis of a chronic disease, fear related to care costs, or the concern of the stigma among peers of having a chronic illness. Early education and support to overcome these barriers in order to achieve health care independence is essential in aiding to reduce the risk of unnecessary medical complications and promote overall personal wellness among young patients.

The physical and mental health symptoms associated with chronic illness in IBD can lead to deleterious effects on QOL. Recognizing symptoms of depression/anxiety along with a focus on overall care related to mental health must be assessed regularly. Prior studies have shown increased rates of internalizing psychological symptoms among young women with chronic disease compared to those without, which poses a challenge to providers in recognizing potential barriers to provide effective care.[23]

In addition, we know that chronic disease poses unique reproductive challenges for women. It is important to be aware that among American women and girls aged 15 to 44 years, approximately 45% of pregnancies are unintended based on a review of pregnancy rates from 2008 to 2011.[24] In particular, it is the experience of the authors that pregnancy is an event that often results in the decision to transfer care. For women who transition due to pregnancy, the fact that they have conceived does not directly prove that they have acquired the skills of self-management, but they will soon be expected in most cases to manage both their care and that of their child in the context of a chronic disease. Developing more focused educational resources for these individuals also may be of benefit. The importance of educating patients on the available options for contraception, safe sex practices, and adherence to routine prophylactic human papillomavirus vaccination is paramount when considering the increased risk of human papillomavirus associated anal, vaginal, and cervical cancer among patients with IBD.[25]

Young women with IBD often transition to adult care and health care independence during a time when their achievement in education, vocation, and development of personal relationships impacts the lives they hope to lead as full adults. Thus, the goal of their health care providers must be to mediate the effect of the disease on their life trajectory.

# Body Image

Body image is defined as the perception that a person has of their physical self and the thoughts and feelings that result from that perception. There is a paucity of data surrounding body image for patients with IBD and in young women with IBD. Negative body image or body image dissatisfaction in IBD patients has been associated with a low QOL, sexual satisfactions, and increased depression and anxiety.[26] A meta-analysis found that body image dissatisfaction was linked to a decreased QOL in IBD patients.[27] Unfortunately, female gender was associated with body image dissatisfaction in 6 out of 10 studies. Women had a 3-fold odds of reporting negative body image. Steroid use, BMI, smoking, and fatigue were also associated with negative impact on body image, while laparoscopic surgery and ileal pouch anal anastomosis were positive.

How IBD impacts body image in children continues to be investigated. The age at which the impact of IBD might be the most influential is unclear, but it is acknowledged that adolescence is a time of great importance. In general, studies of young women suggest that a multitude of societal, psychologic and physiologic forces shape body image between the ages of 12 and 19 years.[28] Investigations evaluating body image among children with chronic disease found an association between earlier onset and longer duration of disease with increased psychological adaptation. Thus highlighting that the differences between the body image of children with and without chronic illness may decline with earlier onset and longer duration of illness.[29] When evaluating age specific effects on perception of body image among children with chronic disease, it is well recognized that adolescence is a vulnerable period. Adolescent development of body image is characterized by a multitude of psychological and physical changes associated with an increased focus on physical appearance among adolescents. Subsequently, any effect on physical appearance related to illness will potentially have substantial negative impact on body image. Examples among patients with IBD include the varied therapy side effects (eg, weight gain, facial edema, acne) essential to disease treatment, such as prednisone. Further visible alterations to physical appearance such as stoma presence can have a significant effect on adolescent perceptions regarding body image. A recent meta-analysis comparing body image perception among young people with and without chronic illness supports the greatest difference in body image perception to be present when there is a visible change in physical appearance obvious to patients and their peers.[30] In studies of children with IBD, patients with a higher symptom index had a lower body image.[31] While studies specifically in female patients transitioning to adult medicine have not been conducted, certainly given these data we can infer that these women are at risk of body image dissatisfaction which can have an important impact on several factors including QOL and mental health. Some factors are those we may hope to improve including steroid use and disease activity along with identifying and providing resources for the psychological impact. Practitioners who provide care to young women with IBD should be attuned to this important aspect of well-being.

# Assessment of Current Transitional Practices

Across the world there are different levels of resource availability and institutional structure as it pertains to transition of care. Since the data on current practices are largely limited to North America and Western Europe, it is our hope that as this process continues to be studied across the globe, practices will be adapted to meet the differing needs of socially diverse populations. Some countries in Europe have published statements of transition policy,[32,33] and the European Crohn's and Colitis Organisation has published a succinct and clear position statement on transition.[34] In the United States, North American Society of Pediatric Gastroenterology Hepatology and Nutrition (NASPGHAN) published a position paper in 2002.[35] In Canada and some countries in Europe, the age of 18 years mandates transition to adult care, whereas in the United States patients are often transitioned later.

## Transition Clinics and Programs

It is a widely held belief that the most successful transitions and development of health care independence should be based on longitudinal efforts to build the groundwork for health care independence and self-efficacy and therefore cannot be achieved in one visit. Usually this would be done predominantly in the pediatric realm prior to the physical transition to adult medicine and would include education and serial assessment of transition readiness. Having a *transition policy* is important to this effort because it formally articulates and identifies the overall goals for both health care providers and patients. The resultant *transition plan* is the execution of that policy. The bare minimum for transition practices in pediatrics have been identified as:

- Portion of visit conducted with patient alone with health care provider
- Health care provider made efforts to promote self-management
- Health care provider discussed the future transition to adult care provider[36]

There are multiple ways transition clinic visits may be structured. The classic, and still seemingly the most common, clinic transition occurs when the patient, once ready (or not), is scheduled with an adult provider. There may be some overlap with final visits to the pediatric provider after the initial introduction to the adult provider, which for some may be optimal if a joint clinic is not available. The joint clinic, where the adult and pediatric provider meet with the patient together, has been identified by some including an European Crohn's and Colitis Organization summary as optimal,[34] although there is limited data to support that belief. This practice varies by country and by region. There are several barriers to a joint clinic. Resources including clinic space may be limited, and economics including billing rules may impact this. Despite the challenges, for those patients who need transition support, the joint clinic continues to be studied and supported as a good means to improve the success of transfer. Another less common model is a unique transition clinic where a patient would attend for the sole intent of addressing the transition needs including assessment and education. Often this is done by a provider that is not the one who will be continuing the patient's chronic care. As the needs of patients vary, it is likely that both single practitioner visit, joint and independent transition education will continue to serve the needs of this population.

The role of a transition clinic coordinator has been reported as a simple yet effective way to assist with the process. Potential activities of such an individual may include assessment, education, follow up to ensure an ongoing connection with the patient and the adult clinic, and other activities. In a retrospective chart review, Gray et al assessed patients who had met with the transition coordinator using Transition Readiness Assessment Questionnaire (TRAQ) scores before and after to monitor. They detected a decrease in the number of patients over the age of 21 years in pediatric clinic and an increase in transition readiness and self-management skills after the intervention.[37] In a systematic review, Eros et al summarized several studies which suggested the efficacy of transition nurses, but the application and outcomes were varied.[14]

Educational programs to assist with the development of self-management skills, and in some cases disease knowledge, have been provided in several ways. When surveyed, patients reported the desire for "individualized and multifaceted" interventions with many choices, including one on one instruction, handouts, and websites.[38] Given suspected variation in preferences for media, it is important not to make assumptions. Huang et al found that an electronic health record based program with annual transition assessments and online delivery of needed resources was well received by young adults with IBD who rated these median utility scores on a scale of 10 as 8 for the transition readiness assessment, 9 for transition resources provided, and 9 for the medical history summary.[39] Of interest, Szeto et al found that adolescents with IBD were less likely to use social media to learn about IBD than adults. Only 17% of the adolescents used the Internet frequently to obtain information about IBD, although almost all accessed the internet for other purposes daily.[40] However, one might attribute this to a lack of interest in learning about the disease and not necessarily the medium. A recent survey study found that young adults identified peer mentoring as important.[41] Formal education programs have also been studied. Schmidt et al reported on the effects of a

2-day transition workshop in sites across Germany for patients with chronic disease including IBD and found that participants had improved transition and self-efficacy scores, but no improvement in QOL.[42] Huang et al assessed the intervention of an intensive web-based approach in a group of patients aged 12 to 20 years with chronic diseases including cystic fibrosis and IBD in a randomized, controlled trial.[43] The intervention was a provision of web-based material provided regarding self-management and communication skills, with short messages service messages and queries to follow up and ensure reception of materials and comprehension. Over 8 months the participants demonstrated improved disease management and self-efficacy scores and an increase in patient-initiated communications with providers.

Intuitively, a successful program for transition will include both the elements of web-based learning, longitudinal visits, and face to face clinic visits. One example of this is a personalized eHealth concept described by Carlsen et al. The concept suggests that in early adolescence, patient reported outcome measures in areas of self-efficacy, knowledge, resilience, and stress would be assessed and used during annual visits with a specialized transition consultation nurse. The transition nurse would focus the visit with dialogue and exercises based on the needs detected by the patient reported outcome measures. Progressively less parent involvement in regular clinic visits would be mandated. This concept involves both longitudinal assessment, use of electronic health assessment, and personalized face to face visits.[44] How to best deliver the resources and education to enhance self-management, disease knowledge, and thus the transition process, remains to be fully understood. Some materials and verbal education should be provided through the clinic. Other forms of delivery including web-based media, written material, and workshops are useful as well. Making use of preparatory interventions via online media such as education or pre-visit surveys would be hoped to enhance the efficacy of the in-person visit. As the needs of transitioning patients are clinical, educational, psychosocial, and economic, addressing these needs will require longitudinal efforts with multiple arms of intervention.

Assessing the effectiveness of these clinics and other transition interventions would optimally include both patient reported outcomes and satisfaction with the process along with clinical outcomes and success of transfer including ongoing reception of care. Most studies focus on only some aspects of these outcomes, and very few report clinical outcomes. Patient reported outcomes that have been assessed by transition intervention studies most commonly include QOL measures, but adherence, self-efficacy, and disease knowledge have also been used as outcomes.[14] In general, there are challenges to these studies because the intervention is not blinded nor easily randomized, and when using historical controls, changes to medical practice can influence outcomes as well. Regarding clinical outcomes, Cole et al designed a study which is fairly unique in reporting clinically relevant outcomes in patients comparing those before and after attending transition clinics.[45] Seventy-two patients were followed from 2006 to 2014. The intervention was a structured transition clinic providing serial visits incorporating disease specific education and assessments of transition readiness. This was followed by actual transfer to adult clinic. Patients in the transition clinic group had higher rates of adherence to medication (89% vs 46%, $P = .002$), recorded lower rates of missed clinic visits (29% vs 78%, $P = .001$), had lower rates of surgery during the reporting period (25% vs 46%, $P = .01$), and fewer hospital admissions (29% vs 61%, $P = .002$. While this is striking and merits further study, it is important to note differences between the 2 groups. The patients in the transition clinic intervention group had shorter duration of disease and a higher rate of anti-tumor necrosis factor therapy (18% vs 7%, $P = .04$) and thiopurine (56% vs 46%) use. Fu et al reported a case-control study of Canadian young adults with IBD referred to a joint pediatric-adult IBD transition clinic to assess the impact of the clinic on attitudes toward medication. While no statistically significant improvement was detected in adherence to medication based on self-reporting, they did detect an improvement in attitudes toward medical therapy and a reduction in skepticism compared to traditional clinic patients.[46] Yerushalmy-Feler et al assessed the outcomes of a structured transitional clinic staffed by both pediatric and adult providers with 4 structured visits over a 6-month period including visits assigned to education and treatment planning. Making use of the "IBD yourself"

self-efficacy scale, they found an increase in self-efficacy, along with disease specific knowledge.[17] Of note, after transfer, females had higher self-efficacy scores than males. It is unfortunate that many transition studies have only been presented as abstracts. Of interest, Eros et al conducted a systematic review and were able to summarize and report the data from several studies, many of which had only been published as abstracts until this time. Four studies have reported on health-related QOL, and in general most studies do report some benefit from a transition program.[14] As transition care advances, further studies should continue to assess patient reported outcomes, but in appropriate settings including clinical outcomes will also support comprehensive assessment of utility.

## Transition Readiness Assessment

Transition readiness assessment is an essential part of transition programs. Transition readiness assessment is necessary both to identify needs of the patient that are not yet addressed in the process of transitioning to health care independence and self-efficacy, and to provide information to the providers as to when the patient and family may be ready to transition. An ideal assessment tool would be age appropriate, easy, and efficient to use for both patients and providers, longitudinal and educational. Use of these measures is varied but widespread, with Gray et al reporting that 79% of NASPGHAN providers reported use of some measure to assess transition readiness.[47] Of note, gender in some studies has been associated with higher score on certain assessments, including the TRAQ.[48] Currently there are no gender specific transition assessments.

There are many measures available to assess transition readiness in young people with IBD (Table 2-2). There is inadequate data currently to directly recommend one assessment over the others. In the survey conducted by Gray et al of NASPGHAN providers, the most commonly used measures were the TRAQ or the NASPGHAN transition checklist.[47] The characteristics of some of these measures are presented in Table 2-2.[48-52] Some tools are generic without disease-specific information such as the TRAQ and some are disease-specific with questions relevant to disease knowledge such as the IBD Self-Efficacy Scale—Adolescent (IBD-SES-A). Some critique of these measures, including TRAQ and IBD-SES-A, is that age impacts scores and in general they are best studied for use in patients in their later teens. At this juncture, the best recommendation is to use one of the assessments of transition readiness longitudinally to assist patients in developing the necessary skills and determine when transfer to adult providers is appropriate.

# Age-Specific Progression of Transitional Skills and Assessment

Ideally, preparing individuals diagnosed with IBD in the pediatric age group for transition to adult medicine and assumption of health care independence and self-efficacy should occur over a period of time. Assessment and promotion of skills should be tailored to the individual's needs based on their maturity and the obstacles they encounter. The understanding of psychosocial development of young women with chronic disease and the challenges that this poses to their QOL and body image still requires further study. Age-specific guidelines for transition skills have been proposed publications by De Silva et al and NASPGHAN Healthcare Provider Transitioning Checklist (https://www.naspghan.org/files/documents/pdfs/medical-resources/ibd/Checklist_PatientandHealthcareProdiver_TransitionfromPedtoAdult.pdf).[53] All of these guidelines and checklists should be utilized with assessment of the emotional age of the individual, understanding that the stated ages are estimates, and there will be marked variation with some individuals functioning at an adult level in adolescence and some at a lower level despite an advanced chronologic age. Table 2-3 provides visualization of the progression of expected skills, barriers, and solutions at these levels.

## Table 2-2. Transition Assessments

| TOOL | DISEASE-SPECIFIC | VALIDATED | NOTES | REPORTED IN AGES (YEARS) |
|---|---|---|---|---|
| TRAQ[48] | No | Yes | Widely used transition readiness assessment. Twenty-question survey that assesses a patient's ability to manage their own disease with questions regarding ability to manage disease and medication knowledge, navigate health care system, and activities of daily living. | 12 to 25 (validated over 14) |
| IBD-SES-A[50] | Yes | Yes | Self-efficacy assessment. Assess 4 domains of ability to manage a) stress, b) medical care, c) symptoms and disease, d) maintaining remission. | 12 to 25 |
| IBD Yourself[51] | Yes | Yes | Assessment of self-efficacy, 59 questions, 12 domains. | 14 to 18 |
| STARx[49] | No | Yes | Questionnaire of 18 questions with correlation to literacy, self-efficacy, and adherence measures. | |
| The NASPGHAN Healthcare Provider Transitioning Checklist | Yes | No | A checklist of transition tasks, disease specific with age-specific categories. (https://www.naspghan.org/files/documents/pdfs/medical-resources/ibd/Checklist_PatientandHealthcareProdiver_TransitionfromPedtoAdult.pdf) | n/a |
| UNC TR(x)ANSITION scale[52] | No | Yes | Scale of 33 questions is administered by a trained health professional who gives patients scores for their answers across 10 domains. | 12 to 22 |

## Table 2-3. Transition Metrics

| | EARLY ADOLESCENCE 12 TO 14 YEARS | MID-ADOLESCENCE 14 TO 17 YEARS | YOUNG ADULT | ADULT |
|---|---|---|---|---|
| | Develop a foundation of knowledge to achieve independent care | Reinforce and solidify health literacy in order to identify gaps in assuming primary health care responsibility | Transfer of primary care responsibilities to patient | Successful transition of care to adult provider |
| PATIENT SKILLS | Name medication/disease<br><br>Participates in health care discussions | Begins to perform independent care actions with support: prescription refills, contacting providers related to care management | Independent care management: communication with providers and medication management | Achieves complete health care independence: appointment scheduling, attending procedures/appointments, medication management/insurance |
| BARRIERS | Lack of educational resources on disease and self-management<br><br>Patient interest/motivation<br><br>Time constraints for family, patient, and provider | Patient discomfort/parental preference leading conversations with providers<br><br>Limited resources to aid in development of skills for health care independence | Reluctance of parent/provider to transfer health related communication to patient<br><br>Identifying adult provider to transfer care<br><br>Facing social/financial barriers | Allotting time for focused time with provider to address potential barriers to health care needs; financial constraints, understanding disease complications, insurance coverage concerns |

*(continued)*

## Early Adolescence (12 to 14 Years)

Most guidelines recommend that the concept of transition be introduced in this age group. Basic expectations would be that the individuals are able to communicate their disease, know their medications, and be able to discuss the impact that IBD has had on their life. Barriers to this initial step include lack of interest or anxiety on the part of the patient and family, and lack of time and resources on the part of the care providers. In newly diagnosed patients, grieving behavior such as

| Table 2-3 (continued). Transition Metrics | | | | |
|---|---|---|---|---|
| | **EARLY ADOLESCENCE 12 TO 14 YEARS** | **MID-ADOLESCENCE 14 TO 17 YEARS** | **YOUNG ADULT** | **ADULT** |
| | Develop a foundation of knowledge to achieve independent care | Reinforce and solidify health literacy in order to identify gaps in assuming primary health care responsibility | Transfer of primary care responsibilities to patient | Successful transition of care to adult provider |
| **SOLUTIONS** | Web-based educational resources<br><br>Time allotment at visits to review primary aims of transition and health care independence | Provider support to families and reinforcing importance of transition goals<br><br>Ongoing reinforcement of available resources to aid in transition<br><br>Address challenges for patient and families at appointments | Involving social work/care coordinators to assist with education and patient support<br><br>Maintaining open communication with adult providers to avoid delays in follow-up/therapies | Schedule follow up appointments focused on discussion of health care and psychosocial needs of the patient<br><br>Involve social work/care coordinators in visits to expedite solutions to identified care needs |

the stage of denial make transition planning particularly difficult. This is an age when the impact of disease on body image may be important and this must be identified. There are no transition assessment tools fully validated in this age group although SES-A and TRAQ have been reported.[48,50] Studies suggest that while individuals of this age may begin to achieve some skills, it is uncommon (and probably unnecessary) for them to master all self-management skills by this age.[54]

## Mid-Adolescence (14 to 17 Years)

At this age, education aimed at improving health care independence should be solidly underway. In those newly diagnosed, part of disease-specific education should include these factors. Skills such as filling one's own prescription and participating in medical decision making should be encouraged. This is an important time for social support to be developed. Barriers include ambivalence on the part of the patient, family, and providers. Interpersonal conflict and parental attitudes will contribute to patient attitudes. As an example, studies in transplant patients in this age group suggest that parental attitudes have significant impact on patient adherence and acceptance of health care recommendations and involvement in care plan.[55] All of the transition assessment tools have been reported in this age group, although those over 16 years may be most well validated, and the checklists such as NASPGHAN and that reported by De Silva et al have skills applicable to patients of this age.

## Young Adult/Adult (18 Years and Older)

In this age group, for most individuals, if the major skills related to health care independence have not been achieved, a focused effort on understanding why and providing resources to address is usually indicated. This would include scheduling and planning appointments and procedures and making decisions. This is not to state that one expects these patients to pursue care alone, as if available, the support and participation of family or friends may be important to IBD patients throughout the extent of their lives. Of import, patients who remain financially dependent on their families to pursue advanced education may delay transition. In 2020 in the United States, the current laws regarding insurance allow for dependents to remain on their parent's insurance until the age of 26, which may affect the development of health care independence. Transition assessment continues through transfer and once the patient has transferred, continued support of self-management skill development is warranted.

# Basic Guidelines for Transition

## For the Pediatric Provider

1. Transition should be introduced much in advance of the actual transfer.
2. Some form of longitudinal assessment of self-efficacy and transition readiness is recommended.
3. For most patients, as patient enters age preceding transfer, conducting part of the clinic visit without parents is indicated.
4. Identification of adult providers willing and able to assume care is important.

## For the Adult Provider

1. Pursue education in regard to health care needs of young adults.
2. Understand the psychosocial and economic challenges faced by patients in this age group.
3. Continue the process of encouraging self-efficacy.

## For the Process Overall

1. Overlap in some form of the pediatric and adult providers is advisable either via joint clinic or communication.
2. Where available, a coordinator may improve outcomes.[14,37]
3. Flexibility in terms of timing and expectations of patient and family enhances the process.
4. An adequate mechanism for transfer of information is necessary.
5. Use of portable health care summaries allows education of the patient along with enhancing information transfer.

# Conclusion

Transitional care includes development of self-management, self-efficacy, and the transfer to adult-centered care. The American Academy of Pediatrics updated clinical report on the state of transition lists the principles of effort to include:

1) importance of youth and young adult centered, strength based focus, 2) emphasis on self-determination and family and/or caregiver, 3) acknowledgement of individual differences and complexities, 4) recognition of vulnerabilities and need for a distinct population health approach for youth and young adults, 5) need for early and ongoing preparation, including the integration into an adult model of care, 6) importance of shared accountability, communication and care coordination between pediatric and adult providers, 7) recognition of influences, cultural beliefs and attitudes as well as socioeconomic status, 8) emphasis on achieving health equity and eliminating health disparities and 9) need for parents and caregivers to support youth and young adults in building knowledge regarding their own health and skills in making health decisions and using health care.[56]

There is still a need across the globe for better programs for young women with IBD to improve the transition process and to enhance the development of disease self-management. Whether specific programs for women with IBD should be developed has not been directly assessed, but several studies suggest that gender does impact the skill set for transition, therefore it is reasonable to conjecture that the transition needs of women might be different.[17-20] Providing specific resources to women who transition at the time of pregnancy is also necessary. Determining better ways to time transfer of care is needed. In studies of patients with chronic disease who transition, one of the most common variables linked to transition readiness is age.[20,50] This should call into question our current transition practices. In countries where the transition age is fluid and not mandated in the late teens, such as the US, the reasons that prompt the transfer to adult medicine should be studied.

Moving forward, use of consistent outcomes in studies of transition programs will improve the additional knowledge gained. Recommended outcomes include adherence to care, disease-specific measures, QOL, self-care skills, satisfaction with care, health care utilization, and health care transition process of care.

Progress has been achieved in developing tools and programs for patients with IBD as they transition to adult providers and disease self-management, but there is still much to be done. Only with commitment to this process by all parties involved including practitioners, patients, and family members will the longitudinal success and health of young women with IBD be achieved.

# Transition Cases

These cases are composite and not reports of actual patients.

## Case Study: Emma

The pediatric gastroenterologist had some reservations about transitioning 22-year-old Emma to adult medicine due to the family dynamic. Emma's mother was a dominating figure in the visits. Emma usually looked at her phone while her mother talked to the doctor. Her mother was somewhat demanding and expected detailed explanations for all results, and treatment plans. Nonetheless, when Emma turned 21, she was fully transferred to an academic, adult gastroenterology practice. She had a joint visit with her mother and the adult and pediatric provider. After this visit, Emma refused to let her mother come back with her for visits. She eventually moved out of her mother's house and had appeared to have achieved independence. After 6 months, Emma let the infusion nurse know she was pregnant. She fell behind in classes at the local community college and dropped out. This led to financial strain from paying back her school loans. Emma gave her child up for adoption. She then started working at a retail store, resulting in restricted flexibility to take time off from work, along with limited means of transportation to get to her appointments. She sporadically made her visits for clinic follow-up with numerous reschedules despite reminder calls, and over time was less adherent with infliximab visits. At one point she had a prolonged delay in her infusions. She felt angry that this happened but was not willing to discuss changing to an injectable biologic to improve adherence if she was not able to make infusions. Emma eventually ended up in the hospital and underwent surgery for an ileal stricture resulting in partial bowel obstruction.

### Case Study Assessment

Emma faced both social and economic challenges. Her mother had directed all her care, but once she sought to release herself from her mother's direction, she did not have the skills and tools to maneuver the worlds of health care and finance alone. A more thorough transition readiness assessment along with resources to teach health care independence such as a clinic, online tools, or a workshop would hope to provide better for these needs. Emma experienced an unintended pregnancy. This is a common occurrence but highlights the need for ongoing discussion and provision of care aimed at avoiding this event. She also struggled financially and likely psychologically after a series of dramatic changes in her life. The assistance of a social worker likely would have benefited this situation. It seems the transfer was identified at the time at which Emma's mother ceased to maintain control, and she then ceased to provide assistance to Emma. How to fully assess economic needs or assist with them is something that care providers struggle with. Of note, economics certainly do impact the success of transition, with McManus et al noting that an income above 400% of the federal poverty level improves increases the likelihood of successful transfer.[18] Emma's adherence was limited by a number of factors, but it resulted unfortunately in progression of her disease.

# Case Study: Maria

Maria was felt to be overdue for transition. She had Crohn's ileitis with quiescent perianal disease and was maintained on infliximab monotherapy. She was assessed for transition readiness and the pediatric provider felt she was appropriate to transfer, but she and her mother were reluctant. She did understand the means of scheduling appointments and filling prescriptions. Finally, at age 24 years she met with the adult practitioner and transitioned. During the clinic visit her mother did most of the talking, but she was able to express her goals and answer questions about her history. For 1 year, Maria presented to clinic visits on her own. She was the one sending messages to the physician on the medical portal. She had a new job and a new girlfriend. Her girlfriend came to one clinic visit. Then she missed a subsequent clinic visit. After 6 months her mother contacted the physician via the online portal stating that Maria was not doing well and asking what the plan was. When the physician was not able to contact Maria by phone, she then contacted the mother out of concern. It seemed Maria had broken up with her girlfriend and was depressed. She had missed a dose of infliximab and felt she might be flaring, complaining of pain and weight loss. After some efforts, and interaction with mental health care providers, Maria continued on infliximab. Her medical workup did not reveal active disease. Maria started coming to clinic by herself again. Her mother accompanied her to procedures.

### Case Study Assessment

Maria made efforts to establish independence, but setbacks in her life as an adult resulted in reversion back to her previous interactions with her mother and her health care providers. This is a behavior that the authors witness commonly in newly transitioned patients. She wanted her mother to manage the care when she did not feel well. She also developed depression, which is an important comorbidity that should be screened for on an ongoing basis. The American College of Gastroenterology Clinical Guidelines in management of Crohn's recommend that assessment and management of stress, depression, and anxiety should be part of routine care.[57] Because the adult provider had worked to develop a functional relationship with Maria's mother, when Maria had her crisis, the team of physician, mother, and patient were able to address the situation in the way that Maria needed at the time, but then kept moving forward toward more complete health care independence in the future. This is fitting with recent studies that suggest that few adult providers are concerned with a patients inability to attend clinic on their own.[58] In regard to programs that might have helped Maria, while she had been assessed and educated serially in transition readiness, she may have benefited from more thorough assessment of her psychological health.

---

## KEY POINTS

1. Transitional care for IBD involves both the discernible transfer of a patient from child-centered to adult-centered care and the transition of the primary responsibility of management of the disease from the family to the patient.

2. Assessment of transition readiness is necessary both to identify needs of the patient in the process of transitioning to health care independence and self-efficacy, and to provide information to the providers as to when the patient and family may be ready to transition. Utilization of recommended transition readiness assessment tools such as TRAQ are recommended.[48]

3. Transition to adult medicine and assumption of health care independence and self-efficacy should occur over a period of time. Assessment and promotion of skills should be tailored to the individual's needs throughout early adolescence to young adulthood based on their maturity and the obstacles they encounter.

4. Awareness of the multifactorial aspects that can impact women with chronic disease and IBD is essential in supporting patients for successful transitions in care.

---

# References

1.  Carlsen K, Haddad N, Gordon J, et al. Self-efficacy and resilience are useful predictors of transition readiness scores in adolescents with inflammatory bowel diseases. *Inflamm Bowel Dis.* 2017;23(3):341-346.

2.  Hughes SA. Promoting self-management and patient independence. *Nurs Stand.* 2004;19(10):47-52; quiz 54, 56.

3.  Matteson-Kome ML, Winn J, Bechtold ML, Bragg JD, Russell CL. Improving maintenance medication adherence in adult inflammatory bowel disease patients: a pilot study. *Health Psychol Res.* 2014;2(1):1389.

4.  Spekhorst LM, Hummel TZ, Benninga MA, van Rheenen PF, Kindermann A. Adherence to oral maintenance treatment in adolescents with inflammatory bowel disease. *J Pediatr Gastroenterol Nutr.* 2016;62(2):264-270.

5.  Eindor-Abarbanel A, Naftali T, Ruhimovich N, et al. Revealing the puzzle of nonadherence in IBD—assembling the pieces. *Inflamm Bowel Dis.* 2018;24(6):1352-1360.

6.  Van Limbergen J, Russell RK, Drummond HE, et al. Definition of phenotypic characteristics of childhood-onset inflammatory bowel disease. *Gastroenterology.* 2008;135(4):1114-1122.

7.  Carroll MW, Kuenzig ME, Mack DR, et al. The impact of inflammatory bowel disease in Canada 2018: children and adolescents with IBD. *J Can Assoc Gastroenterol.* 2019;2(Suppl 1):S49-S67.

8.  Mason A, Malik S, Russell RK, Bishop J, McGrogan P, Ahmed SF. Impact of inflammatory bowel disease on pubertal growth. *Horm Res Paediatr.* 2011;76(5):293-299.

9.  Mackner LM, Greenley RN, Szigethy E, Herzer M, Deer K, Hommel KA. Psychosocial issues in pediatric inflammatory bowel disease: report of the North American Society for Pediatric Gastroenterology, Hepatology, and Nutrition. *J Pediatr Gastroenterol Nutr.* 2013;56(4):449-458.

10. Greenley RN, Hommel KA, Nebel J, et al. A meta-analytic review of the psychosocial adjustment of youth with inflammatory bowel disease. *J Pediatr Psychol.* 2010;35(8):857-869.

11. Malmborg P, Mouratidou N, Sachs MC, et al. Effects of childhood-onset inflammatory bowel disease on school performance: a nationwide population-based cohort study using swedish health and educational registers. *Inflamm Bowel Dis*. 2019;25(10):1663-1673.

12. van der Zaag-Loonen HJ, Grootenhuis MA, Last BF, Derkx HH. Coping strategies and quality of life of adolescents with inflammatory bowel disease. *Qual Life Res*. 2004;13(5):1011-1019.

13. De Boer M, Grootenhuis M, Derkx B, Last B. Health-related quality of life and psychosocial functioning of adolescents with inflammatory bowel disease. *Inflamm Bowel Dis*. 2005;11(4):400-406.

14. Eros A, Soos A, Hegyi P, et al. Spotlight on transition in patients with inflammatory bowel disease: a systematic review. *Inflamm Bowel Dis*. 2020;26(3):331-346.

15. Gray WN, Reed-Knight B, Morgan PJ, et al. Multi-site comparison of patient, parent, and pediatric provider perspectives on transition to adult care in IBD. *J Pediatr Nurs*. 2018;39:49-54.

16. Gray WN, Resmini AR, Baker KD, et al. Concerns, barriers, and recommendations to improve transition from pediatric to adult IBD care: perspectives of patients, parents, and health professionals. *Inflamm Bowel Dis*. 2015;21(7):1641-1651.

17. Yerushalmy-Feler A, Ron Y, Barnea E, et al. Adolescent transition clinic in inflammatory bowel disease: quantitative assessment of self-efficacy skills. *Eur J Gastroenterol Hepatol*. 2017;29(7):831-837.

18. McManus MA, Pollack LR, Cooley WC, et al. Current status of transition preparation among youth with special needs in the United States. *Pediatrics*. 2013;131(6):1090-1097.

19. Gray WN, Holbrook E, Morgan PJ, Saeed SA, Denson LA, Hommel KA. Transition readiness skills acquisition in adolescents and young adults with inflammatory bowel disease: findings from integrating assessment into clinical practice. *Inflamm Bowel Dis*. 2015;21(5):1125-1131.

20. Arvanitis M, Hart LC, DeWalt DA, et al. Transition readiness not associated with measures of health in youth with IBD. *Inflamm Bowel Dis*. 2021;27(1):49-57. doi:10.1093/ibd/izaa026

21. Khoury AJ, Hall A, Andresen E, Zhang J, Ward R, Jarjoura C. The association between chronic disease and physical disability among female Medicaid beneficiaries 18-64 years of age. *Disabil Health J*. 2013;6(2):141-148.

22. Rohan JM, Verma T. Psychological considerations in pediatric chronic illness: case examples. *Int J Environ Res Public Health*. 2020;17(5):1644.

23. Rosina R, Crisp J, Steinbeck K. Treatment adherence of youth and young adults with and without a chronic illness. *Nurs Health Sci*. 2003;5(2):139-147.

24. Finer LB, Zolna MR. Declines in unintended pregnancy in the United States, 2008-2011. *N Engl J Med*. 2016;374(9):843-852.

25. Segal JP, Askari A, Clark SK, Hart AL, Faiz OD. The incidence and prevalence of human papilloma virus-associated cancers in IBD. *Inflamm Bowel Dis*. 2021;27(1):34-39.

26. McDermott E, Mullen G, Moloney J, et al. Body image dissatisfaction: clinical features, and psychosocial disability in inflammatory bowel disease. *Inflamm Bowel Dis*. 2015;21(2):353-360.

27. Beese SE, Harris IM, Dretzke J, Moore D. Body image dissatisfaction in patients with inflammatory bowel disease: a systematic review. *BMJ Open Gastroenterol*. 2019;6(1):e000255.

28. Voelker DK, Reel JJ, Greenleaf C. Weight status and body image perceptions in adolescents: current perspectives. *Adolesc Health Med Ther*. 2015;6:149-158.

29. Newell R. *Body Image and Disfigurement Care*. Routledge: 2000.

30. Pinquart M. Body image of children and adolescents with chronic illness: a meta-analytic comparison with healthy peers. *Body Image*. 2013;10(2):141-148.

31. Perrin JM, Kuhlthau K, Chughtai A, et al. Measuring quality of life in pediatric patients with inflammatory bowel disease: psychometric and clinical characteristics. *J Pediatr Gastroenterol Nutr*. 2008;46(2):164-171.

32. Italian Society of Paediatric Gastroenterology H, Nutrition IAoHG, Endoscopists ISoEISoG, et al. Transition of gastroenterological patients from paediatric to adult care: a position statement by the Italian Societies of Gastroenterology. *Dig Liver Dis*. 2015;47(9):734-740.

33. Brooks AJ, Smith PJ, Cohen R, et al. UK guideline on transition of adolescent and young persons with chronic digestive diseases from paediatric to adult care. *Gut*. 2017;66(6):988-1000.

34. van Rheenen PF, Aloi M, Biron IA, et al. European Crohn's and Colitis Organisation topical review on transitional care in inflammatory bowel disease. *J Crohns Colitis*. 2017;11(9):1032-1038.

35. Baldassano R, Ferry G, Griffiths A, Mack D, Markowitz J, Winter H. Transition of the patient with inflammatory bowel disease from pediatric to adult care: recommendations of the North American Society for Pediatric Gastroenterology, Hepatology and Nutrition. *J Pediatr Gastroenterol Nutr*. 2002;34(3):245-248.

36. Lebrun-Harris LA, McManus MA, Ilango SM, et al. Transition planning among US youth with and without special health care needs. *Pediatrics*. 2018;142(4):e20180194.

37. Gray WN, Holbrook E, Dykes D, Morgan PJ, Saeed SA, Denson LA. Improving IBD transition, self-management, and disease outcomes with an in-clinic transition coordinator. *J Pediatr Gastroenterol Nutr*. 2019;69(2):194-199.

38. Klostermann NR, McAlpine L, Wine E, Goodman KJ, Kroeker KI. Assessing the transition intervention needs of young adults with inflammatory bowel diseases. *J Pediatr Gastroenterol Nutr*. 2018;66(2):281-285.

39. Huang JS, Yueh R, Wood K, et al. Harnessing the electronic health record to distribute transition services to adolescents with inflammatory bowel disease. *J Pediatr Gastroenterol Nutr*. 2020;70(2):200-204.

40. Szeto W, van der Bent A, Petty CR, Reich J, Farraye F, Fishman LN. Use of social media for health-related tasks by adolescents with inflammatory bowel disease: a step in the pathway of transition. *Inflamm Bowel Dis*. 2018;24(6):1114-1122.

41. Maddux MH, Drovetta M, Hasenkamp R, et al. Using a mixed-method approach to develop a transition program for young adults with inflammatory bowel disease. *J Pediatr Gastroenterol Nutr*. 2020;70(2):195-199.

42. Schmidt S, Herrmann-Garitz C, Bomba F, Thyen U. A multicenter prospective quasi-experimental study on the impact of a transition-oriented generic patient education program on health service participation and quality of life in adolescents and young adults. *Patient Educ Couns*. 2016;99(3):421-428.

43. Huang JS, Terrones L, Tompane T, et al. Preparing adolescents with chronic disease for transition to adult care: a technology program. *Pediatrics*. 2014;133(6):e1639-1646.

44. Carlsen K, Hald M, Dubinsky MC, Keefer L, Wewer V. A personalized eHealth transition concept for adolescents with inflammatory bowel disease: design of intervention. *JMIR Pediatr Parent*. 2019;2(1):e12258.

45. Cole R, Ashok D, Razack A, Azaz A, Sebastian S. Evaluation of outcomes in adolescent inflammatory bowel disease patients following transfer from pediatric to adult health care services: case for transition. *J Adolesc Health*. 2015;57(2):212-217.

46. Fu N, Jacobson K, Round A, Evans K, Qian H, Bressler B. Transition clinic attendance is associated with improved beliefs and attitudes toward medicine in patients with inflammatory bowel disease. *World J Gastroenterol*. 2017;23(29):5405-5411.

47. Gray WN, Maddux MH. Current transition practices in pediatric IBD: findings from a National Survey of Pediatric Providers. *Inflamm Bowel Dis*. 2016;22(2):372-379.

48. Wood DL, Sawicki GS, Miller MD, et al. The Transition Readiness Assessment Questionnaire (TRAQ): its factor structure, reliability, and validity. *Acad Pediatr*. 2014;14(4):415-422.

49. Cohen SE, Hooper SR, Javalkar K, et al. Self-management and transition readiness assessment: concurrent, predictive and discriminant validation of the STARx questionnaire. *J Pediatr Nurs*. 2015;30(5):668-676.

50. Izaguirre MR, Taft T, Keefer L. Validation of a self-efficacy scale for adolescents and young adults with inflammatory bowel disease. *J Pediatr Gastroenterol Nutr*. 2017;65(5):546-550.

51. Zijlstra M, De Bie C, Breij L, et al. Self-efficacy in adolescents with inflammatory bowel disease: a pilot study of the "IBD-yourself", a disease-specific questionnaire. *J Crohns Colitis*. 2013;7(9):e375-385.

52. Ferris ME, Harward DH, Bickford K, et al. A clinical tool to measure the components of health-care transition from pediatric care to adult care: the UNC TR(x)ANSITION scale. *Ren Fail*. 2012;34(6):744-753.

53. de Silva PS, Fishman LN. Transition of the patient with IBD from pediatric to adult care-an assessment of current evidence. *Inflamm Bowel Dis*. 2014;20(8):1458-1464.

54. Stollon N, Zhong Y, Ferris M, et al. Chronological age when healthcare transition skills are mastered in adolescents/young adults with inflammatory bowel disease. *World J Gastroenterol*. 2017;23(18):3349-3355.

55. Jakubowska-Winecka A, Biernacka M. Parental attitudes and medication adherence in groups of adolescents after liver and kidney transplantations. *Transplant Proc*. 2018;50(7):2145-2149.

56. White PH, Cooley WC, Transitions Clinical Report Authoring G, American Academy Of Physicians, American Academy Of Family Physicians, American College Of Physicians. Supporting the health care transition From adolescence to adulthood in the medical mome. *Pediatrics*. 2018;142(5):e20182587.

57. Lichtenstein GR, Loftus EV, Isaacs KL, Regueiro MD, Gerson LB, Sands BE. ACG clinical guideline: management of Crohn's disease in adults. *Am J Gastroenterol*. 2018;113(4):481-517.

58. Hait EJ, Barendse RM, Arnold JH, et al. Transition of adolescents with inflammatory bowel disease from pediatric to adult care: a survey of adult gastroenterologists. *J Pediatr Gastroenterol Nutr*. 2009;48(1):61-65.

# 3

# The Role of Diet, Nutrition, and the Microbiome in Women With IBD

Nirupama Bonthala, MD | Kelly Issokson, MS, RD, CNSC

## Introduction

Diet, nutrition, and the microbiome are of increasing interest to patients living with inflammatory bowel disease (IBD). Women with IBD who are pregnant or interested in conception have the additional challenge of ensuring adequate nutrition to support proper fetal growth. In this chapter, we review what is known regarding the microbiome in females, nutritional consequences of IBD, common micronutrient deficiencies, and dietary therapies for active and quiescent disease. We encourage the gastroenterologist to familiarize themselves with these topics to facilitate a productive dialogue with your patient and support them in developing a well-rounded plan of care.

## Microbiome

Emerging data suggest the microbiome plays a critical role and is associated with numerous health outcomes in women and their offspring. Here we review what is known of the role of the microbiome in both the female reproductive organs as well as the female intestinal tract in both those without and with IBD.

Abraham BP, Kane SV, Glassner KL, eds.
*Women's Health in IBD: The Spectrum of Care
From Birth to Adulthood* (pp 39-59).
© 2022 Taylor & Francis Group.

## Overview of the Female Microbiome

The human microbiome consists of bacteria, fungi, archea, and viruses in the intestines, skin, reproductive tract, and oral cavity. The microbiome when functioning optimally works symbiotically with the host but with dysbiosis or an unbalanced microbial system, loses this relationship and disease states may occur. While most of the attention in early microbiome studies focused on the intestinal flora, there is a growing body of research in the female reproductive tract including the vaginal and placental microbiome.

The vaginal microbiome drastically differs throughout a woman's life based on her estrogen level. Prior to puberty, the vaginal microbiome is composed of predominantly gram-negative anaerobic bacteria such as *Bacteroides* and *Fusobacterium* species and a relatively lower abundance of various lactobacilli and *Gardnerella vaginalis*.[1,2] After puberty with the onset of an estrogenic state, there is a preference for glucose fermenting organisms by the thickening vaginal epithelium. Thus the vaginal microbiome after puberty and throughout a woman's childbearing years favors *Lactobacillus* and *Gardnerella* species.[3,4] During menopause, with the cessation of estrogen, the vaginal lining thins and once again shifts to a microbiome similar to that prior to puberty.[4-6]

Until recently, the placenta was thought to be a sterile environment, but several studies now show this to be untrue. A 2014 study on 320 placental samples showed a predominance of *Proteobacteria* which interestingly is most similar to the oral microbiome during pregnancy.[7-9] This relationship may explain why periodontal disease during pregnancy is associated with adverse pregnancy outcomes.[9]

The intestinal microbiome markedly transforms as pregnancy progresses. In the first trimester the intestinal microbiome is relatively similar to the non-pregnant patient. However, by the third trimester, there is an increase in *Proteobacteria* and *Actinobacteria* species as well as a decrease in *Faecalibacterium* species.[9] Interestingly the decrease in *Faecalibacterium* species is similar to the microbiome changes seen in metabolic syndrome associated with weight gain, insulin insensitivity, and a pro-inflammatory response. However, while those changes are maladaptive in non-pregnant patients with metabolic syndrome, the same changes are necessary for a healthy pregnancy.[9,10] Alterations in the pregnancy microbiome from this baseline have also been associated with adverse pregnancy outcomes such as gestational diabetes and preterm birth.[10,11]

Mode of delivery (vaginal delivery or cesarean section) is associated with the neonatal intestinal microbiome. Infants delivered vaginally have an intestinal microbiome similar to their mother's vaginal flora whereas those delivered by cesarean delivery have an intestinal microbiome similar to their mother's skin flora.[12] Cesarean sections have been associated with increased risk of obesity and Type 1 diabetes in the offspring among other disorders.[13,14] These findings beg the question if an early alternation of infant microbiome could be beneficial to reduce the risk of these diseases. An interesting pilot study where the oral cavity of babies born via cesarean delivery were inoculated with mothers' vaginal flora demonstrated that the neonates microbiome was similar to a vaginally born counterpart at 1 month of age.[15] However, the long-term effects of these interventions on the offspring are currently unknown.

## Impact of IBD on the Female Microbiome and Offspring

The microbiome in those with IBD differs from the unaffected population in several ways. In those with IBD, there is a general decrease in microbial diversity compared to healthy gut microbiomes as well as decreases in *Firmicutes* and an increase in *Proteobacteria*.[16] Interestingly, genetics also appear to play a role in bacterial diversity as those with NOD-2 risk allele, which confers a higher risk of developing IBD, have increased abundance of *Enterobacteriaceae* species.[17] The microbiomes also differ between those with ulcerative colitis (UC) and those with Crohn's disease (CD) in regards to relative abundance of the aforementioned bacteria.[18]

How does pregnancy then affect the microbiome of those with IBD? Those with quiescent disease in pregnancy appeared to have the same shifts in the microbiome as pregnant patients without IBD as mentioned in the section previously.[19] In patients with UC in remission during pregnancy, there was a relative abundance of *F prausnitzii* which has been associated with anti-inflammatory processes.[19] However those with IBD flares during pregnancy had significant less diverse microbiomes compared to those who did not flare. In these patients who flared, the *Bilophila* genus, which confers risk for pathologic inflammation, was increased.[19]

The offspring of females with IBD also demonstrate unique intestinal microbiome makeup compared to unaffected controls as demonstrated by the MECONIUM study. Independent of the mode of delivery, for the first 3 months of life infants born to mothers with IBD demonstrated a decrease in Actinobacteriae and an relative abundance of *Gammaproteobacteria* class compared to infants born to unaffected mothers.[20] This same group also demonstrated that placental microbiome and microbial content of cord blood is altered as well in those with IBD compared to unaffected.[20] As this is a longitudinal study, time will tell how these early changes affect these offspring as they grow.

Breastfeeding appears to confer a protective benefit in reducing the incidence of IBD in children in a meta-analysis of 17 studies.[21] There was a decreased risk of developing IBD with a longer duration of breastfeeding up to 12 months.[22] Breastfeeding of any duration was associated with a decreased risk for Crohn's-related surgery.[23] However, the exact reason for these effects has still to be fully elucidated.

# Nutritional Consequences of IBD During Development
## Malnutrition

Nutrition adequacy is a primary concern in an individual whose disease affects the gut. Couple that with the specific nutrient needs required during the different phases of a woman's life and the appreciation of nutrition is hard to ignore. Health care professionals play a pivotal role in identifying patients who need nutritional intervention, which is best delivered by a multidisciplinary team that includes a registered dietitian. Nutrition screening is a Joint Commission requirement, and the National Institute for Health and Care Excellence recommends that all ambulatory patients be screened at their initial visit and repeated when clinically indicated.[24] A skilled and trained health care professional using a standardized screening tool should do nutrition screening. There are several screening tools available such as the Paediatric Yorkhill Malnutrition Score for children, and the Malnutrition Universal Screening Tool for adults.[25,26] While neither are validated specifically in the IBD population, they are widely utilized. The Malnutrition Universal Screening Tool is validated for use in the acute and ambulatory setting and consists of 3 questions relating to body mass index (BMI), weight loss, and the effect of acute disease on oral intake. A positive nutrition screen should elicit a referral to a registered dietitian who can perform a global nutrition assessment to determine if the patient is malnourished and what interventions are appropriate for improving nutrition status.

Malnutrition is common in IBD with studies reporting rates as high as 65% to 75% of those with CD and 18% to 62% of those with UC.[27] The large discrepancy in the prevalence of malnutrition in IBD is largely due to the lack of a universally accepted definition, with some researchers incorrectly using the acute phase protein, albumin, as a marker of malnutrition, and others using anthropometry (BMI, weight loss, percent of ideal weight, decreases in centile channels or falling below the fifth percentile) or micronutrient levels as diagnostic criteria.

## Definition

Malnutrition is most simply defined as an imbalance of nutrients that negatively affects health. An etiology-based definition that considers the effect of inflammation has been proposed by American Society of Parenteral and Enteral Nutrition and the Academy of Nutrition and Dietetics in 2 recently published consensus papers.[28,29] Criteria are proposed for identifying and diagnosing malnutrition in the pediatric and adult populations. In the pediatric population (1 month to 18 years), when one data point is available, the use of z-scores (for weight-for-height, BMI-for-age, length/height-for-age) or mid-upper arm circumference (in those aged 6 to 60 months) is recommended for diagnosing malnutrition, whereas in those with 2 or more data points available, weight gain velocity (in those under 2 years), weight loss (2 to 20 years), deceleration in weight for length/height z-score, and inadequate nutrient intake are recommended to define malnutrition, with greater losses reflecting more severe malnutrition. In adults, American Society of Parenteral and Enteral Nutrition and Academy of Nutrition and Dietetics recommend using a set of 6 criteria for identifying and diagnosing malnutrition, where a patient needs to meet at least 2 criteria for a diagnosis: weight loss, insufficient energy intake, loss of muscle mass, loss of fat mass, fluid accumulation, and diminished functional status as measured by reduced handgrip strength. Using a standardized set of criteria to identify and diagnose malnutrition in clinical practice and research studies will help inform a better understanding of the prevalence, incidence, and global burden of malnutrition in IBD.

## Etiology

Many factors contribute to the development of malnutrition in IBD, including decreased oral intake, malabsorption, increased nutrient losses, increased energy expenditure, and drug-related side effects.[27-30] Patients who are hospitalized are often kept nil per os during the course of their hospitalization, and patients commonly restrict food intake during active disease to help improve symptoms. Bergeron et al. found food restriction in 39% of those with IBD in remission, with the most avoided foods being capsaicin, meat alternatives, and raw vegetables. Significantly higher food avoidance was seen in those with stricturing CD and those with active disease.[31]

Malabsorption can be related to active IBD, bacterial overgrowth, surgical resections, or increased motility. Increased nutrient losses are a consequence of altered epithelial transport (ie, loss of electrolytes and fluids), surgery, or chronic inflammation leading to ulceration of the bowel wall causing blood and protein losses. Biliary salt diarrhea has been seen in patients with terminal ileal disease or resection and may lead to decreased absorption of fat causing steatorrhea and fat-soluble vitamin malabsorption. Active disease increases resting energy expenditure; however, studies show that the total energy expenditure in IBD is similar to other patients, likely due to decreased physical activity in the setting of active disease.[32] Medications can also inhibit nutrient absorption. Methotrexate and sulfasalazine decrease folate absorption and can lead to deficiencies of folate as well as megaloblastic anemia. Glucocorticoids reduce absorption of phosphorus, zinc, and calcium, increasing risk of osteopenia and osteoporosis.[30]

## Complications

In the acute setting, malnutrition leads to an increase in health care utilization, prolonged hospital length of stay, and surgical complications. A recent nationwide study by Nguyen et al. found that patients with IBD and malnutrition have more than double the total health care costs compared to patients without IBD.[33] Those with IBD and malnutrition had more than double the length of stay compared to patients without IBD (11.9 days vs 5.8 days, $P < .00001$).[33] Interestingly, patients with malnutrition who are nutritionally optimized preoperatively are less likely to develop postoperative complications, including development of infection and anastomotic leak.[34]

Malnutrition is common in the pediatric population and can lead to deficits in growth, bone mass, and lean body mass. In a systematic review of children with IBD, 94% of those with CD

## Table 3-1. IBD Select Nutrient Needs for Women Throughout Their Life Span

| LIFE STAGE | FAT (G/D) | PROTEIN (G/D) | CARBOHYDRATE (G/D) | FIBER (G/D) |
|---|---|---|---|---|
| CHILDREN 1 TO 3 YEARS | ND | 13 | 130 | 19* |
| CHILDREN 4 TO 8 YEARS | ND | 19 | 130 | 25* |
| FEMALES 9 TO 13 YEARS | ND | 34 | 130 | 26* |
| FEMALES 14 TO 18 YEARS | ND | 46 | 130 | 26* |
| FEMALES 19 TO 50 YEARS | ND | 46 | 130 | 25* |
| FEMALES 51 TO 70 YEARS | ND | 46 | 130 | 21* |
| FEMALES > 70 YEARS | ND | 46 | 130 | 21* |
| PREGNANCY 14 TO 18 YEARS | ND | 71 | 175 | 28* |
| PREGNANCY 19 TO 50 YEARS | ND | 71 | 175 | 28* |
| LACTATION 14 TO 18 YEARS | ND | 71 | 210 | 29* |
| LACTATION 19 TO 50 YEARS | ND | 71 | 210 | 29* |

*(continued)*

and 48% of those with UC had low lean body mass, with low lean mass levels existing for a longer duration in females.[35] In women of childbearing age, severe disease activity and malnutrition or anorexia may result in secondary amenorrhea and infertility. Inadequate maternal weight gain in pregnancy was associated with adverse outcomes.[36] IBD and older age are independent risk factors for nutritional deficiencies.[37] Hospitalized patients aged 65 years and older have a greater risk of malnutrition, anemia, hypovolemia, higher risk for postoperative complications, and mortality.[38-40] Malnutrition complicates the disease course in all life stages; therefore, nutrition intervention is crucial for helping to improve patient outcomes.

## Common Micronutrient Deficiencies

Micronutrients work as coenzymes and cofactors in metabolism and some are essential for life. Micronutrient needs vary throughout the lifespan (see Table 3-1). IBD increases risk for micronutrient deficiencies due to active disease, medical treatment, or surgical treatment. IBD and older age (60 years and older) are independent risk factors for nutritional deficiencies.[37] Correcting micronutrient deficiencies can help improve quality of life (QOL). It is important to screen for micronutrient deficiencies annually or when deficiencies are clinically suspected. Evaluate micronutrient levels with caution, as micronutrients may increase (ferritin, copper) or decrease (folate, selenium, zinc)[41] in response to inflammation. An Expert Consensus paper published in the *Journal of Parenteral and Enteral Nutrition*[42] recommends considering the effect of inflammation when assessing micronutrients in adults, with a level of 20% below normal range to indicate a deficiency in the setting of inflammation. We will now review several micronutrients, the effect of IBD on their levels, as well as any changes during pregnancy that would require closer monitoring.

## Table 3-1 (continued). IBD Select Nutrient Needs for Women Throughout Their Life Span

| LIFE STAGE | CALCIUM (MG/D) | IRON (MG/D) | ZINC (MG/D) | VITAMIN C (MG/D) |
|---|---|---|---|---|
| *CHILDREN 1 TO 3 YEARS* | 700 | 7 | 3 | 15 |
| *CHILDREN 4 TO 8 YEARS* | 1000 | 10 | 5 | 25 |
| *FEMALES 9 TO 13 YEARS* | 1300 | 8 | 8 | 45 |
| *FEMALES 14 TO 18 YEARS* | 1300 | 15 | 9 | 65 |
| *FEMALES 19 TO 50 YEARS* | 1000 | 18 | 8 | 75 |
| *FEMALES 51 TO 70 YEARS* | 1200 | 8 | 8 | 75 |
| *FEMALES > 70 YEARS* | 1200 | 8 | 8 | 75 |
| *PREGNANCY 14 TO 18 YEARS* | 1300 | 27 | 12 | 80 |
| *PREGNANCY 19 TO 50 YEARS* | 1000 | 27 | 11 | 85 |
| *LACTATION 14 TO 18 YEARS* | 1300 | 10 | 13 | 115 |
| *LACTATION 19 TO 50 YEARS* | 1000 | 9 | 12 | 120 |

*(continued)*

### Iron

Iron is an essential mineral needed to transport oxygen throughout the body, support muscle metabolism, and is necessary for physical growth and neurological development.[43] Dietary iron is available in heme (meat, seafood, poultry) and non-heme (plant-based and iron fortified foods) forms. Iron deficiency can occur because of active IBD, surgical resection or inflammation involving the duodenum (site-specific absorption), inadequate intake (vegetarian diet), and menstruation.

Hepcidin regulates iron absorption and distribution throughout the body and is upregulated during periods of active IBD. This upregulation of hepcidin decreases transport of iron into plasma and extracellular fluid,[44] therefore, in the patient with active IBD and iron deficiency anemia, intravenous iron repletion is recommended over oral iron.[41] Anemia is the most common extraintestinal manifestation in IBD.[41] Iron deficiency anemia is present in about 36% to 90% of those with IBD.[30] Despite high prevalence rates, iron and anemia screening and replacement is poor. Correction of anemia improves QOL in IBD independent of disease activity,[45] therefore, screening and repletion is essential. The European Society for Clinical Nutrition and Metabolism (ESPEN) Practical Guidelines[41] suggest screening for iron in those who are pregnant, anemia in all age groups every 6 to 12 months in those with quiescent or minimally active disease, and every 3 months in those with active disease. Screening should include a complete blood count, serum ferritin, and C-reactive protein. Serum ferritin < 30 ng/mL in quiescent disease, or up to 100 ng/mL in the setting of inflammation can indicate iron deficiency. As iron deficiency progresses, anemia occurs with resulting drop in hemoglobin to < 11 g/dL in children under 6 months to 5 years of age and in females during pregnancy, < 11.5 g/dL in children aged 5 to 11 years, and < 12 g/dL in non-pregnant females aged 12 years and older.[45] A ferritin level > 100 ng/mL and transferrin saturation < 20% indicates anemia of chronic disease.

## Table 3-1 (continued). IBD Select Nutrient Needs for Women Throughout Their Life Span

| LIFE STAGE | VITAMIN D (MG/D)** | VITAMIN B$_6$ (MG/D) | FOLATE (MG/D)*** | VITAMIN B$_{12}$ (MG/D) |
|---|---|---|---|---|
| CHILDREN 1 TO 3 YEARS | 15 | 0.5 | 150 | 0.9 |
| CHILDREN 4 TO 8 YEARS | 15 | 0.6 | 200 | 1.2 |
| FEMALES 9 TO 13 YEARS | 15 | 1.0 | 300 | 1.8 |
| FEMALES 14 TO 18 YEARS | 15 | 1.2 | 400 | 2.4 |
| FEMALES 19 TO 50 YEARS | 15 | 1.3 | 400 | 2.4 |
| FEMALES 51 TO 70 YEARS | 15 | 1.5 | 400 | 2.4 |
| FEMALES > 70 YEARS | 20 | 1.5 | 400 | 2.4 |
| PREGNANCY 14 TO 18 YEARS | 15 | 1.9 | 600 | 2.6 |
| PREGNANCY 19 TO 50 YEARS | 15 | 1.9 | 600 | 2.6 |
| LACTATION 14 TO 18 YEARS | 15 | 2.0 | 500 | 2.8 |
| LACTATION 19 TO 50 YEARS | 15 | 2.0 | 500 | 2.8 |

Table from the Food and Nutrition Board, Institute of Medicine, National Academies, Dietary Reference Intakes (DRI). Note, Recommended Dietary Allowances in regular type, Adequate Intakes indicated by an asterisk (*). **As cholecalciferol. 1 µg cholecalciferol = 40 IU vitamin D. ***As dietary folate equivalents (DFE). 1 DFE = 1 µg food folate = 0.6 µg of folic acid from fortified food or as a supplement consumed with food = 0.5 µg of a supplement taken on an empty stomach. ND, not determined

In pregnancy, iron is necessary for production of fetal and placental tissue as well as to accommodate the expansion of maternal red cell volume by up to 30%. Further iron depletion occurs during blood loss at time of delivery. Iron deficiency anemia in pregnancy increases risk of preterm delivery, low birth weight, and even maternal and fetal mortality.[46,47] Thus it is imperative that adequate replacement is recommended. For all pregnant patients additional supplementation with 30 mg of elemental iron is recommended after week 12 of gestation. For pregnant women who have preexisting anemia, supplementation of 60 mg/day to 100 mg/day of elemental iron is recommended until normalization of anemia is achieved.[47] Common side effects of additional iron supplementation include nausea, which can be mitigated by taking the iron after meals as well as constipation, for which we recommend increasing bowel regimen.

### Vitamin D

Vitamin D is a fat-soluble vitamin that is essential for intestinal calcium absorption, bone metabolism, decreasing risk for colon and breast cancer, and has an immunoregulatory effect.[48] Vitamin D deficiency leads to rickets in children and osteomalacia in adults. Vitamin D deficiency and corticosteroid use increases risk for osteopenia and osteoporosis. Rich food sources of vitamin D include fatty fish (eg, salmon, tuna, mackerel), fish liver oils, egg yolk, and fortified dairy products. Vitamin D is also synthesized endogenously when skin is exposed to sunlight.[48] Risk factors for vitamin D deficiency include malabsorption, ileal disease, and inadequate intakes (vegetarian diet, dairy avoidance).[48]

Vitamin D deficiency is common in IBD, with studies suggesting 55% of adults[41] and 80% of children are deficient.[49] Vitamin D studies in IBD have found deficiency to be associated with an increased need for hospitalization and surgery in both CD and UC.[41] Further, vitamin D may affect disease recurrence, with a recent study showing levels < 35 ng/mL in patients with quiescent UC have an increased risk for a flare in the proceeding 12 months.[50] ESPEN Guidelines[41] recommend monitoring vitamin D in children and adults with active disease and in those who are steroid treated. The Endocrine Society considers serum 25-hydroxyvitamin D levels > 30 ng/mL to be sufficient, < 30 ng/mL insufficient, and < 20 ng/mL deficient.[48] Doses up to 2000 IU/d may be needed in adults to help maintain normal levels. Noncompliance rate of supplementation is high at 40%.[51]

In pregnancy, Vitamin D is essential for growth and development of the fetus, with low levels associated with adverse bone formation and predisposition to fractures.[47] Pregnant patients who are high risk for deficiency, such as those with a vegetarian or vegan diet, should empirically take supplementation. In pregnancy, supplementation doses of vitamin D 1000 IU to 4000 IU were found to be safe.[52]

## Zinc

Zinc is an essential mineral responsible for many metabolic reactions. Zinc plays a role in immunity, wound healing, protein and DNA synthesis, and cell division. Zinc rich foods include oysters, beef, crab, lobster, chicken, and pumpkin seed. Zinc is absorbed throughout the small intestine,[53] but with no means of storage, zinc deficiency can happen rapidly in the setting of excessive gastrointestinal losses (diarrhea, high ostomy output), malabsorption, and inadequate intake (vegetarian diet). Clinical manifestations of zinc deficiency include growth retardation, impaired immune function, altered taste and smell, and hair loss. Prevalence of zinc deficiency in IBD is 15% to 40% in children and adults.[54-56] A prospective study[57] of patients with IBD (n = 996) found zinc deficiency to be associated with an increased risk for hospitalizations, surgery, and increased disease-related complications, with normalization of zinc levels decreasing these risks.

In pregnancy, deficiency is associated with birth defects, intrauterine growth restriction, and fetal mortality.[47] Pregnant women who are vegetarians or vegans may require extra supplementation. Of note, iron competes with zinc for absorption thus those women who are on higher doses of iron supplementation (greater than 60 mg/day of elemental iron) should be also advised to take zinc supplementation.[47]

## Vitamin $B_{12}$

$B_{12}$ is an essential water-soluble vitamin needed for amino acid and fatty acid metabolism, red blood cell production, neurological function, and DNA synthesis. Absorption of $B_{12}$ requires gastric acid and protease to cleave $B_{12}$ from protein, gastric parietal cells to release intrinsic factor and R factor. $B_{12}$ binds with R factor and enters the duodenum, where pancreatic proteases free the $B_{12}$ and allow it to bind to intrinsic factor. This $B_{12}$ and intrinsic factor complex will traverse the small intestine until it is absorbed in the terminal ileum. Vitamin $B_{12}$ comes from animal products and fortified plant-based products, with the richest sources being clams, beef liver, trout, salmon, tuna, and fortified nutritional yeast.

Vitamin $B_{12}$ malabsorption is seen in those with pernicious anemia, reduced gastric acid secretion (due to age or medications), ileostomy, ileal pouch-anal anastomosis (IPAA), and in those with TI disease or resection involving the last 20 cm of ileum. Studies show the prevalence of $B_{12}$ deficiency in CD is up to 38%.[41] Consider sublingual or parenteral $B_{12}$ administration in older adults due to decreased absorptive capacity, in those with terminal ileal disease or resection involving > 20 cm. Serum $B_{12}$ levels do not accurately reflect intracellular $B_{12}$ levels. If $B_{12}$ deficiency is suspected (macrocytic anemia, clinical manifestations of $B_{12}$ deficiency present, such as altered stools, peripheral neuropathy, cognitive impairment), consider checking methylmalonic acid, as this will be elevated in the setting of vitamin $B_{12}$ deficiency.[58]

British Society Guidelines[59] recommend:

- Screening for vitamin $B_{12}$ deficiency as part of initial workup in IBD, in those with acute severe colitis (as part of haematinics with iron and folate) or in those with macrocytosis.

- Monitoring serum $B_{12}$ annually in patients with ileal CD and in those with terminal ileal resection < 20 cm.

- Administering $B_{12}$ parenterally in those with an ileal resection > 20 cm.

## Vitamin $B_6$

Vitamin $B_6$ or *pyridoxine* is an essential water-soluble vitamin. Vitamin $B_6$ is necessary for protein metabolism, synthesis of neurotransmitters, maintaining normal homocysteine levels, immune function, and hemoglobin formation. Foods rich in $B_6$ include chickpeas, beef, tuna, salmon, chicken, potato, and banana. Clinical symptoms of deficiency include microcytic anemia, dermatitis with cheilosis, glositis, depression, and confusion.[60] Deficiency increases risk for venous thromboembolism. $B_6$ deficiency is common in people with IBD, with a recent study finding 29% had subnormal serum values.[54]

In pregnancy, vitamin $B_6$ helps with heme synthesis as well as maternal and fetal antibodies and neurotransmitters. Most commonly, $B_6$ supplementation is used to assist with decreasing nausea and vomiting in pregnancy at a dose of 10 mg to 25 mg 3 times daily.[47,61]

## Folate

Folate, or vitamin $B_9$, is an essential water-soluble vitamin. It is required for nucleic acid synthesis, metabolism of amino acids, and for the conversion of homocysteine to methionine. Folate rich foods include beef liver, spinach, black-eyed peas, fortified grains (required in the United States and Canada), asparagus, and brussels sprouts. Folate deficiency leads to megaloblastic anemia, and hyperhomocysteinemia. Symptoms of folate deficiency include weakness, fatigue, irritability, shortness of breath, and palpitations.[62] Folate deficiency is often assessed through measurement of serum folate, although this is highly influenced by recent intake. Monitoring red blood cell folate may provide a more accurate assessment of long-term folate intake adequacy.

Twenty to 60% of people with IBD have folate deficiency[63] and factors increasing risk for deficiency include malabsorption, medications (sulfasalazine, methotrexate), excess folate utilization due to mucosal inflammation,[41] and may also be due to common avoidance of folate-rich foods (dark, leafy greens). ESPEN Guidelines[41] for folic acid supplementation for adults on methotrexate are in agreement with the European Crohn's and Colitis Organisation/European Society of Pediatric Gastroenterology, Hepatology and Nutrition Guidelines for children on methotrexate: 1 mg daily for 5 days per week or 5 mg once weekly 24 to 72 hours after methotrexate. Those on sulfasalazine or on low-residue diets should also consider daily supplementation with 2 mg daily of folic acid.

Folate deficiency is the most common vitamin deficiency during pregnancy. In pregnancy, folate is essential for fetal cell growth, and inadequate intake of folate during pregnancy increases the risk for neural tube defects.[47] The neural tube closes by 18 to 28 days after conception at a time where many women may not even be aware that they are pregnant. Therefore Centers for Disease Control and Prevention recommendations include that all women of childbearing age should take at least 400 µg/day irrespective of actively attempting for a pregnancy.[64] Once pregnancy occurs, at least 600 µg/day are recommended. Rates of neural tube defects have also been declining since 1998 when the US government began to fortify various grains with folate. Those who avoid grains in their diet may require additional supplementation. Of note, we recommend advising patients to use a separate folate supplement in addition to the prenatal vitamin if higher doses are required rather than increasing the prenatal vitamin, which could inadvertently lead to toxicity of the other vitamins.

## Vitamin C

Vitamin C is a water-soluble vitamin that is essential for synthesis of collagen, L-carnitine, neurotransmitters, and protein metabolism. Vitamin C is important for wound healing, immune function, improves absorption of nonheme iron, and serves as an antioxidant. Rich food sources of vitamin C include bell pepper, citrus, kiwifruit, broccoli, berries, brussels sprouts, and tomato. Symptoms of deficiency include confusion, weakness, myalgia, arthralgia, vascular purpura and hemorrhagic syndrome, bleeding gums, and loss of teeth.[65]

Malabsorption with active IBD and avoidance of fresh fruits and vegetables that is commonly seen in active disease increases risk for vitamin C deficiency. Studies have found that those with IBD who are malnourished have significantly lower intakes of vitamin C,[66] children and adolescents have significantly lower intakes of vitamin C compared to intakes of healthy children,[67] and adults have lower serum vitamin C levels when compared to healthy controls, independent of disease activity.[68] Serum levels of vitamin C < 2.5 mg/L indicate deficiency. In patients with vitamin C deficiency, 1 gram of vitamin C daily for 15 days is recommended as treatment.[69]

In pregnancy, vitamin C is essential for adequate fetal growth but only an extra 10 mg/day are required. There was initial interest that vitamin C via its antioxidative properties would be helpful in reducing rates of preeclampsia, but several trials have not shown this hypothesis to be correct.[47]

# Diet Therapy in IBD

There is increasing interest in the role that diet plays in the onset and management of IBD. A 2016 study[70] found that 60% of patients with IBD feel diet plays an important role in controlling symptoms and disease flares, yet only 36% of patients discuss their nutrition concerns with their providers. Reasons for this include patients' perceptions that the providers lack the time or knowledge to answer their nutrition-related questions. As a result, patients may rely more on social media, friends, family, and other non-medical professionals to answer their diet questions, leading to unnecessary and possibly harmful supplementation regimens or restrictive dieting that can increase risk for malnutrition and decreased QOL. There is growing evidence to support therapeutic diets for reducing risk for IBD development, and for inducing and maintaining remission. Therefore, we encourage providers to educate themselves on these therapeutic diets to allow a more productive conversation with patients, and through shared decision making with the multidisciplinary team, assist patients in choosing the most appropriate and balanced nutrition plan.

## Dietary Factors in the Development of IBD

IBD prevalence has increased globally over the past few decades, particularly in nations that have adopted a westernized lifestyle, therefore, environmental triggers have been hypothesized to modify disease risk.[71] This has led researchers to focus attention on the role that environmental factors play in the onset of IBD. Diet is thought to influence IBD development by modifying the microbiota, altering intestinal permeability, and regulating immune response pathways.[72] Analysis of 2 large prospective Swedish cohorts totaling 83,147 participants aged 45 to 79 years found that those following a Mediterranean diet had a significantly lower risk for CD but not UC.[73]

Population-based studies in adults suggest fiber intake is inversely associated with IBD onset, with intakes of 24 g/day decreasing risk for IBD.[74] Omega-3 fatty acids (FA) may be protective, and omega 6 FA may increase risk of UC. A prospective study of women enrolled in the Nurses' Health study cohorts found that women with higher ratios of omega-3/omega-6 FA had a decreased risk of UC.[75] And a prior prospective cohort found the risk of UC was doubled in females who ate higher intakes of omega 6 FA.[76]

In a female cohort, vitamin D levels were inversely associated with CD risk.[77] Intakes of zinc, resveratrol from grapes and wine, and flavones from thyme, rosemary, and oregano were also found to be inversely related to development of CD.[78,79] In animal studies, emulsifiers (carboxymethyl-cellulose and polysorbate)[80] have been found to increase risk for inflammatory diseases, alter the microbiota, and increase colitis severity,[80-82] therefore, avoidance of these food additives where possible is recommended.

## Diet Therapy in Active Disease

Active disease and surgery can increase nutrient needs. Most patients are encouraged to limit fiber in active disease, yet there is no evidence to support this practice outside of patients with symptomatic stricturing IBD. Further, fiber is metabolized by bacteria to form short chain FA, which enhance fluid and electrolyte absorption, regulate motility, and provide a primary fuel source for colonocytes. Some patients may benefit from reducing lactose intake because of secondary lactase deficiency that can occur in active disease. Personalized dietary modification should be done with the assistance of a registered dietitian to ensure nutrient balance and help with guiding patients in determining the least restrictive diet needed to help with symptom management.

Several exclusion diets have been proposed to help achieve and maintain remission in IBD. Exclusive enteral nutrition (EEN) is effective in inducing remission in pediatric CD, and is recommended as first line therapy by the North American Society of Pediatric Gastroenterology, Hepatology and Nutrition. Studies have found EEN to be less effective in adults but may be able to induce clinical remission in those who are able to adhere to the nutritional therapy. Other diet therapies that have been studied (Specific Carbohydrate Diet [SCD], CD Exclusion Diet [CDED]) have shown positive results for reducing clinical symptoms, but more studies are needed to understand their effects on mucosal healing.[41,83-85] When elective surgery becomes necessary to manage active IBD, studies show patients benefit from nutrition optimization strategies such as carbohydrate loading preoperatively and early feeding postoperatively.

### Children

Corticosteroid therapy is often used in active IBD to help induce remission; however, the side effects of steroids include hyperglycemia, sleep and mood disturbance, osteopenia and osteoporosis, increased risk of infection, and growth impairment.[59] An alternative to corticosteroid therapy is EEN, a form of nutrition therapy whereby all nutrients (macronutrients and micronutrients) are supplied by a formula as the sole source of nutrition. Randomized controlled trials in children have shown EEN to be as effective as corticosteroid therapy for inducing remission in the form of mucosal healing in those with luminal CD irrespective of location, with an overall combined remission rate of 73%.[86-92] EEN was shown to be superior to corticosteroid therapy for mucosal healing.[93,94] Borrelli et al[93] found in their randomized controlled trial that 74% of those on EEN achieved mucosal healing, compared to only 33% on steroids. In another randomized controlled trial[95] 89% of those on EEN had mucosal healing vs 17% in the steroid treated group ($P < .005$). Studies show mucosal healing at around 8 weeks of EEN, therefore, duration of therapy is recommended for a period of at least 8 weeks.[96] Early mucosal healing is associated with reduced relapses, hospitalization, and need for anti–tumor necrosis factor biologic therapy at 1 year.[97]

A Cochrane meta-analysis found polymeric formulas to be as effective as elemental formulas in inducing remission[98] and have the added benefit of being more cost effective and more palatable. Formulas can be administered by mouth or by enteric tube if patient is unable to consume adequate amounts by mouth. Efficacy declines when adherence to EEN falls below 100%. EEN is not recommended as maintenance therapy, and studies show children relapse within 6 to 12 months after EEN cessation without a maintenance medication or strategy in place[99-101]; see next section for diet strategies to help maintain remission. After 8 weeks of EEN, reintroducing foods is recommended.

In a retrospective study, Faiman et al[102] found no significant difference in relapse rates at 1 year with food reintroduction over 3 days vs 5 weeks. The Porto Group of ESPGHAN Guidelines recommend gradually introducing foods paralleled with formula reduction over a period of 2 to 3 weeks.

EEN is effective in inducing mucosal and in some patients transmural healing,[93,94] is generally well tolerated and has the benefit of improving nutrition status, QOL, and improving long-term bone health. Some mild side effects have been reported such as nausea, vomiting, diarrhea, abdominal pain, and bloating that tend to improve with duration of therapy. The only severe adverse event reported has been for refeeding syndrome, a potentially fatal shift of fluids and electrolytes that can happen with rapid infusion of nutrition in a malnourished individual and can lead to respiratory, cardiac, and neurologic complications.[103,104] Consider a slow taper up to EEN goal over 2 to 3 days with close monitoring and replacement of electrolytes (phosphorus, magnesium, potassium) to help mitigate effects of refeeding in the severely malnourished child. There is a paucity of evidence of EEN efficacy for UC, therefore, EEN is not recommended for inducing remission in UC at this time.[105]

EEN can pose a challenge socially and psychologically for patients and families, and partial formula diet is ineffective for inducing remission in CD.[106] This has led researchers to hypothesize if exclusivity of formula intake is needed to achieve remission or if formula combined with a specialized diet can achieve the same clinical benefits. Sigall-Boneh et al developed the CDED, which is a diet comprised of 6 weeks of a restrictive phase with 50% calories coming from a low inflammatory diet and 50% from a polymeric formula (Modulen or Pediasure), followed by a maintenance phase with 75% calories coming from a low inflammatory diet and 25% from a polymeric formula (Modulen or Pediasure). The diet was designed to eliminate foods thought to be associated with inflammation, dysbiosis, and increased gut permeability (emulsifiers, dairy, gluten, red meat, animal fat, processed meats, canned goods). The primary endpoint in their prospective study[107] (n = 47, mean age 16 years) was remission at 6 weeks, defined as Harvey Bradshaw Index < 3 in young adults, and Pediatric CD Activity Index (PCDAI) < 7.5 in children with mild to moderate luminal CD. They found 70% of patients were able to achieve remission, and 70% had normalization of C-reactive protein. In a follow-up study, Levine et al[108] investigated EEN vs CDED, with their primary endpoint being tolerability in children with mild to moderate CD. The CDED was better tolerated than EEN (97% vs 73%, $P$ = .002), and there was no significant difference in corticosteroid-free remission at week 6 on EEN vs CDED. To date, studies investigating mucosal healing on CDED are lacking.

The SCD is a low-carbohydrate, grain-free, soy-free diet that is very popular in both pediatric and adult IBD communities. The diet emphasizes consumption of simple sugars (glucose, fructose) and restricts intake of disaccharide and polysaccharides. A small retrospective study in children with UC and non-stricturing and non-penetrating CD found improvement in PCDAI and Pediatric UC Activity Index within 6 months on SCD.[109] Suskind et al[110] conducted a prospective study in children with mild to moderate IBD (CD and UC) and found 8 out of 12 patients were able to achieve remission when using SCD in combination with medications. Cohen et al[111] prospectively assessed clinical and endoscopic response to SCD in 9 children with CD on SCD for up to 52 weeks and found clinical improvements (significant improvements in Harvey-Bradshaw Index, PCDAI, and Lewis score), as well as mucosal improvements on capsule endoscopy in 2 patients on SCD. Critics of SCD argue that the diet is unbalanced and can lead to weight loss or poor growth. SCD is grain free, soy free, and low in dairy, and therefore foods rich in micronutrients such as B vitamins (folate, thiamine, pyridoxine), calcium, vitamin E, and vitamin D need to be consumed to ensure diet balance. Consultation with a registered dietitian is recommended to help ensure adequate nutrient intake on this or any restrictive diet.

## Adults

EEN is effective for inducing remission in mild to moderate CD in children (see previous section); however, a recent Cochrane meta-analysis[84] of 8 studies (n = 352 patients) in adults concluded only a minimal advantage of steroids compared to EEN in effectiveness for inducing remission, which could be due to intolerance of EEN in the adult cohorts. In adults who can complete the EEN treatment, EEN is effective in inducing clinical remission in CD.[41,84,85] Consider EEN in adults who are highly motivated to use nutrition therapy, in those where corticosteroid therapy is contraindicated, or in the perioperative patient. There are limited studies evaluating the effectiveness of EEN in UC, therefore, it is not recommended for induction therapy at this time.

For those interested in a real-food diet approach, the SCD, the IBD Anti-Inflammatory Diet (IBD-AID), and the CDED are popular and have been studied in adults. The SCD is a grain-free, soy-free diet low in polysaccharides. It is proposed to help reduce inflammation in IBD by limiting intake of foods to those that are easily absorbed in the intestines and altering the microbiota to a more favorable profile that promotes gut healing. In a recent survey[83] of 417 patients (70% female, mean age 34 years), the SCD was reported to lead to clinical remission in 33% at 2 months and 42% at 6 and 12 months. Forty-seven percent reported improvement in abnormal laboratory parameters.

Researchers from the University of Massachusetts adapted SCD based on recent research on dietary factors that affect gut health, and from this, developed the IBD-AID. IBD-AID encourages probiotics and prebiotics, modifying fiber and fat intake based on clinical symptoms, identifying missing nutrients and food intolerances, avoidance of lactose and grains (except oats), and emphasizes intake of omega-3 FA over saturated and trans-fats. In their retrospective review of 11 patients (8 with CD, 3 with UC) who were on IBD-AID for at least 4 weeks, all were able to stop at least one IBD medication, and all had symptom reduction; endoscopic assessments were not performed.[112]

The CDED was developed to help reduce inflammation in active IBD, using a combination of an anti-inflammatory diet and formula from Modulen, Pediasure, or Osmolite (see *Diet Therapy in Active Disease, Children* section for more details). Researchers from Israel investigated the use of CDED in patients (11 adults, 10 children) who failed biologic therapy and found 61% were able to achieve clinical remission at 6 weeks. While these diets may show promise for helping patients achieve clinical remission, none have assessed endoscopic activity, therefore, these diets should only be recommended as complementary therapy and done under the guidance of a registered dietitian.

## Special Considerations for Surgical Patients

Up to 80% of those with CD and 30% of those with UC may need surgery in their lifetime.[59] People with IBD have a greater risk for postoperative complications; furthermore, corticosteroid use and age (> 60 years) increases risk for postoperative infection and mortality.[59] Minimizing steroid use and nutritionally optimizing patients preoperatively can improve postoperative outcomes. Nutrition screening should be done in the pre-op setting, with referral to a registered dietitian for nutrition optimization in all patients, especially in those with significant weight loss (5% in 1 month, 7.5% in 3 months, 10% in 6 months) or inadequate intake. Inadequate intake in patients preoperatively has been shown to be an independent risk factor for postoperative complications.[113]

An oral nutrition supplement (eg, Boost, Ensure, Kate Farms, Orgain) can be used to supplement the diet and provide additional nourishment for those unable to meet nutrition needs through foods alone. Consider nutrition support via tube feeding in those unable to meet > 60% nutrition needs by mouth, with preference to utilizing the gastrointestinal tract if functional, and parenteral nutrition in those with severe IBD, malabsorption, intolerance to enteral feeds, or non-functional gastrointestinal tract. ESPEN Guidelines recommend delaying surgery where possible for 7 to 14 days in malnourished patients to provide intensive medical nutrition support. ESPEN Guidelines[41] also echo the Enhanced Recovery After Surgery guidelines[114] for elective surgical patients and encourage clinicians to minimize fasting times peri-operatively. Consider preoperative carbohydrate loading from a clear liquid beverage (100 g the night before surgery, 50 g the morning of surgery), as this has been shown to improve patient satisfaction, preserve lean body mass, reduce postoperative nausea and vomiting, and help with glycemic control postoperatively.[114] Currently, Ensure Pre-Surgery is the only formula on the market that is designed specifically to meet Enhanced Recovery After Surgery guidelines for preoperative carbohydrate loading; however, Gatorade, Boost Breeze, and even clear fruit juice have been used in clinical practice.

Two meta-analyses have shown benefit in reduction in postoperative complications with early enteral nutrition (within 24 hours).[115,116] Early feeding postoperatively is encouraged, with consideration for additional oral nutrition supplements in addition to a regular diet to help patients meet nutrition needs. In patients who need emergency surgery, consider nutrition support (enteral nutrition vs parenteral nutrition) in those who are malnourished or those who will not be able to consume an oral diet 7 days postoperatively.[41]

## Diet Therapy in Quiescent Disease

Partial enteral nutrition (PEN) can help in the maintenance of remission in CD, with the strongest evidence coming from trials on adults. A semi-vegetarian diet (SVD) or Mediterranean diet (MED) may help in the maintenance of remission in those with UC after IPAA surgery.

### Children

PEN can be effective in maintaining remission in children with mild disease and low risk of relapse,[105] however, duration of therapy and amount needed to classify as PEN is poorly understood in the pediatric population. Most studies on PEN are in adults with CD. A retrospective study in which nasogastric nocturnal feeds were provided to children and allowed free feeding during the daytime found sustained remission an improved linear growth.[117] Another study found similar remission rates in children after EEN remission induction who transitioned to PEN compared to thiopurines at 12 months.[118]

Other diets based on real food and its effect on maintaining remission have been studied more in the adult population; see next section for further details.

### Adults

Adults on PEN receive 30% to 50% of nutrient needs via a standard polymeric formula, and the remainder of nutrition is obtained through a whole foods diet. Verma et al[119] prospectively studied PEN in 39 patients with quiescent CD on PEN using an elemental diet compared to free diet and found 17 (81%) tolerated PEN, with 10 (48%) remaining in remission at 12 months compared to 4 (22%) in the group on a free diet ($P < .0003$); response was independent of age, gender, disease duration, disease location. In 2006, Takagi et al[120] published their randomized controlled study in 51 people who were randomly assigned to a half elemental diet or no diet intervention. Their primary outcome was disease relapse defined as CD Activity Index > 200 or need for therapy to induce remission. They found the half elemental diet significantly reduced relapse of disease when compared to the free diet group (34% vs 64% at 11 months). Further, PEN can be used as combination therapy to help enhance response to biologic therapy. A meta-analysis of 4 studies[121] (n = 342; 3 retrospective and 1 prospective, not randomized controlled trials) found PEN (elemental or polymeric formula combined with a low-fat or regular diet) used in combination with infliximab lead to significantly higher clinical remission rates compared to infliximab monotherapy in adults with CD (clinical remission in 69% vs 45%, respectively; $P < .01$). Further, 74.5% of patients on combination therapy (PEN + infliximab) remained in remission at 1 year, compared to 49.2% on infliximab monotherapy ($P < .01$). A 2018 Cochrane meta-analysis[122] of efficacy of PEN in 4 randomized controlled trials (n = 262) in the maintenance of remission in CD found that no firm conclusions could be made regarding the efficacy and safety of PEN.

A few studies using whole foods have been conducted and proposed to help maintain remission in IBD. Brotherton et al[123] examined dietary intake of 1619 people from the Crohn's and Colitis Foundation of America Partners Internet cohort and found higher intakes of fiber were associated with a decrease risk of disease flare in patients with CD. Chiba et al conducted a prospective single center study (n = 22) in those on SVD with CD who were in medically or surgically induced remission. In those who continued the diet, 94% remained in remission on SVD vs 33% on an unrestricted diet at 2 years.[124] In a prospective study from 2 tertiary IBD centers, Godny et al[125] studied the effect of MED in 153 adults (53% female, mean age 46, mean pouch age 9.5 years) with UC after total proctocolectomy with IPAA. After controlling for IPAA behavior and disease activity, those with highest adherence to a MED had significantly lower fecal calprotectin levels. MED adherence positively correlated with higher intakes of fiber, micronutrients, and antioxidants. When examining risk for relapse of disease over time, adherence to MED showed a trend towards decreased risk for pouchitis over 8 years of follow-up, although this was not statistically significant ($P = .17$).

## Diet and Nutrition Considerations in Preconception, Pregnancy, and Postpartum Period Preconception

We recommend that all IBD patients who are considering pregnancy undergo preconception counseling as this has shown to improve outcomes by increasing medication compliance and decreasing IBD flares during pregnancy.[126] In addition to ensuring that patients are not on harmful medications for their pregnancy such as methotrexate, preconception counseling also allows for an in-depth assessment into their diet, nutrition, and herbal supplementation. For instance, the herbal supplements curcumin, slippery elm, or wormwood are popular among patients for IBD for their perceived anti-inflammatory benefit. However especially in early pregnancy, they have been associated with miscarriages.[127,129,130] Thus it is prudent to screen for these and other herbal supplements to ensure they are safe. Prenatal vitamins should be recommended at that time as well. If the patient is either underweight or overweight, directed diet and exercise advice should be given as both of those extremes can lead to adverse events in pregnancy.[52] Preconception counseling is also an opportunity to screen for the various vitamin deficiencies described in prior sections and address them prior to the patient attempting to conceive.

### Pregnancy

Nutritional guidance during pregnancy should also include the appropriate amount of weight gain for patients. Many patients with IBD can be under or overweight similar to the general population. Pregnancy in patients with a low BMI defined as < 18.5 kg/m$^2$ or who have inadequate weight gain are at risk for complications including preterm birth, small for gestational size infants and even perinatal mortality.[47] Meanwhile pregnancy in patients who are overweight (BMI > 25 kg/m$^2$) or obese (BMI > 30 kg/m$^2$) is also associated with adverse outcomes such as congenital anomalies, preterm birth, gestational hypertension, preeclampsia, and shoulder dystocia among others.[47] Thus it is prudent to discuss with all patients appropriate weight gain recommendations based on BMI. Pregnant patients with low BMI are advised to gain 28 to 40 lbs. Those with normal BMI are advised to gain between 25 to 35 lbs. Patients who are overweight are recommended 15 to 25 lbs weight gain while obese patients are recommended to gain between 11 to 20 lbs.[47]

Energy expenditure certainly increases during pregnancy to support the placenta and the growing fetal tissue, with a need for additional caloric intake as the pregnancy progresses. In the first trimester, no additional caloric intake is required and weight gain is usually minimal. In the second trimester, pregnant women should add an additional 340 kcal/day to their diet. In the third trimester, an additional 452 kcal/day is required for optimal pregnancy outcomes.[128] Additional dietary counseling during pregnancy includes avoiding alcohol, deli meats or other heavily processed foods, unpasteurized dairy products, raw fish/shellfish, and high mercury fish.[47] Caffeine intake should be limited to < 200 mg/day as well.[47]

Pregnant patients on balanced vegetarian diets who consume dairy and eggs have not found to have any significant adverse effects on their offspring. However strict vegan diets have may not have sufficient micronutrients such as those discussed in the above section. Thus, a referral to a dietitian is recommended in patients following strict vegan diets to ensure nutritional adequacy.[47]

## Postpartum

The postpartum period can be a challenging time for many women and it is helpful for the gastroenterologist to offer support during this time period in addition to the obstetrician. Postpartum visits should emphasize continuing IBD medications as was previously discussed. Several herbal supplements are used to assist with lactation. One of the more popular ones is fenugreek but patients with IBD should be counseled to avoid fenugreek as it has been associated with bloody diarrhea.[47]

---

### KEY POINTS

1. The intestinal microbiome in those with IBD is associated with less microbial diversity, general decrease in *Firmicutes,* and an increase in *Proteobacteria*.

2. Those with quiescent IBD in pregnancy appeared to have the same shifts in the microbiome as pregnant patients without IBD.

3. Breastfeeding appears to confer a protective benefit in reducing the incidence of IBD in offspring.

4. Malnutrition is common in IBD and complicates the disease course; screen patients using a validated tool and refer to a registered dietitian for nutrition intervention as needed.

5. Patients with IBD are at an increased risk for micronutrient deficiencies and correcting deficiencies improves clinical course and QOL. Consider monitoring the following: iron, vitamin D, zinc, vitamin $B_{12}$, folate, and vitamin C.

6. Patients have a strong desire to use diet therapy in the management of their IBD. We encourage those taking care of patients with IBD to familiarize themselves with commonly used diets to better support their patients and refer to a knowledgeable gastrointestinal specialized dietitian if necessary.

7. In elective surgical patients, consider carbohydrate loading preoperatively, and early feeding postoperatively to reduce morbidity.

8. Weight gain during pregnancy should be based on pre-pregnancy BMI to optimize pregnancy outcomes.

9. Screen for herbal supplements as you would medications to ensure safety during the pregnancy and postpartum period.

# References

1.  Dei M, Di Maggio F, Paolo GD, Bruni V. Vulvovaginitis in childhood. *Best Pract Res Clin Obstet Gynaecol.* 2010;24(2):129-137.

2.  Randelović G, Mladenović V, Ristić L, Otašević S, Branković S, Mladenović-Antić S, Bogdanović M, Bogdanović D. Microbiological aspects of vulvovaginitis in prepubertal girls. *Eur J Pediatr.* 2012;171(8):1203-1208.

3.  Yamamoto T, Zhou X, Williams CJ, Hochwalt A, Forney LF. Bacterial populations in the vaginas of healthy adolescent women. *J Pediatr Adolesc Gynecol.* 2009;22(1):11-18.

4.  Younes JA, Lievens E, Hummelen R, van der Westen R, Reid G, Petrova MI. Women and their microbes: the unexpected friendship. *Trends in Microbiology.* 2018;26(1):16-32.

5.  Gupta S, Kumar N, Singhal N, Kaur R, Manektala U. Vaginal microflora in postmenopausal women on hormone replacement therapy. *Indian J Pathol Microbiol.* 2006;49(3):457-461.

6.  Hummelen R, Macklaim JM, Bisanz JE, et al. Vaginal microbiome and epithelial gene array in post-menopausal women with moderate to severe dryness. *PLoS One.* 2011;6(11):Article e26602.

7.  Aagaard K, Ma J, Antony KM, Ganu R, Petrosino J, Versalovic J. The placenta harbors a unique microbiome. *Sci Transl Med.* 2014;6(237):237ra65.

8.  Aagaard K, Riehle K, Ma J, et al. A metagenomic approach to characterization of the vaginal microbiome signature in pregnancy. *PLoS ONE.* 2012;7(6):e36466.

9.  Nuriel-Ohayon M, Neuman H, Koren O. Microbial changes during pregnancy, birth, and infancy. *Front Microbiol.* 2016;7:1031. doi:10.3389/fmicb.2016.01031

10.  Koren O, Goodrich JK, Cullender TC, et al. Host remodeling of the gut microbiome and metabolic changes during pregnancy. *Cell.* 2012;150(3):470-480. doi:10.1016/j.cell.2012.07.008

11.  Dahl C, Stanislawski M, Iszatt N, et al. Gut microbiome of mothers delivering prematurely shows reduced diversity and lower relative abundance of *Bifidobacterium* and *Streptococcus*. *PLoS ONE.* 2017;12:e0184336.

12.  Dominguez-Bello MG, Costello EK, Contreras M, Magris M, Hidalgo G, Fierer N, Knight R. Delivery mode shapes the acquisition and structure of the initial microbiota across multiple body habitats in newborns. *Proc Natl Acad Sci.* 2010;107(26):11971-11975.

13.  Cardwell CR, Stene LC, Joner G, et al. Caesarean section is associated with an increased risk of childhood-onset type 1 diabetes mellitus: a meta-analysis of observational studies. *Diabetologia.* 2008;51(5):726-735.

14.  Li HT, Zhou YB, Liu JM. The impact of cesarean section on offspring overweight and obesity: a systematic review and meta-analysis. *Int J Obes (Lond).* 2013;37(7):893-899.

15.  Dominguez-Bello MG, De Jesus-Laboy KM, Shen N, et al. Partial restoration of the microbiota of cesarean-born infants via vaginal microbial transfer. *Nat Med.* 2016;22(3):250-253.

16.  Franzosa EA, Sirota-Madi A, Avila-Pacheco J, et al. Gut microbiome structure and metabolic activity in inflammatory bowel disease [published correction appears in Nat Microbiol. 2019;4(5):898]. *Nat Microbiol.* 2019;4(2):293-305. doi:10.1038/s41564-018-0306-4

17.  Knights D, Silverberg MS, Weersma RK, et al. Complex host genetics influence the microbiome in inflammatory bowel disease. *Genome Med.* 2014;6(12):107.

18.  Mirsepasi-Lauridsen HC, Vrankx K, Engberg J, et al. Disease-specific enteric microbiome dysbiosis in inflammatory bowel disease. *Front Med.* 2018;5:304.

19.  van der Giessen J, Binyamin D, Belogolovski A, et al. Modulation of cytokine patterns and microbiome during pregnancy in IBD. *Gut.* 2020;69(3):473-486. doi:10.1136/gutjnl-2019-318263.

20.  Torres J, Hu J, Seki A, et al. Infants born to mothers with IBD present with altered gut microbiome that transfers abnormalities of the adaptive immune system to germ-free mice. *Gut.* 2019;0:1-10. doi:10.1136/gutjnl-2018-317855

21.  Klement, E, Cohen, RV, Boxman, J, Joseph, A, Reif, S. Breastfeeding and risk of inflammatory bowel disease: a systematic review with meta-analysis. *Am J Clin Nutr.* 2004;80:1342-1352.

22.  Ng SC, Tang W, Leong RW, et al. Environmental risk factors in inflammatory bowel disease: a population-based case-control study in Asia-Pacific. *Gut.* 2015;64(7):1063-1071.

23.  Guo AY, Stevens BW, Wilson RG, et al. Early life environment and natural history of inflammatory bowel diseases. *BMC Gastroenterol.* 2014;14:216.

24.  National Institute of Health and Clinical Excellence (NICE) (2006) Nutritional Support in Adults. Available at: https://pathways.nice.org.uk/pathways/nutrition-support-in-adults (Accessed on 01 February 2020).

25.  Gerasimidis K, Macleod I, Maclean A, et al. Performance of the novel Paediatric Yorkhill Malnutrition Score (PYMS) in hospital practice. *Clin Nutr.* 2011 Aug;30(4):430-435. doi:10.1016/j.clnu.2011.01.015.

26.  Malnutrition Advisory Group (MAG): A Standing Committee of the British Association for Parenteral and Enteral Nutrition (BAPEN). The 'MUST' Explanatory Booklet. A Guide to the 'Malnutrition Universal Screening Tool' ('MUST') for Adults: BAPEN; 2003.

27. Scaldaferri F, Pizzoferrato M, Lopetuso LR, et al. Nutrition and IBD: malnutrition and/or sarcopenia? A practical guide. *Gastroenterol Res Pract*. 2017; 2017: 8646495. Published online 2017 Jan 3. doi:10.1155/2017/8646495

28. White JV, Guenter P, Jensen G, et al. Consensus statement: Academy of Nutrition and Dietetics and American Society for Parenteral and Enteral Nutrition: characteristics recommended for the identification and documentation of adult malnutrition (undernutrition). *JPEN J Parenter Enteral Nutr*. 2012;36(3):275-283. doi:10.1177/0148607112440285

29. Becker P, Carney LN, Corkins MR, et al. Consensus statement of the Academy of Nutrition and Dietetics/American Society for Parenteral and Enteral Nutrition: indicators recommended for the identification and documentation of pediatric malnutrition (undernutrition). *Nutr Clin Pract*. 2015;30(1):147-161. doi: 10.1177/0884533614557642. Epub 2014 Nov 24.

30. Balestrieri P, Ribolsi M, Guarino MPL, Emerenziani S, Altomare A, Cicala M. *Nutritional Aspects in Inflammatory Bowel Diseases Nutrients*. 2020;12(2). pii: E372. doi:10.3390/nu12020372

31. Bergeron F, Bouin M, D'Aoust L, Lemoyne M, Presse N. Food avoidance in patients with inflammatory bowel disease: What, when and who? *Clin Nutr*. 2018;37(3):884-889. doi:10.1016/j.clnu.2017.03.010. Epub 2017 Mar 15.

32. Stokes MA, Hill GL. Total energy expenditure in patients with Crohn's disease: measurement by the combined body scan technique. *JPEN J Parenter Enteral Nutr*. 1993;17(1):3-7.

33. Nguyen GC, Munsell M, Harris ML. Nationwide prevalence and prognostic significance of clinically diagnosable protein-calorie malnutrition in hospitalized inflammatory bowel disease patients. *Inflamm Bowel Dis*. 2008;14(8):1105-1111. doi:10.1002/ibd.20429

34. Grass F, Pache B, Martin D, Hahnloser D, Demartines N, and Hübner M. Preoperative nutritional conditioning of Crohn's patients-systematic review of current evidence and practice. *Nutrients*. 2017;9(6):562.

35. Thangarajah D, Hyde MJ, Konteti VK, Santhakumaran S, Frost G, Fell JM. Systematic review: body composition in children with inflammatory bowel disease. *Aliment Pharmacol Ther*. 2015;42(2):142-157. doi:10.1111/apt.13218. Epub 2015 Jun 4.

36. Schulze H1, Esters P, Dignass A. Review article: the management of Crohn's disease and ulcerative colitis during pregnancy and lactation. *Aliment Pharmacol Ther*. 2014;40(9):991-1008. doi:10.1111/apt.12949. Epub 2014 Sep 9.

37. Eder P, Niezgódka A, Krela-Kaźmierczak I, Stawczyk-Eder K, Banasik E, Dobrowolska A. Dietary support in elderly patients with inflammatory bowel disease. *Nutrients*. 2019;11(6). pii: E1421. doi:10.3390/nu11061421

38. Ananthakrishnan AN, Binion DG. Treatment of ulcerative colitis in the elderly. *Dig Dis*. 2009;27:327-334. doi: 10.1159/000228569

39. Molodecky NA, Soon IS, Rabi DM, et al. Increasing incidence and prevalence of the inflammatory bowel diseases with time, based on systematic review. *Gastroenterology*. 2012;142:46-54. doi:10.1053/j.gastro.2011.10.001

40. Charpentier C, Salleron J, Savoye G, et al. Natural history of elderly-onset inflammatory bowel disease: a population based cohort study. *Gut*. 2014;63:423-432. doi:10.1136/gutjnl-2012-303864

41. Bischoff SC, Escher J, Hébuterne X, et al. ESPEN practical guideline: clinical nutrition in inflammatory bowel disease. *Clin Nutr*. 2020;39(3):632-653.

42. Blaauw R, Osland E, Sriram K, et al. Parenteral provision of micronutrients to adult patients: an expert consensus paper. *JPEN J Parenter Enteral Nutr*. 2019;43 Suppl 1:S5-S23. doi:10.1002/jpen.1525

43. Office of Dietary Supplements (ODS). Iron Fact Sheet For Health Professionals. Updated: October 16, 2019.

44. Nemeth E, Ganz T. The role of hepcidin in iron metabolism. *Acta Haematol*. 2009;122(2-3):78-86. doi:10.1159/000243791

45. Dignass AU, Gasche C, Bettenworth D, et al. European consensus on the diagnosis and management of iron deficiency and anaemia in inflammatory bowel diseases. *Journal of Crohn's and Colitis*. 2015;9(3):211-222.

46. Anemia in Pregnancy. ACOG Practice Bulletin No. 95. American College of Obstetricians and Gynecologists. *Obstet Gynecol*. 2008;112:201-207.

47. Gabbe, SG, Niebyl, JR, Simpson, JL, Anderson, GD (1991). *Obstetrics: Normal and Problem Pregnancies*. Churchill Livingstone.

48. Office of Dietary Supplements (ODS). Vitamin D Fact Sheet For Health Professionals. Updated: August 7, 2019.

49. Kim S, Kang Y, Park S, Koh H, Kim S. Association of Vitamin D with inflammatory bowel disease activity in pediatric patients. *J Korean Med Sci*. 2019;34(32):e204. doi:10.3346/jkms.2019.34.e204

50. Gubatan J, Mitsuhashi S, Zenlea T, Rosenberg L, Robson S, Moss AC. Low serum vitamin D during remission increases risk of clinical relapse in patients with ulcerative colitis. *Clin Gastroenterol Hepatol*. 2017;15(2):240-246. e1. doi:10.1016/j.cgh.2016.05.035. Epub 2016 Jun 4.

51. Kojecký V, Matouš J, Zádorová Z, Gřiva M, Kianička B, Uher M. Vitamin D supplementation dose needs to be higher in patients with inflammatory bowel disease: interventional study. *Vnitr Lek*. 2019;65(7-8):470-474.

52. ACOG Committee on Obstetric Practice. ACOG committee opinion no. 495: vitamin D: screening and supplementation during pregnancy. *Obstet Gynecol*. 2011;118(1):197-198.

53. Lee HH, Prasad AS, Brewer GJ, Owyang C. Zinc absorption in human small intestine. *Am J Physiol*. 1989;256(1 Pt 1):G87-91.

54. Vagianos K, Bector S, McConnell J, Bernstein CN. Nutrition assessment of patients with inflammatory bowel disease. *J Parenter Enteral Nutr.* 2007;31:311-319.

55. Alkhouri RH, Hashmi H, Baker RD, et al. Vitamin and mineral status in patients with inflammatory bowel disease. *J Pediatr Gastroenterol Nutr.* 2013;56:89-92.

56. McClain C, Soutor C, Zieve L. Zinc deficiency: a complication of Crohn's disease. *Gastroenterology.* 1980;78:272-279.

57. Siva S, Rubin DT, Gulotta G, Wroblewski K, Pekow J. Zinc deficiency is associated with poor clinical outcomes in patients with inflammatory bowel disease. *Inflamm Bowel Dis.* 2017;23(1):152-157. doi:10.1097/MIB.0000000000000989

58. Office of Dietary Supplements (ODS). Vitamin B12 Fact Sheet For Health Professionals. Updated: February 19, 2020.

59. Mowat C, Cole A, Windsor A, et al. Guidelines for the management of inflammatory bowel disease in adults. *Gut.* 2011:doi:10.1136/gut.2010.224154

60. Office of Dietary Supplements (ODS). Vitamin B6 Fact Sheet For Health Professionals. Updated: February 24, 2020.

61. ACOG (American College of Obstetrics and Gynecology) Practice Bulletin: nausea and vomiting of pregnancy. *Obstet Gynecol.* 2004;103:803-814.

62. Office of Dietary Supplements (ODS). Folate Fact Sheet For Health Professionals. Updated: July 19, 2019. https://ods.od.nih.gov/factsheets/Folate-HealthProfessional/

63. Rossi RE, Whyand T, Murray CD, et al. The role of dietary supplements in inflammatory bowel disease: a systematic review. *Eur J Gastroenterol Hepatol.* 2016;28:1357-64

64. US Preventive Services Task Force, Agency for Healthcare Research and Quality. Folic acid for the prevention of neural tube defects: US Preventive Services Task Force recommendation statement. *Ann Intern Med.* 2009;150:626.

65. Office of Dietary Supplements (ODS). Vitamin C Fact Sheet For Health Professionals. Updated: February 27, 2020. https://ods.od.nih.gov/factsheets/VitaminC-HealthProfessional/

66. Lim H, Kim HJ, Hong SJ, Kim S. Nutrient intake and bone mineral density by nutritional status in patients with inflammatory bowel disease. *J Bone Metab.* 2014;21(3):195-203. doi:10.11005/jbm.2014.21.3.195. Epub 2014 Aug 31.

67. Hartman C, Marderfeld L, Davidson K, et al. Food intake adequacy in children and adolescents with inflammatory bowel disease. *J Pediatr Gastroenterol Nutr.* 2016;63(4):437-44. doi:10.1097/MPG.0000000000001170

68. Hengstermann S, Valentini L, Schaper L, et al. Altered status of antioxidant vitamins and fatty acids in patients with inactive inflammatory bowel disease. *Clin Nutr.* 2008;27(4):571-8. doi:10.1016/j.clnu.2008.01.007. Epub 2008 Mar 7.

69. Fain O. Vitamin C deficiency. *Rev Med Interne.* 2004;25(12):872-880.

70. Tinsley A, Ehrlich OG, Hwang C, et al. Knowledge, attitudes, and beliefs regarding the role of nutrition in IBD among patients and providers. *Inflamm Bowel Dis.* 2016;22(10):2474-2481.

71. Ananthakrishnan AN, Bernstein CN, Iliopoulos D, et al. Environmental triggers in IBD: a review of progress and evidence. *Nat Rev Gastroenterol Hepatol.* 2018;15(1):39-49. doi:10.1038/nrgastro.2017.136. Epub 2017 Oct 11.

72. Ananthakrishnan AN. Impact of Diet on Risk of IBD. *Crohn's & Colitis 360.* 2020;2(1):otz054.

73. Khalili H, Håkansson N, Chan SS, et al. Adherence to a Mediterranean diet is associated with a lower risk of later-onset Crohn's disease: results from two large prospective cohort studies. *Gut.* 2020;69(9):1637-1644

74. Ananthakrishnan AN, Khalili H, Konijeti GG, et al. A prospective study of long-term intake of dietary fiber and risk of Crohn's disease and ulcerative colitis. *Gastroenterology.* 2013;145(5):970-7. doi:10.1053/j.gastro.2013.07.050. Epub 2013 Aug 2.

75. Ananthakrishnan AN, Khalili H, Konijeti GG, et al. Long-term intake of dietary fat and risk of ulcerative colitis and Crohn's disease. *Gut.* 2014;63:776-84.

76. IBD in EPIC Study Investigators, Tjonneland A, Overvad K, Bergmann MM, et al. Linoleic acid, a dietary n-6 polyunsaturated fatty acid, and the aetiology of ulcerative colitis: a nested case-control study within a European prospective cohort study. *Gut.* 2009;58(12):1606-11. doi:10.1136/gut.2008.169078. Epub 2009 Jul 23.

77. Ananthakrishnan AN, Khalili H, Higuchi LM, et al. Higher predicted vitamin d status is associated with reduced risk of Crohn's disease. *Gastroenterology.* 2012;142:482-9.

78. Ananthakrishnan AN, Khalili H, Song M, et al. Zinc intake and risk of Crohn's disease and ulcerative colitis: a prospective cohort study. *Int J Epidemiol.* 2015;44:1995-2005.

79. Lu Y, Zamora-Ros R, Chan S, et al. Dietary polyphenols in the aetiology of Crohn's disease and ulcerative colitis-a multicenter European Prospective Cohort Study (EPIC). *Inflamm Bowel Dis.* 2017;23:2072-2082.

80. Viennois E, Chassaing B. First victim, later aggressor: how the intestinal microbiota drives the pro-inflammatory effects of dietary emulsifiers? *Gut Microbes.* 2018;9:289-291. doi:10.1080/19490976.2017.1421885. [Epub ahead of print]

81. Chassaing B, Van de Wiele T, De Bodt J, Marzorati M, Gewirtz AT. Dietary emulsifiers directly alter human microbiota composition and gene expression ex vivo potentiating intestinal inflammation. *Gut.* 2017;66(8):1414-1427. doi:10.1136/gutjnl-2016-313099. Epub 2017 Mar 21.

82. Chassaing B, Koren O, Goodrich JK, et al. Dietary emulsifiers impact the mouse gut microbiota promoting colitis and metabolic syndrome. *Nature.* 2015;519:92-6.

83. Suskind DL, Wahbeh G, Cohen SA, et al. Patients perceive clinical benefit with the specific carbohydrate diet for inflammatory bowel disease. *Dig Dis Sci.* 2016;61:3255-60.
84. Narula N, Dhillon A, Zhang D, Sherlock ME, Tondeur M, Zachos M. Enteral nutritional therapy for treatment of active Crohn's disease. Cochrane Database of Systematic Reviews 2018, Issue 4. Art No.: CD000542. doi: 10.1002/14651858.CD000542.pub3
85. Wall CL, Day AS, Gearry RB. Use of exclusive enteral nutrition in adults with Crohn's disease: a review. *World J Gastroenterol.* 2013;19:7652-7660.
86. Zachos M, Tondeur M, Griffiths AM. Enteral nutritional therapy for induction of remission in Crohn's disease. Cochrane Database Syst Rev. 2007:Cd000542.
87. Heuschkel RB, Menache CC, Megerian JT, et al. Enteral nutrition and corticosteroids in the treatment of acute Crohn's disease in children. *J Pediatr Gastroenterol Nutr.* 2000;31:8-15.
88. Dziechciarz P, Horvath A, Shamir R, et al. Meta-analysis: enteral nutrition in active Crohn's disease in children. *Aliment Pharmacol Ther.* 2007;26:795-806.
89. Rubio A, Pigneur B, Garnier-Lengline H, et al. The efficacy of exclusive nutritional therapy in paediatric Crohn's disease, comparing fractionated oral vs. continuous enteral feeding. *Aliment Pharmacol Ther.* 2011;33:1332-1339.
90. Levine A, Turner D, Pfeffer Gik T, et al. Comparison of outcomes parameters for induction of remission in new onset pediatric Crohn's disease: evaluation of the porto IBD group "growth relapse and outcomes with therapy" (GROWTH CD) study. *Inflamm Bowel Dis.* 2014;20:278-285.
91. Lee D, Baldassano RN, Otley AR, et al. Comparative effectiveness of nutritional and biological therapy in North American children with active Crohn's disease. *Inflamm Bowel Dis.* 2015;21:1786-1793.
92. Day AS, Whitten KE, Lemberg DA, et al. Exclusive enteral feeding as primary therapy for Crohn's disease in Australian children and adolescents: a feasible and effective approach. *J Gastroenterol Hepatol.* 2006;21:1609-1614.
93. Borrelli O, Cordischi L, Cirulli M, et al. Polymeric diet alone versus corticosteroids in the treatment of active pediatric Crohn's disease: a randomized controlled open-label trial. *Clin Gastroenterol Hepatol.* 2006;4:744-753.
94. Berni Canani R, Terrin G, Borrelli O, et al. Short- and long-term therapeutic efficacy of nutritional therapy and corticosteroids in paediatric Crohn's disease. *Dig Liv Dis.* 2006;38:381-387.
95. Pigneur B, Lepage P, Mondot S, et al. Mucosal healing and bacterial composition in response to enteral nutrition vs steroid-based induction therapy: a randomized prospective clinical trial in children with Crohn's disease. *J Crohn's Colitis.* 2019;13:846-855.
96. Fell JM, Paintin M, Arnaud-Battandier F, et al. Mucosal healing and a fall in mucosal pro-inflammatory cytokine mRNA induced by a specific oral polymeric diet in paediatric Crohn's disease. *Aliment Pharmacol Ther.* 2000;14:281-289.
97. Grover Z, Muir R, Lewindon P. Exclusive enteral nutrition induces early clinical, mucosal and transmural remission in paediatric Crohn's disease. *J Gastroenterol.* 2014;49:638-645.
98. Akobeng AK, Thomas AG. Enteral nutrition for maintenance of remission in Crohn's disease. Cochrane Database Syst Rev 2007:CD005984.
99. Knight C, El-Matary W, Spray C, et al. Long-term outcome of nutritional therapy in paediatric Crohn's disease. *Clin Nutr.* 2005;24:775-779.
100. Cameron FL, Gerasimidis K, Papangelou A, et al. Clinical progress in the two years following a course of exclusive enteral nutrition in 109 paediatric patients with Crohn's disease. *Aliment Pharmacol Ther.* 2013;37:622-629.
101. Frivolt K, Schwerd T, Werkstetter KJ, et al. Repeated exclusive enteral nutrition in the treatment of paediatric Crohn's disease: predictors of efficacy and outcome. *Aliment Pharmacol Ther.* 2014;39:1398-1407.
102. Faiman A, Mutalib M, Moylan A, et al. Standard versus rapid food reintroduction after exclusive enteral nutritional therapy in paediatric Crohn's disease. *Eur J Gastroenterol Hepatol.* 2014;26:276-281.
103. Afzal NA, Addai S, Fagbemi A, et al. Refeeding syndrome with enteral nutrition in children: a case report, literature review and clinical guidelines. *Clin Nutr.* 2002;21:515-520.
104. Akobeng AK, Thomas AG. Refeeding syndrome following exclusive enteral nutritional treatment in Crohn disease. *J Pediatr Gastroenterol Nutr.* 2010;51:364-366.
105. Miele E, Shamir R, Aloi M, et al. Nutrition in paediatric inflammatory bowel disease: a position paper on behalf of the porto IBD group of ESPGHAN. *J Pediatr Gastroenterol Nutr.* 2018;66(4):687-708.
106. Johnson T, Macdonald S, Hill S, et al. Treatment of active Crohn's disease in children using partial enteral nutrition with liquid formula a randomised controlled trial. *Gut.* 2006;55:356-361.
107. Sigall-Boneh R, Pfeffer-Gik T, Segal I, et al. Partial enteral nutrition with a Crohn's disease exclusion diet is effective for induction of remission in children and young adults with Crohn's disease. *Inflamm Bowel Dis.* 2014;20:1353-1360.
108. Levine A, Wine E, Assa A, et al. Crohn's disease exclusion diet plus partial enteral nutrition induces sustained remission in a randomized controlled trial. *Gastroenterology.* 2019;157(2):440-450.e8. doi:10.1053/j.gastro.2019.04.021. Epub 2019 Jun 4.
109. Obih C, Wahbeh G, Lee D, et al. Specific carbohydrate diet for pediatric inflammatory bowel disease in clinical practice within an academic IBD center. *Nutrition.* 2016;32:418-425.

110. Suskind DL, Cohen SA, Brittnacher MJ, et al. Clinical and fecal microbial changes with diet therapy in active inflammatory bowel disease. *J Clin Gastroenterol.* 2018;52:155-163.

111. Cohen SA, Gold BD, Oliva S, et al. Clinical and mucosal improvement with specific carbohydrate diet in pediatric Crohn disease. *J Pediatr Gastroenterol Nutr.* 2014;59:516-521.

112. Olendzki BC, Silverstein TD, Persuitte GM, et al. An anti-inflammatory diet as treatment for inflammatory bowel disease: a case series report. *Nutr J.* 2014;13:5.

113. Kuppinger D, Hartl WH, Bertok M, et al. Nutritional screening for risk prediction in patients scheduled for abdominal operations. *Br J Surg.* 2012;99(5):728-737.

114. Gustafsson UO, Scott MJ, Hubner M, et al. Guidelines for perioperative care in elective colorectal surgery: Enhanced Recovery After Surgery (ERAS®) Society recommendations: 2018. *World J Surg.* 2019;43(3):659-695. doi:10.1007/s00268-018-4844-y

115. Andersen HK, Lewis SJ, Thomas S. Early enteral nutrition within 24h of colorectal surgery versus later commencement of feeding for postoperative complications. *Cochrane Database Syst Rev.* 2006;18(4):CD004080

116. Lewis SJ, Andersen HK, Thomas S. Early enteral nutrition within 24 h of intestinal surgery versus later commencement of feeding: a systematic review and meta-analysis. *J Gastrointest Surg.* 2009;13(3):569-575.

117. Wilschanski M, Sherman P, Pencharz P, et al. Supplementary enteral nutrition maintains remission in paediatric Crohn's disease. *Gut.* 1996;38:543-548.

118. Duncan H, Buchanan E, Cardigan T, et al. A retrospective study showing maintenance treatment options for paediatric CD in the first year following diagnosis after induction of remission with EEN: supplemental enteral nutrition is better than nothing! *BMC Gastroenterol.* 2014;14:50.

119. Verma S, Kirkwood B, Brown S, Giaffer MH. Oral nutritional supplementation is effective in the maintenance of remission in Crohn's disease. *Dig Liver Dis.* 2000;32(9):769-774.

120. Takagi S, Utsunomiya K, Kuriyama S, et al. Effectiveness of an 'half elemental diet' as maintenance therapy for Crohn's disease: a randomized-controlled trial. *Aliment Pharmacol Ther.* 2006;24(9):1333-1340.

121. Nguyen DL, Palmer LB, Nguyen ET, et al. Specialized enteral nutrition therapy in Crohn's disease patients on maintenance infliximab therapy: a meta-analysis. *Therap Adv Gastroenterol.* 2015;8:168-175

122. Akobeng AK, Zhang D, Gordon M, MacDonald JK. Enteral nutrition for maintenance of remission in Crohn's disease. Cochrane Database Syst Rev. 2018;8:CD005984. doi:10.1002/14651858.CD005984.pub3

123. Brotherton CS, Martin CA, Long MD, Kappelman MD, Sandler RS. Avoidance of fiber is associated with greater risk of Crohn's disease flare in a 6 month period. *Clin Gastroenterol Hepatol.* 2016;14(8):1130-1136.

124. Chiba M, Abe T, Tsuda H, Sugawara T, Tsuda S, Tozawa H, et al. Lifestyle-related disease in Crohn's disease: relapse prevention by a semi-vegetarian diet. *World J Gastroenterol.* 2010;16:2484-2495.

125. Godny L, Reshef L, Pfeffer-Gik T, et al. Adherence to the Mediterranean diet is associated with decreased fecal calprotectin in patients with ulcerative colitis after pouch surgery. *Eur J Nutr.* 2020;59(7):3183-3190. doi:10.1007/s00394-019-02158-3

126. de Lima A, Zelinkova Z, Mulders AG, van der Woude CJ. Preconception Care Reduces Relapse of Inflammatory Bowel Disease During Pregnancy. *Clin Gastroenterol Hepatol.* 2016;14:1285-1292.e1

127. https://naturalmedicines.therapeuticresearch.com/databases/commercial-products/commercial-product.aspx?cpid=150165

128. Trumbo P, Schlicker S, Yates AA, Poos M. Dietary reference intakes for energy, carbohydrate, fiber, fat, fatty acids, cholesterol, protein and amino acids. Food and Nutrition Board of the Institute of Medicine, The National Academies. *J Am Diet Assoc.* 2002;102(11):1621-1630.

129. https://naturalmedicines.therapeuticresearch.com/databases/food,-herbs-supplements/professional.aspx?productid=978

130. https://naturalmedicines.therapeuticresearch.com/databases/food,-herbs-supplements/professional.aspx?productid=729

# 4

# Mental Health Issues Affecting Women With IBD

Laurie Keefer, PhD  |  Jordyn Feingold, MD

## Introduction

It is virtually impossible to disentangle the medical experience of living with inflammatory bowel disease (IBD) from its psychosocial context. The nature of the disease, including its incurability, unpredictability, severity of symptoms, stigmatization, as well as medication and surgical side effects, may severely impair one's quality of life (QOL), contributing to significant psychological burden.[1,2] Women with IBD may experience unique challenges to their mental health, given that mental illnesses including depression and anxiety are more prevalent in women in the general population, and that transition periods including pregnancy and the postpartum period when mental illnesses spike are unique to the female experience.

The burden of living with IBD is determined both by symptom and disease severity, and also by a patient's ability to cope with her symptoms while minimizing interruptions into daily life.[3] In recent decades, research and practice spanning the fields of gastroenterology, psychology, and psychiatry have converged, with a large body of research elucidating the comorbidity of IBD and psychiatric diagnoses and supporting the promise of psychological and behavioral interventions for symptoms and QOL in patients with IBD.

In this chapter specifically about women's mental health and IBD across the life span, we focus on recommendations from the emerging field of *psychogastroenterology* that infuses integrated mental health care into routine gastroenterology care for patients with digestive disorders. We discuss the mental health issues that differentially affect women with IBD, as well as protective factors that promote psychological resilience, optimism, coping, and self-regulation. We highlight the promise of both medical therapies and behavioral interventions that have shown promise in improving

- 61 -

Abraham BP, Kane SV, Glassner KL, eds.
*Women's Health in IBD: The Spectrum of Care
From Birth to Adulthood* (pp 61-81).
© 2022 Taylor & Francis Group.

the mental health and QOL in patients with IBD and discuss who should receive such therapies. Additionally, we provide several basic recommendations for how gastroenterologists and IBD providers can specifically address patient's psychological needs and mental health concerns within the clinical setting.

It is important to note upfront that the absence of a psychiatric diagnosis in a woman with IBD does not mean that she is optimally functioning or coping with her disease. Conversely, the presence of a comorbid psychiatric diagnosis in a patient with IBD does not necessarily mean that she lacks resilience, self-regulation, or the ability to cope with her illness. Approaches to maximizing the mental health and well-being of patients with IBD should therefore be specific to the individual and may target the elimination or treatment of a particular diagnosis as well as the promotion of skills aimed at enhancing human strengths relevant to gastrointestinal health. We end this chapter by highlighting the promise of strengths-based approaches to evaluating and tracking the mental health of patients with IBD, and the role of integrated mental health care in the clinical setting for the prevention of psychiatric diagnosis in women with IBD.

# IBD Self-Management: A Window Into Mental Health

Disease self-management is essential for successful long-term QOL in IBD, and is certainly mediated by psychological and psychiatric factors. Principles of self-management are mediated by the presence of a mental illness, social support, and support from integrated clinical teams. Three primary self-management tasks have been described in the literature as essential for patients living with Crohn's disease (CD) and ulcerative colitis (UC)[4,5]:

1. Medical management, including adherence to therapies, medical decision making, disease knowledge, and the quality of relationships and communication with medical teams

2. Preservation or creation of meaningful life roles and adjustment to the limitations that one's disease presents

3. Acknowledgment and management of the emotional and psychological impacts of IBD

Sub-optimal self-management, or failure to achieve these 3 self-management tasks, can be both a driver of and a consequence of mental illness. In fact, it is estimated that approximately 15% of patients with IBD account for nearly half of health care expenditures attributable to this disease, driven by chronic pain, depression, and poor social support.[3,6,7] As the chronicity of IBD requires constant shifts in coping and self-management skills over time, it makes sense that patients with IBD are at an increased risk for the development of mental health issues. Analogously, mental well-being, the presence of positive psychosocial characteristics that enable people to thrive, can both lead to and result from better disease management. Indeed, a patient's capacity to self-manage is optimized in the context of strong support from an interdisciplinary care team, including gastroenterologists, nurses, dieticians, and mental health professionals.

It is well established that patients with IBD are at increased risk for mental health disorders, including depression, anxiety, and opioid use disorders.[1,5] Women in the general population are also at an increased risk for both depression and anxiety compared with their male counterparts, with females experiencing 1.5- to 3-fold higher rates of depression than males, beginning in early adolescence, and 2-fold higher rates of anxiety.[8,9] While these trends exist within the general population, the majority of studies examining the rates of comorbid mental illness in IBD populations are not powered to examine differences across genders. Furthermore, much of the evidence that we cite in this chapter regarding the relationship between mental health and inflammatory bowel diseases is not necessarily specific to only women. Therefore, this is an area ripe for future research and inquiry.

Irrespective of sex differences, systematic reviews reveal that rates of anxiety and depression are higher in patients with IBD relative to healthy controls. Rates of anxiety and depression are higher in those with active disease compared with inactive IBD, and rates of anxiety and depression may be modestly higher in patients with CD compared with UC.[1] We discuss the purported mechanisms of such findings in a later section, including the bidirectional relationship between IBD and depression.

When untreated, depression and anxiety have been linked to more severe symptoms of IBD and more frequent flares,[10] higher rates of hospitalization,[11] and lower treatment adherence[12] than those without a mental illness.[1]

Notably, rates of anxiety and depression have been shown to be lower in patients with IBD compared with those with other chronic illnesses (irritable bowel syndrome [IBS], chronic liver disease, celiac disease, food allergy, gastroesophageal reflux disease, juvenile idiopathic arthritis, multiple sclerosis, rheumatoid arthritis, or self-limited colitis). However, in some patients, there may be a great deal of symptom overlap between IBD and some of these other autoimmune conditions. Regarding temporality, there is a high level of evidence to suggest that adults with IBD are more likely to develop anxiety and depression before the onset of an IBD diagnosis, though there may be a substantial portion of adults developing depression after disease onset. In children, it appears that there is a higher risk of developing anxiety or depression after IBD onset compared with controls.[1] Due to these varying temporal effects between the onset of a mental illness and a diagnosis of IBD, it is critical that gastroenterologists inquire about and screen for mental illness upon first meeting a patient with suspected IBD, and at regular intervals afterwards to monitor for the potential onset of psychopathology.

Substance use, particularly chronic opioid use that is typically initiated in the setting of acute pain management, is also more prevalent in patients with IBD compared with individuals in the general population. Among patients with IBD, women, youth and young adults, those with CD or indeterminate colitis, and those with a mental illness are at disproportionate risk for an opioid use disorder.[13] As chronic opioid use is an independent predictor of poor outcomes in IBD, and rates of opioid dependence are rising in the United States, it is essential that gastroenterologists be attuned to these patterns, including substance use monitoring in their mental health assessments, and avoiding reliance on chronic opioid use for pain management.

When discussing "depression" in IBD, we often refer specifically to 1 of 3 separate psychiatric diagnoses: major depressive disorder (MDD; diagnostic criteria in Table 4-1), depressive disorder due to another medical condition, and/or adjustment disorder.

Depressive disorder due to another medical condition is defined as "prominent and persistent period of depressed mood or markedly diminished interest or pleasure in all, or almost all, activities with evidence from patient history, physical examination, or laboratory findings that the disturbance is the direct pathophysiologic consequence of another medical condition."[14] In IBD, a direct pathophysiologic consequence might include vitamin malabsorption due to inflammation in a patient's gastrointestinal tract or systemic inflammation.

The *adjustment disorders*, defined as the "development of emotional or behavioral symptoms in response to an identifiable stressor(s) occurring within 3 months of the onset of the stressor(s)" might refer to psychiatric symptoms that result as a consequence of physiologic discomfort from active symptoms of IBD, or from receiving the diagnosis itself. In this case, the stress-related disturbance does not meet criteria for another mental disorder and is not an exacerbation of a preexisting mental disorder. Symptoms of an adjustment disorder must last less than 6 months from the onset of the stressor. This acute period of distress and adjustment reflects a window of opportunity to capture patients at risk and provide interventions to build resilience around transitions in medical care.

Additionally, some patients may not fully reach criteria for MDD or one of these other diagnoses, but still manifest psychological distress, depressed mood, or other concerning behaviors. Provided that such diagnostic accuracy in depression is perhaps beyond the scope of a gastroenterologist, when possible IBD providers should refer patients for more complete and comprehensive evaluations with a mental health provider.

## Table 4-1. *Diagnostic and Statistical Manual of Mental Disorders, Fifth Edition* Criteria for Major Depressive Disorder

Must have one of the following:
- Depressed most of the day, nearly every day as indicated by subjective report (eg, feels sad, empty, hopeless) or observation made by others (eg, appears tearful, flat)
- Markedly diminished interest or pleasure in all, or almost all, activities most of the day, nearly every day (as indicated by subjective account or observation)

May also have:
- Significant weight loss when not dieting or weight gain (eg, change of more than 5% of body weight in a month), or decrease or increase in appetite nearly every day
- Insomnia or hypersomnia nearly every day
- Psychomotor agitation or retardation nearly every day (observable by others, not merely subjective feelings of restlessness or being slowed down)
- Fatigue or loss of energy nearly every day
- Feelings of worthlessness or excessive or inappropriate guilt (which may be delusional) nearly every day (not merely self-reproach or guilt about being sick)
- Diminished ability to think or concentrate, or indecisiveness, nearly every day (either by subjective account or as observed by others)
- Recurrent thoughts of death (not just fear of dying), recurrent suicidal ideation without a specific plan, or a suicide attempt or a specific plan for committing suicide

Timing and duration:
- These symptoms must be present during the same 2-week period and represent a change from previous functioning
  - The symptoms must cause clinically significant distress or impairment in social, occupational, or other important areas of functioning
  - The episode is not attributable to the physiological effects of a substance or to another medical condition

Gender differences:
- Females experience MDD at 1.5- to 3-fold higher rates than males, beginning in early adolescence; there are no clear differences in symptom presentation, course, treatment response, or functional consequences
- There is a higher risk of suicide attempts in women relative to men in the general population, but the risk of suicide completion is lower in women than men

## Rates of Depression in IBD

A systematic review of data published between 2005 and 2014 reveals that rates of depression are as high as 21.2% in patients with quiescent IBD, compared with 13.4% in healthy controls. Rates of depression can be almost twice as high (34.7%) with active IBD. Notably, the definition of active disease differs across studies. Female patients with IBD seem to be more prone to develop depression.[15,16]

When comorbid with IBD, depression has been associated with worse disease outcomes including increased risk for hospital readmission within 90 days,[17] increased risk of surgery, and unnecessary computed tomography scans and colonoscopies.[18]

# Mechanisms of Depression and IBD

It has become increasingly clear that there is more at play connecting IBD and depression than simply the burden of coping with the symptoms and chronic nature of CD or UC. The modern conceptualizations in chronic care recognize the bidirectional relationship between IBD and depression in which 1) poor self-management leads to poor disease outcomes just as much as poor disease outcomes including active disease leads to poor self-management,[19] and 2) inflammation associated with the chronic inflammatory process of IBD drives depression, and depression drives heightened inflammation.[20] Both hypotheses serve to explain why depression is known to be more severe in active disease vs inactive disease; not only are flares associated with greater systemic inflammatory burden, they also pose greater demands for enhanced coping. Additionally, the inflammatory hypothesis might explain the slightly lower incidence of mental illness in patients with UC compared to CD, as CD has a more systemic pattern of inflammation than UC, whereas UC inflammation is localized to the colon.[21] Here we explain the bidirectionality of the relationship and mechanisms of both purported pathways.

## Pathway 1

IBD requires a shift in coping skills ↔ poor adjustment increases risk of both depression and worse disease outcomes

*Behavioral activation theory*, a dominant conceptualization of depression, posits that people become depressed with a lack of environmental reinforcement (joy in life) or excessive environmental punishment (pain, symptoms, flares). As discussed previously with differential rates of depression with active disease, there is clearly a link between disease-free intervals and protection from depression. Similarly, when symptoms due to IBD result in an inability to function in daily life—experiencing pain, staying home from school or work, periods of hospitalization or nutritional support—depression is more likely.[5]

Similarly, another risk factor for the onset of depression in women with IBD is the degree to which IBD (the diagnosis or its ensuing medical or surgical needs) impacts her body image, self-esteem, or perceived disability.[22,23] Patients with IBD who have difficulty adapting to the disease report more systemic and gut symptoms, higher perceived stress, higher health care utilization, and a greater emotional representation of illness. Active depression further lowers patient's ability to positively reframe illness, plan for the future, tolerate distress, and adhere to medications, and increases the likelihood of denial and dependency on others for care. Ultimately, comorbid depression can impact a woman's ability to self-manage her disease through diet, sleep, exercise, and maintaining positive social relationships with one's treatment team or caregivers.[24] Through various studies on both women and men, it is clear that depression undermines a patient's ability to cope with illness, and that poor coping, mediated by active disease, further increases the chances of becoming depressed.

## Pathway 2

Depression drives inflammation ↔ inflammation drives IBD

The second mechanism underpinning a bidirectional relationship between IBD and depression involves inflammation as an independent driver of both depression and IBD. Growing data support increased inflammation in depressed patients compared with healthy controls, with specific increases in interleukin (IL)-1, IL-6, IL-12, and tumor necrosis factor-alpha, and possible alterations in IL-12 pathways, particularly in depression dominated by vegetative symptoms (eg, flat affect, excessive sleeping, eating).[25] C-reactive protein, another marker of inflammation, has also been reported to be elevated in adults with depression[26] and can be used as a marker of depression severity and likeliness of recurrence.[27] There is also evidence that individuals with depression are able to activate their immune systems similarly to the immune response seen with acute infection, which might explain the propensity to flare in IBD.[25]

Data from the *Nurse's Health Study*, one of the most valuable sources of women-specific health information, reveal that women aged 29 to 72 years with depression may have a 2-fold increased risk for the development of CD compared with their non-depressed counterparts.[28] Additionally, in a Swiss study of more than 2000 Swiss patients with IBD (both male and female), depression was associated with physician-reported clinical recurrence of disease. IBD patients with depression have significantly shorter times to clinical recurrence, particularly in CD when compared to UC.[29]

# Effects of IBD Treatment on Mood

Another bidirectional relationship between IBD and depression pertains to treatments for IBD. Indeed, the treatment of IBD can impact mood, and mood can also mediate treatment response. In patients with CD, anti–tumor necrosis factor-alpha administration with infliximab or adalimumab has been shown to specifically reduce visceral sensitivity and improve central features of depression, including cognitive-affective biases linked to negative attributions about self, the world, and the future and alterations in limbic (amygdala) function.[30]

Other studies reveal that the presence of MDD before starting infliximab predicts a lower IBD remission rate at 1 month later. Depressive disorder is shown to be an independent determinant of active disease both at baseline and at reevaluation.[31] There is also evidence that treatment with infliximab may have a positive impact on depression, potentially by modifying the shared inflammatory pathways that underlie both IBD and depression.[5,32]

Whereas corticosteroids are some of the most widely used drug therapies in disease flare, as many as 40% of adults experience mood or anxiety symptoms on corticosteroids, with those on high doses or with histories of mood disorders at highest risk.[33]

# Anxiety

Anxiety is a general term that refers to feelings of panic, worry, or nervousness. An anxiety disorder occurs when patients are unable to control their feelings of unease, worry, and/or fear. Anxiety may be mild or severe and can last for periods up to 6 months' duration.[34]

Anxiety may manifest as one of several distinct psychiatric diagnoses, ranging from subclinical worry and stress to specific phobias to panic disorder, to generalized anxiety disorder (GAD) to agoraphobia, the fear of and avoidance of places or situations that might lead to panic, feeling trapped, helpless, or embarrassed. Notably, many patients with IBD may avoid situations in which they may not have access to a bathroom, but do not qualify for a diagnosis of agoraphobia.

GAD is the most common anxiety disorder, defined as persistent and excessive anxiety and uncontrollable worry about various life domains, including health, safety, work, and school performance. Physical symptoms accompany uncontrolled worry, including restlessness, feeling on edge, being easily fatigued, difficulty concentrating or mind going blank, irritability, muscle tension, and sleep disturbance. GAD in IBD, for example, can present as excess, uncontrollable worry around disease uncertainty, such as one's need for surgery/ostomy in the future, biologics causing cancer, or passing along IBD to one's children; these concerns often impact treatment decision making, the doctor-patient relationship, disability, and QOL. Additionally, there is a specific diagnosis in the DSM-5 known as "anxiety due to another medical condition" similar to its "depression due to another medical condition" counterpart as described previously. Additionally, the shorter-lived adjustment disorders can also take on an anxiety, rather than a depressive form.

## Table 4-2. Somatic Manifestations of Anxiety by Body System

| GENERAL AND AUTONOMIC SYMPTOMS | • Chills<br>• Hot flashes<br>• Trembling<br>• Sweating<br>• Exaggerated startle response<br>• Passing out |
|---|---|
| NEUROLOGIC AND PSYCHIATRIC SYMPTOMS | • Dizziness<br>• Lightheadedness<br>• Numbness or tingling<br>• Headache<br>• Dissociation<br>• Sense of impending doom<br>• Impaired concentration<br>• Irritability<br>• Insomnia |
| CARDIAC AND PULMONARY SYMPTOMS | • Shortness of breath<br>• Chest pain or discomfort<br>• Choking or globus sensation<br>• Heart palpitations |
| GASTROINTESTINAL SYMPTOMS | • Nausea<br>• Diarrhea<br>• Abdominal pain |
| MUSCULOSKELETAL SYMPTOMS | • Muscle tension<br>• Muscle spasms<br>• Body aches |

Indeed, IBD patients may possess general *gastrointestinal-specific anxiety*, defined as cognitions, emotions, and behaviors resulting from fear and anxiety about gastrointestinal sensations, symptoms, and the context in which the sensations and symptoms appear.[36] While gastrointestinal-specific anxiety has been proposed to influence symptom severity and QOL in patients with IBS,[37] patients with IBD—especially those with functional overlap—may suffer from this type of symptom-related anxiety as well. Additionally, women with IBD in particular have demonstrated IBD-related concerns regarding the impact of having IBD, the effects of treatments such as medications, surgery, and having an ostomy, developing cancer, and personal or interpersonal concerns regarding sexual impact, being a burden on caregivers, and bodily stigma.[38] Simply eliciting and addressing patient concerns and symptom-specific anxieties with female patients is postulated to have therapeutic value.

## Rates of Anxiety in IBD

Less is known about the prevalence or incidence of anxiety disorders in IBD in part because of the difficulty in defining anxiety. Abnormal levels of anxiety have been estimated to be between 29% and 35% during periods of remission, and up to 80% in active disease or clinical relapses.[39] Rates of anxiety may be more prevalent in those with CD compared to UC[1] and rates of anxiety are rising.[40] It is controversial whether female sex in IBD is a risk factor for anxiety, as the evidence is mixed.[41,42] In some studies, older age (being 40 years or older) has been shown to be an independent risk factor for the development of anxiety disorders and impaired QOL.[34,43] Surgery or hospitalization is another known risk, explained by both side effects of surgical intervention, medications, and the intimidating hospital environment.[44]

## Mechanisms of Anxiety and IBD

Just as in depression, the relationship between anxiety and IBD is bidirectional. The experience of anxiety or stress in women with IBD can also contribute to disease flares in active IBD,[45-48] or manifest clinically as functional gastrointestinal symptoms such as abdominal pain, diarrhea, nausea, and vomiting even when IBD is in remission.[49] Conversely, IBD symptoms, mediated by inflammatory cytokines and visceral pain can contribute to increasing levels of symptom-specific anxiety, including fear to leave the house, go to school or work due to pain, or use public transportation. Side effects of medications including corticosteroids used to treat disease flares can also induce or exacerbate anxiety levels,[34] and the timing of such effects can be quite variable, from early stages of treatment, during or even at the end of therapy.[33]

As with all emotional disturbance symptoms, it is important to disentangle whether IBD is causing the anxiety symptoms, or whether these are merely associated. Many studies that look at the symptom overlap of anxiety symptoms in IBD use symptom inventories that capture general symptoms of anxiety or worry. Fewer look at disease-specific or gastrointestinal-specific anxiety, which would clearly be a helpful clinical indicator of disease coping and help to accurately classify patients.

However, just as in depression in which precise diagnostic accuracy is out of the scope of the gastroenterologist, doctors with high suspicion that their patients might be suffering from a clinical anxiety disorder should refer patients for more comprehensive evaluation with a mental health provider.

# Stress

Even in the absence of a psychiatric disorder, acute and chronic stress can affect gastrointestinal symptoms. The effect of stress on the gut—and conversely, the gut on stress—is mediated by multiple afferent and efferent pathways comprising the brain-gut axis, including the enteric nervous system of the gastrointestinal tract, the autonomic nervous system with efferent branches modulating gastrointestinal sensorimotor function, and the hypothalamic-pituitary-adrenal axis with its neuroendocrine mediators, particularly the "stress hormone" cortisol.[50] When the brain perceives acute stress, transient yet pronounced increases in psychological and biological stress markers circulate through the body, evidenced by increased cortisol levels, heart rate, and blood pressure. Gastrointestinal motor function, local inflammatory processes, and gut permeability may also result,[50] which may cause disturbing gastrointestinal symptoms in patients with IBD, even those considered to be in remission. Stress-induced mucosal mast cell activation and epithelial damage have been shown to be more pronounced in patients with IBD than in healthy controls, a purported mechanism connecting stress with disease relapse.[51]

Strong evidence from prospective studies reveals a genuine link between stressful life events and IBD disease activity, supporting the notion that chronic stress, major life events, and negative affect are associated with an increased risk of disease relapse and exacerbations in patients with quiescent IBD.[50] Perceived stress has been shown to triple the risk of disease exacerbation,[46,52] and is associated with rectal mucosal abnormalities in UC patients.[53] While the directionality of the relationship among perceived stress, intestinal inflammation, and IBD symptoms remains elusive, it is most likely bidirectional, just as the relationships are between anxiety and depression, and symptoms of IBD.[5,54] Most available evidence supports a complex interplay among stress, psychological changes, and changes in gastrointestinal symptoms in terms of a vicious cycle, with chronic IBD symptoms causing both acute and chronic stress, and such stress leading to more disease activity.[55] Ultimately, it is important to keep these interactions in mind when treating women with IBD who may not meet criteria for a psychiatric disturbance but still may experience symptoms due to stress and brain-gut dysregulation.

# Comorbid Functional Disorders in Patients With IBD, Depression, and Anxiety

Underlying symptoms in many women who experience brain-gut dysregulation are often attributable to comorbid functional gastrointestinal disorders (ie, disorders of gut-brain interaction), particularly IBS. Patients with IBD, especially CD with comorbid depression and anxiety, are more likely to endorse symptoms of IBD in the absence of active inflammation. This suggests that patient-reported IBD severity might be influenced by psychopathology, and what patients might actually be experiencing is functional rather than organic disturbance.[56] This effect poses a risk for overtreatment of IBD and poor health care delivery.[57] Such patients, who experience debilitating functional symptoms on top of their IBD, are ideal candidates for brain-gut–directed therapies, described in a later section.

# Opioid Use and Disorder in Women With IBD

Pain related to disease activity, acute flares, complications, or surgeries in IBD is often treated, at least temporarily, with opioid analgesics. Long-term use of opioid analgesia is not recommended due to gastrointestinal side effects, including narcotic bowel syndrome, the paradoxical development of or increases in abdominal pain associated with continuous or increasing doses of opioids,[58] constipation, tolerance, and the possibility of addiction.[59,60] However, it is well established that the prevalence of chronic opioid use in IBD is rising, as it is in the general US population with approximately 6% of youth and 3% to 13% of adults receiving chronic opioid therapy for uncontrolled disease activity and chronic pain.[13,59,61]

Studies reveal that women are more likely than men to be prescribed opioids in both inpatient[62] and outpatient settings,[61,63] raising particular concern in the female population. Emerging evidence suggests that adolescents and young adults with IBD are at particular risk of becoming chronic opioid users and experiencing adverse effects.[13] A landmark population-based study in Manitoba, Canada, demonstrated that patients with IBD, particularly children and young adults, are nearly 3 times more likely than controls to become heavy opioid users, concluding that IBD is an independent risk factor for developing on opioid use disorder.[64] Risk factors for persistent opioid use post-flare in previously opioid naïve patients include a prior history of depression and substance use, chronic obstructive pulmonary disease, and CD or indeterminate colitis compared with UC.[65] It is also hypothesized that the presence of psychiatric disease may increase one's likelihood of opioid-seeking behavior.[65]

Opioid use, specifically in CD is associated with a known increased risk in mortality. One prospective cohort study of more than 6000 patients found a 1.5-fold increased mortality and a 3-fold increased risk of serious infections among patients with IBD on opioid treatment.[66] Indeed, clinicians should look for risk factors and evaluate heavy opioid use in their patients with IBD, especially women and young adults, including those with psychiatric comorbidities. Efforts to provide patients on opioids with behavioral interventions and multi-disciplinary pain management could support opioid weaning, which can be critical in enhancing QOL and outcomes for patients with IBD[13] and preventing opioid misuse into adulthood.[67,68] Additionally, it is essential that patients with comorbid depression and anxiety, who are more likely to be on chronic opioids, be effectively treated for these underlying conditions. Experts in psychogastroenterology endorse a growing body of literature for non-opioid pharmacologic agents for pain, including several anti-depressant agents, as well as behavioral interventions such as cognitive behavioral therapies (CBTs) and mindfulness trainings discussed in a later section.[60]

# Pregnancy and Peripartum Effects on Mood and Substance Use Disorders

Women with IBD are at a small but significantly elevated risk of new-onset perinatal mental illness, particularly mood and anxiety disorders, and substance use disorders.[21] The elevated risk appears to be in the postpartum period, particularly the early postpartum period (0 to 90 days postpartum), not during pregnancy, and in particular in women with CD. This may be attributable to the presence of pro-inflammatory cytokines that alter brain function and increase the risk of mental illness in patients with IBD.[21,69] Anecdotally, women often report lack of sleep, unpredictability/change in schedule, and physical demands (breast feeding, holding/carrying baby) as precipitating factors of emotional distress. Predictors of developing a perinatal psychiatric disorder among women with IBD are similar to those in the general population, and include young maternal age, infant morbidity and mortality, and health service use that increases the likelihood of detection of a psychiatric disorder.[21] These findings are consistent with studies showing that other chronic medical illnesses (diabetes, heart disease, migraine, and neurological disorders) are also associated with increased risk for depression in pregnancy and the postpartum period.[70]

It is certainly possible that one mechanism behind these findings is that women with IBD have greater comfort with accessing the health system due to their chronic disease, and therefore, they are more likely to be detected as having a mental illness compared with women in the perinatal period who do not have IBD. The absolute increased risk of developing a mood or substance use disorder for women with IBD in the peripartum period is modest; however, given the substantial association between perinatal mental illness and maternal and child morbidity and mortality, this increased risk warrants efforts at prevention, monitoring, and prompt treatment in women who are affected.[21]

Importantly, none of the screening measures for anxiety and depression that have been developed and validated in patients with IBD or drug screening tools have been validated specifically for postpartum and pregnant women with IBD.

# Assessment and Treatment of Depression and Anxiety in IBD Patients

Psychogastroenterology experts recommend that depression be part of IBD assessment, given the strong, negative impact on disease outcomes.[3,5,6] While such an evaluation is not recommended for general gastrointestinal practice, it may be helpful in special, high-risk populations such as IBD.[71]

Validated and easy-to-use metrics to assess the clinical significance of patient's symptoms may be helpful to have on-hand and integrated into IBD care. For depression, the Patient Health Questionnaire-9 is useful and has the highest sensitivity when compared with other depression scales in an IBD sample.[72] For anxiety, the National Institutes of Health Patient-Reported Outcomes Measurement Information System[73] screening tool for anxiety has the highest sensitivity among patients with IBD, and the tool is also widely accessible and free to use.[72]

Once depression or anxiety is identified, psychotherapy and/or medications can be extremely effective. Such therapies would generally warrant referral to a specific mental health provider and collaboration with the gastroenterologist to manage these patients. On the other hand, for patients who experience symptom-specific anxiety, mood disturbances, or reliance on substances related to their IBD, but do not necessarily qualify as having a clinical mood or substance use disorder, evidence-based brain-gut psychotherapies are recommended.

# Brain-Gut Psychotherapies

Brain-gut psychotherapies (BGP) are defined as therapies that leverage the brain's ability to bring under voluntary control the symptom processes that seem, at first, to be driven exclusively by the gut.[3] Such therapies differ from traditional psychotherapeutic approaches in that they are typically short-term, primarily focused on improving gastrointestinal symptoms, and skills based, focused specifically on the down-regulation of unpleasant gastrointestinal sensations, decreasing avoidance behaviors associated with fear of having symptoms, and building coping and resilience to stress or lifestyle changes imposed by a chronic condition. In fact, those with comorbid depression and anxiety are not the best candidates for BGP.

BGPs are optimally delivered by mental health professionals such as health psychologists or social workers who specialize specifically in psychogastroenterology (see Table 4-3 for a description of different mental health providers who may deliver psychogastroenterology treatments). These therapies have been shown to reduce health care utilization and symptom burden,[74] especially when they are integrated directly into gastrointestinal practice settings.[7,75] Psychotherapies in IBD work on 2 related pathways:

1. They target abdominal pain, visceral hypersensitivity, and gastrointestinal motility by reducing arousal of the autonomic nervous system, decreasing the stress-response, and even reducing inflammation. The physiologic effects are due to correction of dysregulation in the brain-gut axis.[74]

2. Such therapies also facilitate improved coping, acceptance, resilience, and self-regulation skills that patients practice and implement throughout their lives, to lessen stress during disease flare, and promote self-management behaviors to reduce the likelihood of flare in the first place.

The following describes the 3 BGP with the most robust evidence base, including CBT, gut-directed hypnotherapy, and mindfulness-based stress reduction.[74]

## Cognitive Behavioral Therapies

CBTs help patients examine the relationship among situations, thoughts, behaviors, emotions, and physical sensations in the body. Working with a therapist or even through online modules, patients develop insight into how these factors interact with one another and learn skills to intervene on unhelpful thinking patterns, behaviors, or to engage in relaxation techniques in service of eliminating psychological and physical distress.

While in IBS, CBTs have been shown to improve physical symptoms or overall disease status in adult patients, the same has not yet been shown in IBD, but likely apply at least to patients with functional overlap. CBTs in IBD have been linked to improved QOL and coping skills in patients

## Table 4-3. Mental Health Professionals Who May Deliver Brain-Gut Psychotherapies and Serve as Therapists for Patients With Mental Illness

| MENTAL HEALTH PROVIDER | DEGREE/LICENSURE | DESCRIPTION |
| --- | --- | --- |
| Psychiatrist | Doctor of Medicine (MD), or Doctor of Osteopathic Medicine (DO), with completion of residency training in psychiatry<br><br>Psychiatrists are licensed by licensure boards in the state where they practice | Psychiatrists are medical doctors who specifically treat patients with psychopathology. They can evaluate patient's mental health, make diagnoses, administer medications, and provide psychotherapy. |
| Psychologist<br>Health psychologist | Doctor of Philosophy (PhD) or Doctor of Psychology (PsyD)<br><br>Psychologists are licensed by licensure boards in each state where they practice | Psychologists are trained to evaluate patient's mental health, make diagnoses, and provide psychotherapy.<br>Health psychologists are specifically trained in the connection between physical health, mental health, and behavior change. They work with medically sick patients to promote well-being and healthy living through psychotherapy. |
| Social worker | Master's degree in social work (MSW), or doctorate in social work (DSW or PhD)<br><br>Examples of licensure include: Licensed Clinical Social Worker (LCSW), Licensed Independent Social Worker (LICSW), and others | Social workers are trained to evaluate patient's mental health and provide psychotherapy. They are also specifically trained in case management and advocacy services. |

*(continued)*

with comorbid psychiatric symptoms and those without psychiatric distress who possess concerning disease-modifying behaviors (eg, smoking, obesity, poor adherence, excessive stress).[74,76]

Trials of CBT[77] including those adapted specifically for adolescent populations[78-80] show particular promise. CBTs have shown effectiveness among patients with IBD in ameliorating symptoms of depression, and improving QOL in adolescents, including those with active disease. Both CBTs and supportive psychotherapy may actually be associated with reduced IBD activity.[80] Online CBT delivery can be an acceptable model for adults with IBD,[81] and CBT via self-guided books have been shown to reduce depression and anxiety.[82]

Among patients who do not possess psychiatric symptoms or are not interested in traditional psychotherapy, experts recommend behavioral or self-management therapies, which are informed by CBTs but lack the cognitive component of traditional CBTs (examining maladaptive thinking patterns). Rather, such therapy focuses specifically on targeting negative health behaviors that

## Table 4-3 (continued). Mental Health Professionals Who May Deliver Brain-Gut Psychotherapies and Serve as Therapists for Patients With Mental Illness

| MENTAL HEALTH PROVIDER | DEGREE/LICENSURE | DESCRIPTION |
|---|---|---|
| Psychiatric/mental health nurse practitioner (NP) | Master of Science (MS) or Doctor of Philosophy (PhD) in nursing, with specialized focus in psychiatry<br><br>NPs are licensed nurses in states where they practice | Psychiatric or mental health NPs can assess, diagnose, and provide psychotherapy for patients with mental health conditions. In some states, they may prescribe and monitor medications. They typically work under the direct supervision of a psychiatrist. |
| Physician assistant (PA) | PAs are licensed by licensure boards in the state where they practice | Psychiatric PAs practice psychiatry in collaboration with a psychiatrist. They diagnose and treat mental health disorders, provide psychotherapy, and may prescribe medications. |
| Licensed professional counselor | Master's degree (MS or MA) in mental health-related field such as psychology, counseling psychology, or others<br><br>Licensure varies by state | Licensed Professionals Counselors are master's-level professionals trained to evaluate mental health and administer psychotherapy. |

"Therapist" is a general term for a provider who helps patients better cope with thoughts, feelings, and behaviors; depending on the type of provider, they may or may not be able to assess and diagnose mental illness, or provide medications to treat mental illness. Depending on state or region, professional roles and specialties may vary.

contribute to poor disease management, including medication non-adherence, poor diet, and others. Such therapies have shown evidence for improvement in disease outcomes and QOL.[76,83]

### Hypnotherapy

Gut-directed hypnotherapy is a type of medical hypnosis that delivers post-hypnotic suggestions specifically tailored to symptoms of the gastrointestinal tract. The treatment course typically involves 7 to 12 weekly sessions in which patients progress from learning to achieve and deepen a hypnotic state, to being led through gut-focused imagery with hypnotic suggestions. Patients often practice these exercises at home using audio recordings, and self-monitor progress and symptoms.[74]

Hypnotherapy has been shown to have a more positive impact on disease severity than psychiatric symptoms or QOL. Studies in patients with UC reveal hypnotherapy has led to reductions in rectal mucosal inflammatory responses in just one session.[84] With 7 sessions, UC patients randomized to hypnotherapy demonstrates prolonged clinical remission of ~2.5 months longer than controls.[85] One study with a 5-year follow-up shows that 27% of patients with IBD who received 12 sessions of hypnotherapy maintained remission for the entire follow-up period and 60% required no corticosteroid therapy in the follow-up period.[86] Gut-directed hypnotherapy has also been found to be highly efficacious in patients with IBS, including refractory IBS[87,88] and thus, such a treatment might be ideal for patients with IBD who have IBS overlap.[89]

## Mindfulness-Based Therapy

Mindfulness-based therapy (MBT), primarily based in the mindfulness-based stress reduction,[90] uses formal exercises in meditation and deliberate breathing to help patients purposefully pay attention to the present moment. Patients are taught to practice observing details about their surroundings without passing judgment or reacting to environmental triggers.[74] The goal of MBT is to help patients cultivate non-judgmental awareness in their daily activities.

Such therapies are effective for a wide range of psychiatric and medical diagnoses.[91,92] In both CD and UC and with both active and inactive disease, mindfulness has led to significant improvements in anxiety, QOL, and depression compared with a waitlist control.[93] Mindfulness might also be protective for patients enduring disease flare.[94] Mindfulness has great evidence specifically in female patients with IBS to decrease hypervigilance to visceral sensations, decrease catastrophizing in active IBS symptoms, and leading to improvement in overall QOL.[95] Thus, while the evidence for MBT is sparser than that of CBT and hypnosis in patients with IBS, such a therapy shows promise for women with IBD and IBS overlap and warrants further study.

# Medications

Antidepressants are now considered *central neuromodulators*, as their effects exceed simply treating psychiatric disorders. While antidepressants have been established in treating comorbid anxiety, depression, pain, and impaired sleep associated with chronic gastrointestinal conditions, recent evidence is emerging for off-label treatment of gastrointestinal symptoms in IBD and disorders of gut-brain interaction.[96] It is believed that these medications work on gut motility and sensation via modulation of serotonin, norepinephrine, and corticotropin releasing factor,[97] have an analgesic effect[98] by modulating efferent and afferent signals between the brain and gut[99,100] and have a role in neurogenesis.[100,101] Three classes of antidepressants are commonly used in disorders of gut-brain interaction and may be considered in IBD: tricyclic antidepressants (TCAs), selective serotonin reuptake inhibitors (SSRIs), and serotonin-norepinephrine reuptake inhibitors (SNRIs).[96]

TCAs (amitriptyline, imipramine), which inhibit serotonin and norepinephrine reuptake in the synaptic cleft, even at low "non-psychiatric doses," have been shown to reduce pain and rectal hypersensitivity, increase appetite and weight gain, and are useful in patients with early satiation and weight loss.[96] Anticholinergic side effects including dry mouth, drowsiness, insomnia, agitation, orthostatic hypotension, arrythmias, and coma and seizure with overdose, warrant caution with patients with cardiac conditions or who may be at risk for overdose.

SSRIs (sertraline, fluoxetine, citalopram, escitalopram), which work by inhibiting serotonin uptake and dopamine reuptake, have less benefit with gastrointestinal pain compared with TCAs,[102] possibly because they do not act on norepinephrine.[96] However these drugs are firstline in treating anxiety and depression, may augment the analgesic effects of the TCAs, and have more favorable side effect profiles compared with the TCAs. Side effects that are particularly bothersome to patients include headache, sexual dysfunction, and insomnia.[96] While there are limited prospective studies on the use of SSRIs in IBD, one national Danish cohort study looking at SSRI use in IBD patients with comorbid depression found a decrease in relapse rates, steroid use, and number of endoscopies.[103] No positive randomized controlled trials have shown efficacy of SSRIs on clinical IBD symptoms to date.

SNRIs (venlafaxine, duloxetine), which inhibit serotonin and norepinephrine reuptake, are used for pain-related conditions with fewer side effects than the TCAs. They are associated with improvements in pain, slowing of gastrointestinal transit, and are useful in patients with diarrhea due to their anticholinergic effects. Side effects include dry mouth, palpitations, sweating, sleep disturbance, blurred vision, and increased diastolic blood pressure.[96] They also might be more activating for patients with anxiety due to their effects on norepinephrine reuptake. In one placebo-controlled study, duloxetine lowered anxiety and depression, improved QOL, and reduced clinical disease activity in 44 patients with IBD compared with placebo.[96,104]

While more evidence is certainly needed beyond the 3 randomized controlled trials to date looking at antidepressants in IBD, there is great promise for use of these medications in managing psychiatric comorbidities, comorbid functional gastrointestinal disorders like IBS, improving chronic pain and sleep quality, and reducing inflammation.[96] It is important for IBD providers to become familiar with a few reliable medications (eg, one SSRI/SNRI and one TCA) that they can administer to patients with depression and anxiety, either as a bridge to more robust mental health services, or if such services are not available.[3]

# A New Paradigm:
# Early, Effective Psychological Interventions

It is essential for gastroenterologists treating women with IBD to be well versed in the potential mental health concerns that may arise, to normalize the challenges that living with IBD may pose for patient's mental health, and to be well versed in how to optimally manage such cases early in disease course (eg, knowing when to prescribe medications, when to refer out to mental health providers in the community who can augment psychosocial care, social support services). Often, unless gastroenterologists provide strong, compelling recommendations for effective behavioral therapies for their patients with IBD, many patients suffering will go without treatment, or receive treatment only after psychological distress or a psychiatric condition becomes refractory. Given the significance of the impact of psychiatric comorbidities and psychological distress on disease outcomes, the goal of psychological interventions should primarily be about prevention, early identification, and harm reduction.

Additionally, mental health is not solely about the absence of psychopathology, but also the presence of positive psychological characteristics that improve one's mental state and QOL. Such characteristics include optimism, social support and positive relationships, spirituality, engagement in life, school and work, the cultivation of one's unique character strengths, among others.[105,106] These positive psychology (the study of why people thrive) constructs, which focus on outcomes such as resilience and subjective well-being, are currently underutilized in the gastroenterology setting, especially among patients with IBD.[105]

A shift toward integrating psychology and mental health resources into gastroenterology practices can and should facilitate access to early, effective psychological care, well before patients develop maladaptive coping habits, chronic stress, high physical and psychiatric symptom burden, and poor, costly disease outcomes.[106] Such integration will enable women with IBD to thrive and cultivate the human strengths and coping styles that will protect against the negative effects of living with a chronic gastrointestinal disease.

# KEY POINTS

1. Routinely assess patients for their health-related QOL, symptom-specific anxiety, and consider screening for depression, anxiety, and substance use disorders.

   - Use 1 to 2 open-ended questions to invite your patient to provide how IBD impacts physical symptoms. For example: "What areas of your life are affected most by IBD?" or "How do your symptoms interfere with your ability to do what you want to do in your everyday life?"

   - Consider administering the Patient Health Questionnaire-9 to screen for depression and the Patient-Reported Outcomes Measurement Information System-Anxiety scale, as these scales have been shown to have the highest sensitivity in capturing depression and anxiety in patients with IBD.

   - Once a mental illness is identified, a strong recommendation and referral from an IBD provider to seek mental health support can be extremely effective in getting patients the support they need.

2. Spend time with patients explaining in simple terms the bidirectional relationship among stress, depression, anxiety, and IBD (see Box 4-1). Attention to this topic has the potential to reduce stigma and increase buy-in for treatment, should it be warranted. It can also help contextualize for patients why a referral to a mental health provider in the community might be necessary to augment their care.

3. Identify and establish direct referral pathways and ongoing communication with a handful of highly qualified mental health providers in the community to whom you might refer patients with specific mental needs. Collaborate with these providers to optimally care for your patients with comorbid IBD and mental illness. Additionally, familiarize yourself with 1 to 2 antidepressants (1 SSRI/SNRI, 1 TCA) that you are comfortable prescribing for patients who suffer from depression and/or anxiety as a bridge to mental health services, or if these services are unavailable.

## BOX 4-1. LANGUAGE TO USE WHEN TALKING TO PATIENTS ABOUT THE BRAIN-GUT CONNECTION, AND HOW TO REFER TO MENTAL HEALTH SERVICES WHILE REDUCING STIGMA

1. Explaining the brain-gut connection to patients:

   • The relationship among IBD, depression, and anxiety is not completely understood, but we do know that patients with IBD are significantly more likely to experience depression, anxiety, and chronic stress compared to people without IBD. We also know that depression and anxiety are more likely to manifest when disease is active, and that stress can make disease activity worse. Experts in this area believe that there are many reasons for this. Firstly, depression and anxiety share several common pathways with IBD on a biological level that make these illnesses occur together. Secondly, people with IBD frequently have to modify their usual activities, avoid certain foods, and change up their routines because of their illness. This can lead to frustration, stress, and low mood. Additionally, when we feel anxious or acutely stressed out, our bodies put us into "fight or flight" mode, which redirects blood flow that would normally go to our intestines, toward our heart, lungs, and extremities to prepare us to run away. Fight or flight responses were very helpful throughout our evolution when we had to run away from life-threatening danger in order to survive, but today, especially in patients with IBD whose intestines are already very sensitive, this alteration in blood flow can lead to us feeling symptoms like diarrhea, nausea, and vomiting. Do you feel that any of these experiences might apply to you and your experience with IBD?

2. Encouraging patient referral to a mental health provider:

   • It seems to me that things have been particularly difficult for you lately. It is my job to ensure that in addition to getting your intestines and body well, we are taking care of your mind and whole self. Many patients with IBD who experience fatigue, depression, and/or anxiety benefit a great deal from short-term counseling or even medication to move forward in light of everything that is going on. It is very common, and I think you would be a great candidate. Would you like me to make a referral to someone who specializes in this? I'm happy to talk to you more about what this might look like and answer any questions you may have.

Adapted from Keefer L, Kane SV. Considering the bidirectional pathways between depression and IBD: recommendations for comprehensive IBD care. *Gastroenterol Hepatol (N Y)*. 2017;13(3):164-169.

# References

1. Mikocka-Walus A, Knowles SR, Keefer L, Graff L. Controversies revisited: a systematic review of the comorbidity of depression and anxiety with inflammatory bowel diseases. *Inflamm Bowel Dis*. 2016;22(3):752-762.

2. Panara AJ, Yarur AJ, Rieders B, et al. The incidence and risk factors for developing depression after being diagnosed with inflammatory bowel disease: a cohort study. *Aliment Pharmacol Ther*. 2014;39(8):802-810.

3. Keefer L, Palsson OS, Pandolfino JE. Best practice update: incorporating psychogastroenterology into management of digestive disorders. *Gastroenterology*. 2018;154(5):1249-1257.

4. Reusch A, Weiland R, Gerlich C, et al. Self-management education for rehabilitation inpatients suffering from inflammatory bowel disease: a cluster-randomized controlled trial. *Health Educ Res*. 2016;31(6):782-791.

5. Keefer L, Kane SV. Considering the bidirectional pathways between depression and IBD: recommendations for comprehensive IBD care. *Gastroenterol Hepatol (N Y)*. 2017;13(3):164-169.

6. Click B, Ramos Rivers C, Koutroubakis IE, et al. Demographic and clinical predictors of high healthcare use in patients with inflammatory bowel disease. *Inflamm Bowel Dis*. 2016;22(6):1442-1449.

7. Regueiro MD, McAnallen SE, Greer JB, Perkins SE, Ramalingam S, Szigethy E. The inflammatory bowel disease specialty medical home: a new model of patient-centered care. *Inflamm Bowel Dis*. 2016;22(8):1971-1980.

8. Piccinelli M, Wilkinson G. Gender differences in depression. Critical review. *Br J Psychiatry*. 2000;177:486-492.

9. Bekker MH, van Mens-Verhulst J. Anxiety disorders: sex differences in prevalence, degree, and background, but gender-neutral treatment. *Gend Med*. 2007;4 (Suppl B):S178-193.

10. Mittermaier C, Dejaco C, Waldhoer T, et al. Impact of depressive mood on relapse in patients with inflammatory bowel disease: a prospective 18-month follow-up study. *Psychosom Med*. 2004;66(1):79-84.

11. van Langenberg DR, Lange K, Hetzel DJ, Holtmann GJ, Andrews JM. Adverse clinical phenotype in inflammatory bowel disease: a cross sectional study identifying factors potentially amenable to change. *J Gastroenterol Hepatol*. 2010;25(7):1250-1258.

12. Nigro G, Angelini G, Grosso SB, Caula G, Sategna-Guidetti C. Psychiatric predictors of noncompliance in inflammatory bowel disease: psychiatry and compliance. *J Clin Gastroenterol*. 2001;32(1):66-68.

13. Wren AA, Bensen R, Sceats L, et al. Starting young: trends in opioid therapy among US adolescents and young adults with inflammatory bowel disease in the Truven MarketScan database between 2007 and 2015. *Inflamm Bowel Dis*. 2018;24(10):2093-2103.

14. American Psychiatric Association. *Diagnostic and Statistical Manual of Mental Disorders 5th ed*; 2013.

15. Trachter AB, Rogers AI, Leiblum SR. Inflammatory bowel disease in women: impact on relationship and sexual health. *Inflamm Bowel Dis*. 2002;8(6):413-421.

16. Fuller-Thomson E, Lateef R, Sulman J. Robust association between inflammatory bowel disease and generalized anxiety disorder: findings from a nationally representative Canadian study. *Inflamm Bowel Dis*. 2015;21(10):2341-2348.

17. Allegretti JR, Borges L, Lucci M, et al. Risk factors for rehospitalization within 90 days in patients with inflammatory bowel disease. *Inflamm Bowel Dis*. 2015;21(11):2583-2589.

18. Ananthakrishnan AN, Gainer VS, Perez RG, et al. Psychiatric co-morbidity is associated with increased risk of surgery in Crohn's disease. *Aliment Pharmacol Ther*. 2013;37(4):445-454.

19. Katon WJ, Lin EH, Von Korff M, et al. Collaborative care for patients with depression and chronic illnesses. *N Engl J Med*. 2010;363(27):2611-2620.

20. Martin-Subero M, Anderson G, Kanchanatawan B, Berk M, Maes M. Comorbidity between depression and inflammatory bowel disease explained by immune-inflammatory, oxidative, and nitrosative stress; tryptophan catabolite; and gut-brain pathways. *CNS Spectr*. 2016;21(2):184-198.

21. Vigod SN, Kurdyak P, Brown HK, et al. Inflammatory bowel disease and new-onset psychiatric disorders in pregnancy and post partum: a population-based cohort study. *Gut*. 2019;68(9):1597-1605.

22. van der Have M, Fidder HH, Leenders M, et al. Self-reported disability in patients with inflammatory bowel disease largely determined by disease activity and illness perceptions. *Inflamm Bowel Dis*. 2015;21(2):369-377.

23. McDermott E, Mullen G, Moloney J, et al. Body image dissatisfaction: clinical features, and psychosocial disability in inflammatory bowel disease. *Inflamm Bowel Dis*. 2015;21(2):353-360.

24. Trivedi MH, Lin EH, Katon WJ. Consensus recommendations for improving adherence, self-management, and outcomes in patients with depression. *CNS Spectr*. 2007;12(8 Suppl 13):1-27.

25. Martin-Subero M, Anderson G, Kanchanatawan B, Berk M, Maes M. Comorbidity between depression and inflammatory bowel disease explained by immune-inflammatory, oxidative, and nitrosative stress; tryptophan catabolite; and gut–brain pathways. *CNS Spectrums*. 2016;21(2):184-198.

26. O'Brien SM, Scott LV, Dinan TG. Antidepressant therapy and C-reactive protein levels. *Br J Psychiatry*. 2006;188:449-452.

27. Liukkonen T, Silvennoinen-Kassinen S, Jokelainen J, et al. The association between C-reactive protein levels and depression: results from the northern Finland 1966 birth cohort study. *Biol Psychiatry*. 2006;60(8):825-830.

28. Ananthakrishnan AN, Khalili H, Pan A, et al. Association between depressive symptoms and incidence of Crohn's disease and ulcerative colitis: results from the Nurses' Health Study. *Clin Gastroenterol Hepatol.* 2013;11(1):57-62.

29. Mikocka-Walus A, Pittet V, Rossel JB, von Kanel R, Swiss IBDCSG. Symptoms of depression and anxiety are independently associated with clinical recurrence of inflammatory bowel disease. *Clin Gastroenterol Hepatol.* 2016;14(6):829-835.e1

30. Gray MA, Chao CY, Staudacher HM, Kolosky NA, Talley NJ, Holtmann G. Anti-TNFalpha therapy in IBD alters brain activity reflecting visceral sensory function and cognitive-affective biases. *PLoS One.* 2018;13(3):e0193542.

31. Persoons P, Vermeire S, Demyttenaere K, et al. The impact of major depressive disorder on the short- and long-term outcome of Crohn's disease treatment with infliximab. *Aliment Pharmacol Ther.* 2005;22(2):101-110.

32. Lichtenstein GR, Bala M, Han C, DeWoody K, Schaible T. Infliximab improves quality of life in patients with Crohn's disease. *Inflamm Bowel Dis.* 2002;8(4):237-243.

33. Ciriaco M, Ventrice P, Russo G, et al. Corticosteroid-related central nervous system side effects. *J Pharmacol Pharmacother.* 2013;4(Suppl 1):S94-98.

34. Bannaga AS, Selinger CP. Inflammatory bowel disease and anxiety: links, risks, and challenges faced. *Clin Exp Gastroenterol.* 2015;8:111-117.

35. Organization WH. The ICD-10 classification of mental and behavioural disorders: clinical descriptions and diagnostic guidelines. World Health Organization. https://apps.who.int/iris/handle/10665/37958.

36. Labus JS, Bolus R, Chang L, et al. The Visceral Sensitivity Index: development and validation of a gastrointestinal symptom-specific anxiety scale. *Aliment Pharmacol Ther.* 2004;20(1):89-97.

37. Jerndal P, Ringstrom G, Agerforz P, et al. Gastrointestinal-specific anxiety: an important factor for severity of GI symptoms and quality of life in IBS. *Neurogastroenterol Motil.* 2010;22(6):646-e179.

38. Drossman DA, Leserman J, Li ZM, Mitchell CM, Zagami EA, Patrick DL. The rating form of IBD patient concerns: a new measure of health status. *Psychosom Med.* 1991;53(6):701-712.

39. Bennebroek Evertsz F, Thijssens NA, Stokkers PC, et al. Do inflammatory bowel disease patients with anxiety and depressive symptoms receive the care they need? *J Crohns Colitis.* 2012;6(1):68-76.

40. Goodhand JR, Wahed M, Mawdsley JE, Farmer AD, Aziz Q, Rampton DS. Mood disorders in inflammatory bowel disease: relation to diagnosis, disease activity, perceived stress, and other factors. *Inflamm Bowel Dis.* 2012;18(12):2301-2309.

41. Magalhaes J, Castro FD, Carvalho PB, Moreira MJ, Cotter J. Quality of life in patients with inflammatory bowel disease: importance of clinical, demographic and psychosocial factors. *Arq Gastroenterol.* 2014;51(3):192-197.

42. Nahon S, Lahmek P, Durance C, et al. Risk factors of anxiety and depression in inflammatory bowel disease. *Inflamm Bowel Dis.* 2012;18(11):2086-2091.

43. Kim ES, Cho KB, Park KS, et al. Predictive factors of impaired quality of life in Korean patients with inactive inflammatory bowel disease: association with functional gastrointestinal disorders and mood disorders. *J Clin Gastroenterol.* 2013;47(4):e38-44.

44. Ananthakrishnan AN, Gainer VS, Cai T, et al. Similar risk of depression and anxiety following surgery or hospitalization for Crohn's disease and ulcerative colitis. *Am J Gastroenterol.* 2013;108(4):594-601.

45. Walker EA, Roy-Byrne PP, Katon WJ, Li L, Amos D, Jiranek G. Psychiatric illness and irritable bowel syndrome: a comparison with inflammatory bowel disease. *Am J Psychiatry.* 1990;147(12):1656-1661.

46. Levenstein S, Prantera C, Varvo V, et al. Stress and exacerbation in ulcerative colitis: a prospective study of patients enrolled in remission. *Am J Gastroenterol.* 2000;95(5):1213-1220.

47. Bitton A, Dobkin PL, Edwardes MD, et al. Predicting relapse in Crohn's disease: a biopsychosocial model. *Gut.* 2008;57(10):1386-1392.

48. Mawdsley JE, Rampton DS. Psychological stress in IBD: new insights into pathogenic and therapeutic implications. *Gut.* 2005;54(10):1481-1491.

49. Filipovic BR, Filipovic BF. Psychiatric comorbidity in the treatment of patients with inflammatory bowel disease. *World J Gastroenterol.* 2014;20(13):3552-3563.

50. Labanski A, Langhorst J, Engler H, Elsenbruch S. Stress and the brain-gut axis in functional and chronic-inflammatory gastrointestinal diseases: a transdisciplinary challenge. *Psychoneuroendocrinology.* 2020;111:104501.

51. Farhadi A, Keshavarzian A, Van de Kar LD, et al. Heightened responses to stressors in patients with inflammatory bowel disease. *Am J Gastroenterol.* 2005;100(8):1796-1804.

52. Singh S, Graff LA, Bernstein CN. Do NSAIDs, antibiotics, infections, or stress trigger flares in IBD? *Am J Gastroenterol.* 2009;104(5):1298-1313; quiz 1314.

53. Levenstein S, Prantera C, Varvo V, et al. Psychological stress and disease activity in ulcerative colitis: a multidimensional cross-sectional study. *Am J Gastroenterol.* 1994;89(8):1219-1225.

54. Gracie DJ, Guthrie EA, Hamlin PJ, Ford AC. Bi-directionality of brain-gut interactions in patients with inflammatory bowel disease. *Gastroenterology.* 2018;154(6):1635-1646 e1633.

55. Elsenbruch S, Enck P. The stress concept in gastroenterology: from Selye to today. *F1000Res.* 2017;6:2149.

56. Gracie DJ, Williams CJM, Sood R, et al. Poor correlation between clinical disease activity and mucosal inflammation, and the role of psychological comorbidity, in inflammatory bowel disease. *Am J Gastroenterol.* 2016;111(4):541-551.

57. Gracie DJ, Ford AC. Psychological comorbidity and inflammatory bowel disease activity: cause or effect? *Clin Gastroenterol Hepatol.* 2016;14(7):1061-1062.

58. Keefer L, Drossman DA, Guthrie E, et al. Centrally mediated disorders of gastrointestinal pain. *Gastroenterology.* 2016.

59. Buckley JP, Cook SF, Allen JK, Kappelman MD. Prevalence of chronic narcotic use among children with inflammatory bowel disease. *Clin Gastroenterol Hepatol.* 2015;13(2):310-315 e312.

60. Szigethy E, Knisely M, Drossman D. Opioid misuse in gastroenterology and non-opioid management of abdominal pain. *Nat Rev Gastroenterol Hepatol.* 2018;15(3):168-180.

61. Cross RK, Wilson KT, Binion DG. Narcotic use in patients with Crohn's disease. *Am J Gastroenterol.* 2005;100(10):2225-2229.

62. Long MD, Barnes EL, Herfarth HH, Drossman DA. Narcotic use for inflammatory bowel disease and risk factors during hospitalization. *Inflamm Bowel Dis.* 2012;18(5):869-876.

63. Hanson KA, Loftus EV, Jr., Harmsen WS, Diehl NN, Zinsmeister AR, Sandborn WJ. Clinical features and outcome of patients with inflammatory bowel disease who use narcotics: a case-control study. *Inflamm Bowel Dis.* 2009;15(5):772-777.

64. Targownik LE, Nugent Z, Singh H, Bugden S, Bernstein CN. The prevalence and predictors of opioid use in inflammatory bowel disease: a population-based analysis. *Am J Gastroenterol.* 2014;109(10):1613-1620.

65. Noureldin M, Higgins PDR, Govani SM, et al. Incidence and predictors of new persistent opioid use following inflammatory bowel disease flares treated with oral corticosteroids. *Aliment Pharmacol Ther.* 2019;49(1):74-83.

66. Lichtenstein GR, Feagan BG, Cohen RD, et al. Serious infections and mortality in association with therapies for Crohn's disease: TREAT registry. *Clin Gastroenterol Hepatol.* 2006;4(5):621-630.

67. Miech R, Johnston L, O'Malley PM, Keyes KM, Heard K. Prescription opioids in adolescence and future opioid misuse. *Pediatrics.* 2015;136(5):e1169-1177.

68. McCabe SE, West BT, Veliz P, McCabe VV, Stoddard SA, Boyd CJ. Trends in medical and nonmedical use of prescription opioids among US adolescents: 1976-2015. *Pediatrics.* 2017;139(4):e20162387.

69. Hauser W, Schmidt C, Stallmach A. Depression and mucosal proinflammatory cytokines are associated in patients with ulcerative colitis and pouchitis—a pilot study. *J Crohns Colitis.* 2011;5(4):350-353.

70. Brown HK, Qazilbash A, Rahim N, Dennis CL, Vigod SN. Chronic medical conditions and peripartum mental illness: a systematic review and meta-analysis. *Am J Epidemiol.* 2018;187(9):2060-2068.

71. Farraye FA, Melmed GY, Lichtenstein GR, Kane SV. ACG clinical guideline: preventive care in inflammatory bowel disease. *Am J Gastroenterol.* 2017;112(2):241-258.

72. Bernstein CN, Zhang L, Lix LM, et al. The validity and reliability of screening measures for depression and anxiety disorders in inflammatory bowel disease. *Inflamm Bowel Dis.* 2018;24(9):1867-1875.

73. Pilkonis PA, Choi SW, Reise SP, et al. Item banks for measuring emotional distress from the Patient-Reported Outcomes Measurement Information System (PROMIS(R)): depression, anxiety, and anger. *Assessment.* 2011;18(3):263-283.

74. Ballou S, Keefer L. Psychological interventions for irritable bowel syndrome and inflammatory bowel diseases. *Clin Transl Gastroenterol.* 2017;8(1):e214.

75. Kinsinger SW, Ballou S, Keefer L. Snapshot of an integrated psychosocial gastroenterology service. *World J Gastroenterol.* 2015;21(6):1893-1899.

76. Keefer L, Doerfler B, Artz C. Optimizing management of Crohn's disease within a project management framework: results of a pilot study. *Inflamm Bowel Dis.* 2012;18(2):254-260.

77. Knowles SR, Monshat K, Castle DJ. The efficacy and methodological challenges of psychotherapy for adults with inflammatory bowel disease: a review. *Inflamm Bowel Dis.* 2013;19(12):2704-2715.

78. Szigethy E, Kenney E, Carpenter J, et al. Cognitive-behavioral therapy for adolescents with inflammatory bowel disease and subsyndromal depression. *J Am Acad Child Adolesc Psychiatry.* 2007;46(10):1290-1298.

79. Szigethy E, Bujoreanu SI, Youk AO, et al. Randomized efficacy trial of two psychotherapies for depression in youth with inflammatory bowel disease. *J Am Acad Child Adolesc Psychiatry.* 2014;53(7):726-735.

80. Szigethy E, Youk AO, Gonzalez-Heydrich J, et al. Effect of 2 psychotherapies on depression and disease activity in pediatric Crohn's disease. *Inflamm Bowel Dis.* 2015;21(6):1321-1328.

81. McCombie A, Gearry R, Mulder R. Preferences of inflammatory bowel disease patients for computerised versus face-to-face psychological interventions. *J Crohns Colitis.* 2014;8(6):536-542.

82. Hunt MG, Loftus P, Accardo M, Keenan M, Cohen L, Osterman MT. Self-help cognitive behavioral therapy improves health-related quality of life for inflammatory bowel disease patients: a randomized controlled effectiveness trial. *J Clin Psychol Med Settings.* 2020;27(3):467-479.

83. Hommel KA, Herzer M, Ingerski LM, Hente E, Denson LA. Individually tailored treatment of medication nonadherence. *J Pediatr Gastroenterol Nutr.* 2011;53(4):435-439.

84. Mawdsley JE, Jenkins DG, Macey MG, Langmead L, Rampton DS. The effect of hypnosis on systemic and rectal mucosal measures of inflammation in ulcerative colitis. *Am J Gastroenterol.* 2008;103(6):1460-1469.

85. Keefer L, Taft TH, Kiebles JL, Martinovich Z, Barrett TA, Palsson OS. Gut-directed hypnotherapy significantly augments clinical remission in quiescent ulcerative colitis. *Aliment Pharmacol Ther.* 2013;38(7):761-771.

86. Miller V, Whorwell PJ. Treatment of inflammatory bowel disease: a role for hypnotherapy? *Int J Clin Exp Hypn.* 2008;56(3):306-317.

87. Gholamrezaei A, Ardestani SK, Emami MH. Where does hypnotherapy stand in the management of irritable bowel syndrome? A systematic review. *J Altern Complement Med.* 2006;12(6):517-527.

88. Palsson OS. Hypnosis treatment of gastrointestinal disorders: a comprehensive review of the empirical evidence. *Am J Clin Hypn.* 2015;58(2):134-158.

89. Szigethy E. Hypnotherapy for inflammatory bowel disease across the lifespan. *Am J Clin Hypn.* 2015;58(1):81-99.

90. Kabat-Zinn J. *Full Catastrophe Living: Using the wisdom of your body and mind to face stress, pain, and illness.* Bantam Doubleday Dell Publishing; 1990.

91. Lakhan SE, Schofield KL. Mindfulness-based therapies in the treatment of somatization disorders: a systematic review and meta-analysis. *PLoS One.* 2013;8(8):e71834.

92. Chiesa A, Serretti A. Mindfulness based cognitive therapy for psychiatric disorders: a systematic review and meta-analysis. *Psychiatry Res.* 2011;187(3):441-453.

93. Neilson K, Ftanou M, Monshat K, et al. A controlled study of a group mindfulness intervention for individuals living with inflammatory bowel disease. *Inflamm Bowel Dis.* 2016;22(3):694-701.

94. Jedel S, Hoffman A, Merriman P, et al. A randomized controlled trial of mindfulness-based stress reduction to prevent flare-up in patients with inactive ulcerative colitis. *Digestion.* 2014;89(2):142-155.

95. Gaylord SA, Palsson OS, Garland EL, et al. Mindfulness training reduces the severity of irritable bowel syndrome in women: results of a randomized controlled trial. *Am J Gastroenterol.* 2011;106(9):1678-1688.

96. Mikocka-Walus A, Ford AC, Drossman DA. Antidepressants in inflammatory bowel disease. *Nat Rev Gastroenterol Hepatol.* 2020;17(3):184-192.

97. Gershon MD, Tack J. The serotonin signaling system: from basic understanding to drug development for functional GI disorders. *Gastroenterology.* 2007;132(1):397-414.

98. Tracey I, Mantyh PW. The cerebral signature for pain perception and its modulation. *Neuron.* 2007;55(3):377-391.

99. Drossman DA. Beyond tricyclics: new ideas for treating patients with painful and refractory functional gastrointestinal symptoms. *Am J Gastroenterol.* 2009;104(12):2897-2902.

100. Morgan V, Pickens D, Gautam S, Kessler R, Mertz H. Amitriptyline reduces rectal pain related activation of the anterior cingulate cortex in patients with irritable bowel syndrome. *Gut.* 2005;54(5):601-607.

101. Perera TD, Park S, Nemirovskaya Y. Cognitive role of neurogenesis in depression and antidepressant treatment. *Neuroscientist.* 2008;14(4):326-338.

102. Bomholt SF, Mikkelsen JD, Blackburn-Munro G. Antinociceptive effects of the antidepressants amitriptyline, duloxetine, mirtazapine and citalopram in animal models of acute, persistent and neuropathic pain. *Neuropharmacology.* 2005;48(2):252-263.

103. Kristensen MS, Kjærulff TM, Ersbøll AK, Green A, Hallas J, Thygesen LC. The influence of antidepressants on the disease course among patients with Crohn's disease and ulcerative colitis-a Danish nationwide register-based cohort study. *Inflamm Bowel Dis.* 2019;25(5):886-893.

104. Daghaghzadeh H, Naji F, Afshar H, et al. Efficacy of duloxetine add on in treatment of inflammatory bowel disease patients: a double-blind controlled study. *J Res Med Sci.* 2015;20(6):595-601.

105. Feingold J, Murray HB, Keefer L. Recent advances in cognitive behavioral therapy for digestive disorders and the role of applied positive psychology across the spectrum of GI care. *J Clin Gastroenterol.* 2019;53(7):477-485.

106. Keefer L. Behavioural medicine and gastrointestinal disorders: the promise of positive psychology. *Nat Rev Gastroenterol Hepatol.* 2018;15(6):378-386.

# 5

# Medications and Alternative Treatments in Women With IBD

Emilie S. Kim, MD | Dana J. Lukin, MD, PhD | Ryan Warren, RD | Ellen J. Scherl, MD

## Introduction

This chapter is intended to underscore the challenge of personalized medicine in treating and diagnosing inflammatory bowel disease (IBD) in women. IBD is a chronic, lifelong, interrupting, and sapping illness characterized by recurrences and remissions.[1-4] Only around half of IBD patients are in clinical remission each year. Up to 60% of patients with IBD use complementary and alternative medicine to control both inflammatory and non-inflammatory symptoms.[5,6] The great variability among individuals defines medicine as both precision science and personalized art.[7] Remembering that personalizing medicine is ultimately about the person, it is helpful to use objective measures to define whether an individual's symptoms are related to active IBD or overlap with non-inflammatory, functional, obstructive, gynecologic, or nutritional symptoms.

# Inflammatory and Non-Inflammatory Symptoms in Women With IBD

The diagnosis of IBD activity should be confirmed to ensure appropriate treatment. Women with overlapping non-inflammatory symptoms may be overtreated for IBD rather than being evaluated for non-inflammatory symptoms.[8] Many of the symptoms of active bowel inflammation, including abdominal pain, bloating, diarrhea, nausea, vomiting, anorexia, rectal bleeding, weight loss, food intolerance, and body aches, may also be components of other gastrointestinal

Abraham BP, Kane SV, Glassner KL, eds.
*Women's Health in IBD: The Spectrum of Care
From Birth to Adulthood* (pp 83-113).
© 2022 Taylor & Francis Group.

disorders. The differential diagnosis for non-inflammatory conditions mimicking IBD is broad, including irritable bowel syndrome (IBS), hemorrhoids, bile salt diarrhea, small intestinal bacterial overgrowth,[9,10] overgrowth of methane-producing organisms,[11] gallbladder disease, maldigestion, and intestinal obstruction. Gynecologic disorders such as endometriosis, polycystic ovarian syndrome, vulvovaginal disorders,[12] pelvic floor dyssynergia, ovarian cancers, or tumors, in addition to celiac disease,[13] pancreatitis,[14-17] Hashimoto's thyroiditis, rheumatoid arthritis, and other arthridites should be included in the differential. Disordered eating, including the anorexia and bulimia spectrum, and laxative use may masquerade as IBD but also may confound the diagnosis of disease flares in women with confirmed diagnoses of IBD.[18,19] Diet-related symptoms also arise in patients experiencing fructose-, sucrose-, and lactose-malabsorption.[20-22] It is important to recognize the increased likelihood of non-inflammatory symptoms confounding IBD flares, and this underscores the need to elucidate the immunobiology of post-infectious gut dysfunction as well as ruling out intercurrent enteric infections.[8,23] Fecal calprotectin, C-reactive protein (CRP), and erythrocyte sedimentation rate may be increased in infectious enterides and active IBD but will distinguish between inflammatory and non-inflammatory symptoms.[24,25] The physician who understands IBD understands medicine. This chapter will discuss each of the entities described above within the context of the female patient with IBD.

# IBD Activity and Progression in Women

Women's disease activity may be linked to their menstrual cycle and pregnancy, as well as peri- and post-menopause. It is important to consider both disease activity and disease progression (disease activity over time) in the distinction of inflammatory and functional symptomatology. In a study of 1203 women, over half reported a worsening of symptoms during menses.[26] IBD has been associated with delayed menarche and a variety of menstrual irregularities, possibly related to cyclical variation in gastrointestinal microbiota.[27] Active IBD has been found to be associated with increased vulvovaginal discomfort, compared to women in remission.[12] IBD activity is frequently impacted by pregnancy and may in turn influence pregnancy outcomes, such as adverse perinatal events (Figure 5-1).[28-30] Preconception counseling may reduce disease relapse during pregnancy.[31] Early therapeutic intervention may reverse the natural history[18] of IBD, stricturing fistulizing Crohn's disease (CD), stricturing ulcerative colitis (UC), as well as long-term risks of dysplasia,[32,33] malignancy, and nutritional complication.

# Medication Overview

As with all patients with IBD, an essential goal of therapy in women with active IBD is the achievement of corticosteroid-free remission. While steroids are effective in the induction of remission, they are not safe or effective as maintenance agents (see Figure 5-1). Therefore, whenever steroid therapy is initiated, a plan for subsequent steroid-sparing therapy should be also developed. Optimizing dosage of aminosalicylates, immunomodulating drugs, and biologic medications may help achieve this goal of steroid-free remission (Table 5-1).[34] While the majority of therapeutic management of IBD is independent of gender, it is important to address the unique clinical considerations in treating a female patient.

Gender-related differences likely exist regarding attitude toward IBD medication. While adherence to medical treatment was generally not influenced by gender,[35] use and attitudes may differ by IBD drug due to concerns specific to women. Female CD patients have been identified to have higher Rating Form of IBD Patient Concerns scores than male patients, suggesting greater concerns about their disease and its management.[36] Therefore, it is important that the physician discuss potential concerns prior to treatment initiation to maximize confidence in treatment decisions and

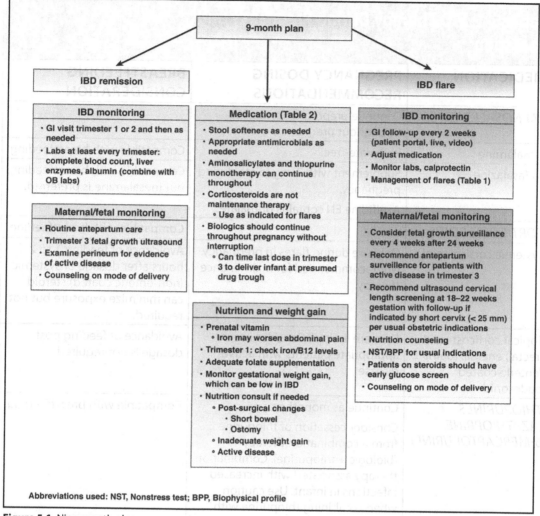

**Figure 5-1.** Nine-month plan.

to minimize possible medication non-adherence, whether intentional or non-intentional. This may be addressed with patient education, employment of motivational counseling, or simplification of therapeutic regimens used in treatment of women with IBD.[37,38] Such measures may improve adherence and help prevent and delay the need for therapeutic escalation, hospitalization, and surgery.[39] Shared decision making and patient engagement should address the use of early biologic intervention, surgical and medical therapy, as well as complementary and conventional strategies.[40]

## Effect of Iron Replacement Therapy and Menses on Women With IBD

Fatigue, both emotional and physical, among women living with IBD is underappreciated. In addition to anemia resulting from chronic gastrointestinal bleeding and malabsorption in IBD, women are at risk for anemia related to menstruation and associated fatigue. In the absence of active gastrointestinal inflammatory disease, women with menorrhagia may be responsive to oral iron preparations if tolerated. However, women with active IBD and iron deficiency anemia due to chronic blood loss or women with inactive IBD who do not tolerate oral iron therapy should be considered for intravenous (IV) iron preparations. Oral iron should be avoided in active IBD due to

## Table 5-1. IBD Therapy During Pregnancy and Lactation

| MEDICATION | PREGNANCY DOSING RECOMMENDATIONS | BREASTFEEDING CONSIDERATION |
|---|---|---|
| *AMINOSALICYLATES* | Continue prepregnancy dosing throughout pregnancy. | |
| Mesalamine | Phthalate-free. | Compatible with breastfeeding. |
| Sulfasalazine | Supplement with 2-mg folate during pregnancy. Azulfidine EN contains phthalate. | Compatible with breastfeeding, but mesalamine is preferred. |
| *CORTICOSTEROIDS* | | Compatible with breastfeeding. |
| Systemic corticosteroid | Only use during flares in pregnancy. Not recommended for maintenance therapy. | Avoidance of feeding 1 to 2 hours after dosage of systemic (non-enteric coated) steroid can minimize exposure but not required. |
| Topical corticosteroid (rectal, enema, foam) /enteric-coated budesonide | Data are limited. Consider use in appropriate patients with active disease. | Avoidance of feeding post dosage is not required. |
| *THIOPURINES (AZATHIOPRINE, 6-MERCAPTOPURINE)* | Continue as monotherapy. Consider cessation of thiopurine from a combination therapy (biologic + thiopurine). Combination therapy associated with increased infections in infant. Use caution when combining thiopurine with allopurinol, with possibility of toxic effects on embryo. | Compatible with breastfeeding. |
| *METHOTREXATE* | Contraindicated in pregnancy and medication must be terminated 3 months prior to conception. | Breastfeeding not advised. |
| *CYCLOSPORINE* | Only use as salvage therapy. Cyclosporine use is associated with hypertension, gestational diabetes, preterm birth, low birthweight/ small for gestational age. | Compatible with breastfeeding. Transfer of cyclosporine in breast milk is minimal. |
| *NOVEL SMALL MOLECULES: TOFACITINIB* | Limited human data. Not advised during pregnancy, especially in first trimester. | Limited human data. Not advised. |

*(continued)*

## Table 5-1 (continued). IBD Therapy During Pregnancy and Lactation

| MEDICATION | PREGNANCY DOSING RECOMMENDATIONS | BREASTFEEDING CONSIDERATION |
|---|---|---|
| *BIOLOGICS* | Continue prepregnancy dosing through all 3 trimesters of pregnancy. Plan administering final dose according to drug half-life so to minimize transfer. | All biologics are compatible with breastfeeding. |
| Adalizumab | Plan final injection 2 to 3 weeks before expected delivery date. Resume postpartum. | |
| Certolizumab pegol | Continue scheduled dosing throughout pregnancy. | |
| Golimumab | Plan final injection 4 to 6 weeks before expected delivery date. Resume postpartum. | |
| Infliximab | Plan final pregnancy infusion 6 to 10 weeks before expected delivery date. Resume postpartum. (If every-4-week dosing, then 4 to 5 weeks before expected delivery date. Resume postpartum.) Continue prepregnancy dosing through pregnancy. | |
| Ustekinumab | Plan final pregnancy dose 6 to 10 weeks before expected delivery date. Resume postpartum. (If every-4-week dosing, then 4 to 5 weeks before expected delivery date.) | |
| Natalizumab | Plan final pregnancy infusion 4 to 6 weeks before expected delivery date and resume postpartum. | |
| Vedolizumab | Plan final pregnancy dose 6 to 10 weeks before expected delivery date and resume postpartum. (If every-4-week dosing, then 4 to 5 weeks before expected delivery date.) | |

*(continued)*

## Table 5-1 (continued). IBD Therapy During Pregnancy and Lactation

| MEDICATION | PREGNANCY DOSING RECOMMENDATIONS | BREASTFEEDING CONSIDERATION |
|---|---|---|
| *ANTIBIOTICS* | Used only with perianal disease and pouchitis. Not recommended for planned maintenance therapy. | |
| Amoxicillin-clavulanate | Preferred antibiotic for use during pregnancy. No harm observed with first trimester use. | Compatible with breastfeeding. |
| Metronidazole | Preferred antibiotic for use during pregnancy. Can be used throughout all trimesters. | |
| Fluoroquinolones (ciprofloxacin) | Not recommended during pregnancy. Effects of fluoroquinolones on long-term bone and cartilage development of infant is unknown. | Preferred over metronidazole during breastfeeding. |
| Rifaximin | Avoid during pregnancy. Associated with teratogenicity. | Not compatible with breastfeeding. |

Adapted from Mahadevan U, Robinson C, Bernasko N, et al. Inflammatory bowel disease in pregnancy clinical care pathway: a report from the American Gastroenterological Association IBD Parenthood Project Working Group. *Gastroenterology.* 2019;156(5):1508-1524.

poor tolerability and impaired absorption. Women with inactive IBD may not tolerate oral iron due to constipation and IBS-like overlap symptoms frequently elicited by these preparations.[41]

## Effect of Hormonal Therapy on IBD

It is important to consider estrogen and progesterone in the life cycle of women living with IBD.[42-44] This will be further addressed in Chapters 7 and 10.

## Anticoagulation Prophylaxis

Risk of venous thromboembolism (VTE) is elevated in women with IBD. Therefore, in hospitalized patients who have active inflammation or patients receiving a caesarean section, anticoagulative prophylaxis and mechanical thromboprophylaxis should be considered, especially in the postpartum period for up to 3 to 6 weeks wherein the risk of VTE is high.[45-47] While the risk of VTE is higher among pregnant women in the general population, it is further increased 2-fold among women with IBD.[48] Tofacitinib has been implicated with increased VTE in rheumatoid arthritis at the 10 mg twice daily dosage[49]; therefore, patients with deep vein thrombosis and pulmonary embolism risks should be monitored. However, at this time such associations have not been observed in the UC population (where active inflammation poses its own significant risk of thrombosis) and we do not suggest that the patient stop oral contraceptives with progesterone due to tofacitinib use. Further phase IV studies are needed to determine the VTE risk pertaining to tofacitinib within the IBD population.

Some women with IBD are at increased risk for Budd-Chiari syndrome related to hormonal contraception and hypercoagulability due to active IBD.[50] A case study has suggested that the development of Budd-Chiari syndrome may be complicated by active disease flares in IBD patients.[50] This condition should also be considered in women with IBD.

# 5-Aminosalicylic Acid Medications/Mesalamine

5-aminosalicylic acid (5-ASA) and related aminosalicylate medications include sulfasalazine, mesalamine, olsalazine, and balsalazide. All 5-ASA drugs work through the common active metabolite, N-acetyl-5-aminosalicylate. There are no significant gender-related differences regarding the use of 5-ASA medication. Female patients may be managed with 5-ASA drugs in alignment with evidence-based clinical practice guidelines for treatment and maintenance of remission of all adult IBD patients. However, while all patients receiving sulfasalazine should be supplemented with 1 mg of folic acid as folate absorption is impaired by this medication, female IBD patients on sulfasalazine planning for pregnancy should be increased from 1 mg to 2 mg prior to conception[51,52] and throughout all 3 trimesters of pregnancy to promote healthy neural development of the fetus (see Figure 5-1). Mesalamine is deemed safe in women of all ages. In women, topical 5-ASA preparations such as suppositories, foams, and enemas are well tolerated throughout a woman's life, including pregnancy (see Table 5-1).[53] Two studies examining 5-ASA medications found no significant gender-related treatment outcomes.[54,55] However, non-adherence to 5-ASA therapy has been found to be more likely in male UC patients than female patients ($P < .05$).[56]

# Corticosteroids

Corticosteroids are powerful anti-inflammatory medications that work in part by counteracting the abnormal activation of the immune system and are frequently used as short-term treatment for IBD. Due to the lack of data demonstrating a long-term benefit as a maintenance therapy as well as the well-established risks associated with long-term use of corticosteroids, these agents should be used only during induction therapy with a focus on the use of steroid-sparing therapies (see Figure 5-1). Complications associated with systemic corticosteroids are numerous and include risk of bone loss due to bone remodeling and Cushing's syndrome. Though these conditions are not limited to female IBD patients, steroid-related adverse effects may have specific implications in women (see Table 5-1).

Women are especially vulnerable to osteopenia and osteoporosis as they age, and steroids increase this risk significantly.[57,58] While systemically acting steroids are associated with a risk of osteoporosis and a greater fracture risk, in a case-control study[59] and a separate multicenter randomized trial[60] of 272 patients, locally acting steroids like budesonide were found to have a lesser risk of osteoporosis than conventional steroids.[57,59] To avoid risk of bone fracture, it is important to assess bone density frequently, and administer calcium and vitamin D, as well as bisphosphonates to at-risk women treated with steroids, as indicated. Additionally, as catabolic steroids may promote the breakdown of both bone and muscle, physical therapy may be required to compensate for these losses, especially among women requiring prolonged steroid courses.

Metabolic changes due to use of corticosteroids may manifest as Cushingoid features in IBD patients. In women, such metabolic changes result in weight gain, stretch marks, hirsutism, moon facies, hair loss, and fat deposition on the back. A poor body image, associated with these changes, may contribute to the psychosocial concerns of female patients. These body image disturbances may possibly affect the disordered eating practices that occur frequently in IBD populations,[19,61,62] which are especially relevant in women, as positive screens for maladaptive eating have been associated with females with IBD.[63] Additionally, in patients undergoing prolonged steroid therapy, it is important to monitor blood sugar and vision, and minimize intake of sugar and salt. Addisonian crisis should be recognized in women after steroid withdrawal following long-term use, including with budesonide. This risk may be minimized by using a supervised steroid taper, but if arises may require administration of IV fluids and dexamethasone or hydrocortisone.[64]

Steroid use is associated with psychological side effects and emotional lability, including the potential for suicidality.[65] Women need to be aware of the potential for these events and a monitoring plan for support from family, friends, and/or mental health providers should be considered for at-risk patients. Providers may advise anger and stress management techniques, as well as outlets for stress such as yoga, adjunctive medication, and regular routine exercise.[65]

# Immunomodulators

## Azathioprine/Mercaptopurine

Azathioprine (AZA) and mercaptopurine (often referred to as "6"-mercaptopurine; MP) are thiopurine antimetabolite immunomodulators. The strategies for administration and management of disease with thiopurines for female patients follow the guidelines set for all patients with IBD (see Figure 5-1). A specific concern in use of thiopurines in women relates to a possible link with human papillomavirus-associated cervical dysplasia, although results of studies have been inconsistent. While some studies have observed a positive association of thiopurine use with risk of cervical cancer,[66,67] others have found that AZA and 6-MP, as well as corticosteroids, do not significantly contribute to abnormal cervical Papanicolou smear results.[68-70] Despite these inconclusive results, cervical cancer surveillance and vaccination of at-risk adolescents and adults is recommended as outlined in Chapter 6 and 1, respectively.

A recent prospective cohort study based on the SAPPHIRE registry analyzed the risk of immunosuppressant use on subsequent cancers in patients who have histories of solid, gastrointestinal, dermatologic, or hematologic malignancies.[71] This study identified no increase in risk of a new or recurrent malignancy in patients with IBD who have received immunomodulator monotherapy after a prior cancer diagnosis, compared to patients not exposed to immunosuppressants (risk ratio 4.94, 95% confidence interval [CI] 0.50 to 48.6).[71] However, there was an increased risk of new or recurrent cancers among patients receiving thiopurines in combination with tumor necrosis factor (TNF) antagonists. A retrospective study of 333 patients in 8 academic medical centers showed similar results, wherein treatment with antimetabolites (thiopurines and methotrexate) in patients with IBD with histories of cancer was not associated with increased risk of incident cancer.[72] Such data could guide us in consideration of thiopurine therapy in female patients having a history of cancer; however, long-term prospective studies are warranted for a more robust analysis of the safety of these drugs within this population.

Gender difference in adherence to AZA and MP were studied in a cohort of 112 IBD patients in Portugal. In the self-administered questionnaire, male patients had higher nonadherence than female patients (odds ratio [OR] 3.79, 95% CI 1.2 to 11.95, $P = .023$).[38] Although adherence was improved in women, overall nonadherence to immunomodulator therapy for all patients was extremely high (70.5%) and there were no differences in adherence to immunomodulator as monotherapy vs dual immunomodulator-biologic therapy. Other studies also saw greater non-adherence of thiopurines in male patients.[73] Younger age and depression have been identified as independent predictors of nonadherence to thiopurines in several studies.[38,39] Thus, physicians should emphasize patient education in younger women (ie, patients transferring from pediatric to adult care)[39] and be aware of psychosocial needs to optimize adherence to immunomodulators.

## Methotrexate

Methotrexate is a folate antagonist and a well-established teratogenic and abortifacient agent (see Table 5-1). While it is an effective therapy for CD and in combination with biologic agents, use in women of childbearing age should be carefully considered on an individualized basis for those patients with moderate to severe and refractory IBD. Women within this age group should be counseled to use effective methods of contraception and to stop therapy with methotrexate 3 to 6 months before trying to conceive (see Table 5-1).[74]

### Cyclosporine

Cyclosporine may be used in women with UC as a steroid-refractory rescue therapy. It should not be used for long-term maintenance therapy for women, especially during pregnancy (see Table 5-1).[75] However, given the risk of severe disease during pregnancy among higher risk patients who have severe disease and/or prior exposure to multiple IBD medications, cyclosporine may be considered during pregnancy as a salvage therapy for steroid-refractory acute severe UC (see Table 5-1).[52] Currently, cyclosporine use is extremely limited given the availability of newer therapies.

## Novel Small Molecules: Tofacitinib, Filgotinib, Upadacitinib

Tofacitinib is a novel small molecule used to treat UC. It is a pan-Janus kinase (JAK) inhibitor used in moderate to severe UC. Gender differences pertaining to tofacitinib therapy have not been identified within the UC population, although the possibility for as yet unknown adverse events exists given the relatively short time since its US Food and Drug Administration approval. In the rheumatoid arthritis literature, a post-marketing study showed that tofacitinib may be associated with thromboembolic events, with pulmonary embolism more frequently observed in patients on higher dosages.[76] In a post-hoc analysis of 1157 UC patients with tofacitinib exposure, 5 patients but all with other VTE risk factors had thromboembolic events.[77] Further investigations are necessary to determine the link between VTE and tofacitinib use. While much of the VTE risk in IBD stems from active inflammation, other risks include comorbid hypercoagulable states, concomitant corticosteroid use, and estrogen containing oral contraceptive pill. Women with these risk factors should be aware of tofacitinib's potential role in thromboembolism and caution must be used when considering its use.

Filgotinib is a JAK1-selective inhibitor. In the FITZROY study, filgotinib was found to have increased induction of clinical remission compared to placebo for moderate to severe CD patients.[78,79]

Upadacitinib is a selective JAK inhibitor that may treat moderate to severe CD and UC, especially in patients with disease refractory to TNF-alpha (TNF-α) inhibitors. In a double-blind placebo-controlled study, induction treatment with upadacitinib in UC has shown significant improvement in mucosal healing compared to placebo when observed endoscopically and histologically.[80] A CD study showed statistically significant steroid-free endoscopic and clinical improvements in patients taking upadacitinib.[81]

## Tumor Necrosis Factor–Alpha Antagonists

TNF-α is a cytokine involved in systemic inflammation that is produced by lymphocytes. TNF-α antagonists are monoclonal antibodies that mainly function by neutralizing TNF and inhibiting pro-inflammatory downstream signaling pathways in patients with IBD. Agents within this class include the IV infliximab (CD and UC) and subcutaneous adalimumab (CD and UC), certolizumab pegol (CD), and golimumab (UC). These agents are approved for moderate to severe IBD refractory to conservative therapies including corticosteroids. These agents appear to be most effective in women with objective signs of inflammation such as elevated biologic markers or endoscopically visible inflammatory lesions.[82]

TNF-α inhibitors show differences in pharmacokinetics and efficacy between sexes. Despite weight-based dosing of infliximab, a study found the volume of distribution of the central compartment, consisting of plasma and tissues where there is rapid drug distribution, was higher in male patients and those with increased weight.[83] However, in patients with low body weight, the weight-based dosing for infliximab became non-linear with patients less than 40 kg being more likely to have low infliximab troughs.[84] Therefore, patients with low body mass index may benefit from increased or individualized infliximab dosing,[84] such as women with severe weight loss due to malnutrition or eating disorders, and those with low albumin. A personalized approach focusing on appropriate dose and infusion intervals guided by serum levels of infliximab and anti-drug antibodies should be considered.[85]

Next, the use and discontinuation of anti-TNF-α therapy may differ between the sexes. In a multicenter retrospective study of 349 IBD patients receiving TNF-α inhibitors (155 female), women were found to have a significantly higher rate of discontinuation of adalimumab than men ($P = .03$).[86] Though not significant, the rate of infliximab discontinuation was also numerically higher in women than in men.[86] Similarly, another study found that female CD patients were more likely to be on infliximab therapy for a shorter period than male patients.[87] In terms of response to therapy, several studies associated a decreased response to adalimumab among female patients.[88,89] However, a separate retrospective study of patients with CD determined that women had a better response to the TNF-α inhibitors adalimumab and infliximab.[84] Though these sex-based discrepancies are far from elucidated and warrant more research, it should be considered as part of a personalized therapeutic approach to care for female patients.

Though anti-TNF-α drugs are recommended as a safe medicine to use during pregnancy, young women with IBD may have fears and concerns regarding potential risks to the fetus (see Table 5-1; discussed in Chapter 8). In a Swedish cohort of patients with IBD, 33% more men were found to have received TNF-α inhibitors than women in the 20 to 40 years age group.[90] This gender difference was not seen in other age groups—less than 20 years old, 40 to 60 years old, or 60 to 80 years old—and could be explained by matters of fertility and pregnancy. Counseling regarding updated safety data from several large cohorts and registry studies of TNF-α inhibitors should be performed early with female patients to assuage common concerns and misconceptions.[91]

## Combination Therapy (Anti-Tumor Necrosis Factor-Alpha + Immunomodulator)

In the ongoing prospective cohort study using the SAPPHIRE registry, there was an increase in risk for new or recurrent cancer to arise in IBD patients who have experienced previous cancers using both a biologic agent and an immunomodulator (risk ratio 6.81, 95% CI 1.40 to 33.2). However, the sample size of combination therapy users (n = 29; 52% female) is small and needs further enrollment to assess safety.[71] Another retrospective study yielded similar results with no difference in risk of incident cancer in patients who had prior cancers using an anti-TNF agent vs those not using immunosuppression.[72]

In the SONIC study, receiving infliximab and azathioprine combination therapy was more effective and had better clinical response than infliximab or azathioprine monotherapy among treatment naïve patients with ileal CD.[82] Combination therapy (in patients previously naïve to azathioprine) was also found more effective than infliximab monotherapy at achievement of steroid-free remission. In contrast, patients with CD without active inflammation did not see this benefit; when post-hoc subgroup analyses were performed for patients with normal CRP or without endoscopic lesions, there were no significant differences in clinical response when treated with infliximab monotherapy or combination therapy than with azathioprine monotherapy.[82]

The effectiveness of combination therapy should not be the only factor guiding the use of this therapeutic strategy. Due to the increased risk of non-melanoma skin cancer and other malignancies associated with combination therapy compared to the general population as well as those receiving anti-TNF-α monotherapy, the potential risks of combination therapy should be weighed carefully against the benefits in women with IBD.[92]

## Anti-Integrins: Natalizumab and Vedolizumab

Natalizumab and vedolizumab (VDZ) prevent leukocyte trafficking via targeting cell surface integrins. Natalizumab is an alpha-4 integrin inhibiting IgG1 monoclonal antibody lacking specificity for beta integrins, which is approved for the treatment of moderate to severe CD.[93] VDZ is an IgG1 monoclonal antibody selectively modulating intestinal lymphocyte trafficking via antagonism of alpha-4 beta-7 integrin and its interaction with mucosal addressin cell adhesion molecule-1 on vascular endothelium approved for the treatment of both UC [94] and CD.[95] Due to its gut specificity, VDZ has a favorable safety profile. Unlike natalizumab, it does not target systemic lymphocyte trafficking in other organs, such as the brain which has been associated with progressive multifocal leukoencephalopathy, a rare and often fatal viral disease characterized by progressive damage of the white matter in patients harboring the John Cunningham virus. In addition to its overall safety profile, VDZ is perceived as lower risk than systemic anti-integrins for the mother, fetus, and infant during pregnancy and lactation (see Table 5-1).

VDZ has been associated with weight gain in some studies.[96] This change is more likely the result of clinical improvement with increases in appetite and intestinal absorption rather than a direct effect on weight gain. Therefore, it is important to discuss the possibility of weight gain within the context of therapeutic efficacy in women planning to start therapy with VDZ.

In women with IBD and a history of recent cancer, exposure to anti-integrins (natalizumab and VDZ) was not associated with a significant increased risk of recurrence or new cancer in the SAPPHIRE prospective cohort study.[71] While other prospective data are lacking, a case report of a young woman with CD and recurrent genital dysplasia under treatment with TNF-α inhibitors showed favorable results with disappearance of dysplasia after switching from TNF-α inhibitor to gut-selective anti-integrin therapy.[97] While far from high-level evidence, this case sheds light on the theoretical advantages of long-term therapy with gut-selective VDZ for young human papillomavirus.

## Ustekinumab

Ustekinumab is a monoclonal IgG1 antibody binding the common p40 subunit of the interleukin (IL)-12 and -23 receptors inhibiting IL-12 and IL-23 signaling. In the SAPPHIRE prospective cohort study, ustekinumab monotherapy was not associated with increased recurrence or new cancers.[71] In a retrospective monocenter study, male sex was associated as a predictor of nonresponse to ustekinumab therapy.[98]

## New Therapies

Etrolizumab is a beta-7 integrin inhibitor that blocks the mucosal addressin cell adhesion molecule-1 that can limit the inflammatory response.[99] It is currently undergoing clinical trials and there is a dearth of literature on its effects specific to women.

Rizankinumab is a selective inhibitor of IL-23.[100] It is currently in clinical trials for safety and efficacy. No literature specific to women with IBD is currently available.

Ozanimod is a sphingosine 1-phosphate receptor modulator. Further study should be implemented to assess the benefit of its use in patients with UC and CD.[101]

Etrasimod is a sphingosine 1-phosphate receptor modulator currently in clinical trials for moderate to severe UC. In phase 2 trials, it was found as more effective for clinical and endoscopic improvements than placebo.[78]

## Stem Cell Therapy

Hematopoietic and mesenchymal stem cells are currently being investigated as treatment modalities for IBD.[102-104] Stem cell–based therapies have been used effectively to treat perivaginal and perianal fistula.[105] Recently, mesenchymal stem cells have also been successfully used to treat rectovaginal fistulae in CD following surgical diversion.[106] It is also been found as a safe option for local treatment in women who desire to conceive, with no impact of mesenchymal stem cells injection therapy on ability to conceive or pregnancy outcomes in a retrospective study.[107]

## Antibiotics

Antibiotics may play an important role in active disease.[108] Antibiotics including antimycobacterial therapy, macrolides, quinolones, and rifaximin have been shown to have positive effects in active disease in certain patients. Amoxicillin-clavulanate and metronidazole may be used during pregnancy, whereas fluoroquinolones should be avoided due to unknown effects on infant bone growth and rifaximin should be avoided due to associated teratogenicity (see Table 5-1).

# Complementary and Alternative Therapies

In addition to the conventional therapies described in the first part of this chapter, many patients turn to complementary or alternative medicines (CAM) due to the limited efficacy of conventional medical therapies, concern for adverse effects, or the wish for a "natural" approach to treatment.[5,6] In this section we will review the complementary and alternative therapies currently used in the treatment of IBD and related gastrointestinal disorders.

## Hydration and Laxatives

Women with stricturing CD or postoperative dysmotility may find laxatives to be helpful in facilitating bowel movements. Additionally, the achievement of remission in patients with previously active inflammatory disease may unmask a tendency for constipation. However, we should consider the possibility of laxative abuse and disordered eating when taking a medical history in this patient population. While laxatives may help treat constipation and improve motility issues, they are also associated with weight loss, diarrhea, and abdominal pain. Women who have body image issues may also abuse laxatives. Inclusion of a nutritionist in the care team of women with suspected disordered eating and inappropriate laxative use is important. We favor the use of osmotic laxatives such as polyethylene glycol over stimulant laxatives in patients with IBD, as they will be effective in the presence of stricturing disease and carry minimal potential for abuse.

Dehydration is a sequela of laxative use as well as active intestinal inflammation or postoperative anatomy. Additional causes of dehydration within the IBD patient population include comorbid alcohol abuse, caffeine use, and diuretic medications. Asian women may be more susceptible to alcohol use as rapid metabolizers, and the effects of dehydration should be discussed with them. Therefore, a thorough dietary, social, and medication history is important in assessing the risk of dehydration. Women with an ileostomy, ileal pouch, or active ileal disease have increased risks of dehydration and should be encouraged to increase water intake and minimize their use of coffee and alcohol, which are diuretics. Oral and IV rehydration in select cases is an effective measure to consider in at-risk patients.[109] Symptoms of overhydration should be considered as well and patients should be educated as to oral hydration strategies.

# Pain Management
## *Opioids*

Patients with IBD may experience both abdominal pain and musculoskeletal pain related to extraintestinal manifestations (EIMs) or associated rheumatologic conditions. Pharmacologic management of these types of pain includes the use of a variety of analgesic formulations, nonsteroidal anti-inflammatory drugs (NSAIDs), and opioids. While effective in treating severe pain, narcotic medications are associated with a risk of dependency and other serious complications. Within the IBD population, chronic opioid use has been associated with many adverse outcomes, including increased overall mortality and post-surgical infections.[110,111] The TREAT registry, which assessed the safety of infliximab, also found that the rate of mortality was doubled in CD patients taking narcotic analgesics.[112] Another study showed that exposure to opioid medications, both IV and oral, in hospitalized IBD patients was associated with increased risk of future opioid use, with a dose-dependent effect.[113] Therefore, extreme caution should be used when prescribing opioid analgesics and efforts should be made to limit the quantities used and length of treatment. An emphasis on treatment of the underlying inflammatory disease and using narcotic-sparing strategies, often within a multi-disciplinary framework, is essential to promoting favorable outcomes in IBD. There should be efforts to minimize exposure to opioids in the inpatient setting and alternative pain management therapies should be considered.

Patients with IBD are overall more likely to exhibit heavy opioid use (OR 2.91; 95% CI 2.19 to 3.85), and females may have an overall higher risk than males (OR 1.18; 95% CI 0.82 to 1.70).[114] A separate study found females with IBD to have an increased likelihood of opioid medication use as compared to males (OR 2.4; 95% CI 1.3 to 4.4).[115] Therefore, it is imperative to address concerns regarding narcotic use with female patients and to develop a shared decision-making approach toward minimizing unnecessary use.

## *Nonsteroidal Anti-Inflammatory Drugs and Aspirin*

NSAIDs are readily available as over-the-counter therapies used to treat pain. Given the lack of a need for prescription, many patients with IBD take these medications readily for pain without awareness that they may pose a harm with regard to gastrointestinal bleeding and their IBD. Women may be particularly more inclined to use preparations containing NSAIDs during or prior to menses. The potential for gastrointestinal irritation or bleeding[116] should limit the use of NSAID medications even in the event of premenstrual symptoms or intermittent headaches in the presence of IBD. NSAIDs play a role in inhibition of cyclooxygenase (COX) -1 and -2 enzymes. COX-2 is expressed in the inflamed bowel in response to pro-inflammatory cytokine stimulation, and its inhibition can therefore lead to favorable anti-inflammatory sequelae. However, COX-1 has been implicated in gastrointestinal maintenance, and its inhibition is thought to contribute to gastric and intestinal ulcers, bowel strictures,[117-119] and enteritis as well as worsening clinical disease in IBD patients.[120] NSAIDs have been linked with the development of both CD and UC in some studies. In a case-control study, NSAID use was correlated with exacerbation of disease activity in UC and CD patients, compared to their use in the IBS population.[116] In a prospective cohort study of women in the United States using NSAIDs, frequent use (of at least 15 days/month) was associated with increased absolute incidence of CD (6 cases per 100,000 person-years [95% CI 0 to 13]; multivariate hazard ratio, 1.59 [CI 0.99 to 2.56]) and UC (absolute difference, 7 cases per 100,000 person-years [CI 1 to 12]; multivariate hazard ratio, 1.87 [CI 1.16 to 2.99]) compared to NSAID non-users.[121] Such association was not seen between aspirin usage and IBD.[121] This could reveal a possible mechanistic role of NSAIDs in contribution to inflammation and exacerbation of disease in a woman with IBD. However, other studies such as a prospective population-based study of symptomatic flares in IBD found that there are no differential rates of NSAID use associated with IBD flares.[122] With the conflicting literature on the possibility of flare due to NSAIDs and aspirin, more studies are warranted. The role of limited use of aspirin and other NSAIDs should be discussed with the provider prior to use for pain relief and anti-inflammation. Alternatives to NSAID analgesics, such as acetaminophen or curcumin, should therefore be considered for regular use in women requiring ongoing anti-inflammatory therapy, such as athletes or those with prior injuries.

## Low-Dose Naltrexone

Low-dose naltrexone (LDN) is an opioid antagonist that is frequently used for IBD refractory to conventional therapy or among patients seeking a CAM approach. It has been found to improve wound healing and decreased endoplasmic reticulum stress levels.[123] Case reports have noted some effectiveness and clinical improvement with use of LDN.[124] A prospective study of 47 IBD patients using LDN observed increased clinical improvement as well as cases of remission in its cohort.[123] However, a meta-analysis of 2 small randomized controlled trials found that though there may be some improved clinical and endoscopic response in active CD and adverse events are not increased compared to placebo, the evidence was inconclusive in determining the safety and efficacy of therapeutic LDN in CD due to the small sample size.[125] Larger randomized controlled trials are needed using more objective endpoints in order determine any potential role for LDN in treating IBD. Additionally, LDN can be problematic for the female IBD patient as it may mask pelvic pain and abdominal pain potentially leading to missed diagnosis of pelvic pathology, such as rupture of ovarian cysts or torsion. Furthermore, without clear evidence of benefit, use of LDN places patients at risk for disease progression and complications which might be prevented by the use of FDA-approved therapies.

## Cannabis/Cannabinoids

Medical marijuana and cannabinoids, derived from the *Cannabis sativa* plant, are currently used as a complementary and alternative medicine in IBD. These agents target the cannabinoid receptors in the gut. Studies of the endogenous cannabinoid system have found cannabinoid-1 receptors expressed in the gut have functions related to pain, nausea, and vomiting, while cannabinoid-1 and -2 receptors are related to modulation of inflammation.[126-128] Accordingly, exogenous cannabis and cannabinoids have been observed to alleviate subjective symptoms of pain and nausea and improve appetite, but not objective improvement in intestinal inflammation in patients with IBD.

In a small prospective, randomized, placebo-controlled study of inhaled cannabis in patients with CD, a significantly improved clinical response was observed.[129] While this study was placebo controlled, the inhaled control did not reproduce the "high" seen with the cannabis, and it is unclear how this impacted the results. There was no change in serum inflammatory markers seen between groups. In a prospective trial of patients with IBD, use of cannabis significantly improved quality of life (QOL), increased weight, and decreased disease activity.[130] Another retrospective observational study of patients with CD showed a significant improvement in disease activity after treatment with cannabis.[131] Despite the potential benefit in QOL, these trials have not clearly demonstrated evidence of efficacy in terms of objective improvement in inflammatory biomarkers or endoscopic disease activity.[128]

In women specifically, the endogenous cannabinoid system has been implicated in the menstrual cycle and the proliferation of the endometrium in molecular studies, but there are no clinical studies associating cannabis use with fertility.[132-135] More human studies are needed to understand the role of cannabis use in female fertility, hormone production, regulation of the menstrual cycle, and reproductive health. Currently, due to lack of data, marijuana use is not recommended during pregnancy as possible adverse neurodevelopmental effects may present in the development of the fetus and child even years after the exposure in utero.[136]

In a study examining treatment-seeking cannabis users, cannabis withdrawal symptoms were greater in women than in men, with increased mood symptoms such as irritability, anger, restlessness, and violent outbursts as well and increased gastrointestinal symptoms like nausea and pain.[137] Though this may not apply to patients who do not have cannabis use disorder, it is an important consideration for the safety of women with IBD who already experience gastrointestinal symptoms due to their disease.

## Curcumin

Curcumin, a derivative of *Curcuma longa*, has been identified as an anti-inflammatory bioactive substance studied for use in many inflammatory conditions. Its effects include inhibition of cyclooxygenase-2, lipoxygenase, TNF-α, interferon gamma, inducible nitric oxide synthase, and transcription nuclear factor kappa B. In experimental models of IBD, curcumin has been shown to suppress induced colitis with a decreased level of pro-inflammatory Th1-type cytokines and increased level of anti-inflammatory Th2-type cytokines.[138] In a human pilot study in which patients were dosed with 360 mg of curcumin in an open label fashion 3 to 4 times/day for a total of 3 months, clinical relapse in patients with quiescent IBD was not observed.[139] A prospective, randomized, placebo controlled study in 50 patients with UC[140] found curcumin in combination with oral mesalamine maintenance therapy was associated with clinical and endoscopic remission as compared to mesalamine alone.[138] However, in a systematic review and meta-analysis of randomized controlled trials of oral curcumin in patients with UC, curcumin administration was found not significantly superior to placebo for attaining remission in UC using an intention-to-treat analysis, but a per-protocol analysis did favor curcumin (OR = 5.83; 95% CI 1.24 to 27.43).[138] Further randomized controlled trials are warranted to clarify curcumin's role in remission. As curcumin is a medical food, preparations are not standardized as to curcumin content and more knowledge regarding dosing and safety are required. However, due to the relative safety in IBD trials to date and a likely benefit, curcumin is a non-immunosuppressive option which should be considered in women with IBD who are interested in CAM approaches.

# Anti-Inflammatory Nutritional Supplements
## Vitamin E

Vitamin E, which encompasses biologically active tocopherols and tocotrienol, has been identified to have anti-inflammatory properties. In a rat experimental colitis model, vitamin E reversed the effects of colitis-induced rises in TNF-α, IL-18, and IL-6 (all $P < .001$).[141] Its use also had antioxidant properties such as decreasing levels of the oxidizing agents myeloperoxidase and malondialdehyde while increasing antioxidants such as glutathione and superoxide dismutase (all $P < .001$).[141] Vitamin E has been associated with decreased risk of colon cancer, which may be of additional benefit to patients with IBD.[142] It may be therefore considered as a complementary therapy due to these properties, however, due to its anticoagulant effects, women with IBD should discuss with their physicians in order to minimize risk of gastrointestinal and other bleeding.

## Vitamin C

Vitamin C has been associated with several anti-inflammatory properties. Oxidative stress causes damage to tissue in IBD. Ascorbic acid is a potent antioxidant and functions as a cofactor in enzymatic reactions that activate molecular pathways reducing oxidative stress.[143,144] In a murine experimental colitis model, ascorbic acid treatment was associated with significantly reduced levels of inflammatory cytokines, myeloperoxidase, malonaldehyde, as well as clinical signs.[144] A randomized controlled trial examining treatment with antioxidants (vitamins C and E) in patients with CD observed significantly decreased oxidative damage, as observed by serologic markers, in the supplemented group compared to placebo.[145] It is important to recognize that low ascorbic acid levels or even scurvy is underappreciated in women with IBD.[146,147] As patients with active disease may be oxidatively stressed, vitamin C should be supplemented with supervision from the nutrition team and clinician.

## Vitamin D

Vitamin D is a fat-soluble vitamin essential to many pathways whose biology is implicated in several pathologic conditions. Although it is possible that low vitamin D levels are both the cause of disease, or the end results of chronic inflammation, numerous studies have implicated low vitamin D levels with increased inflammatory activity. There is strong evidence of low serum 25-OH vitamin D levels among patients with more severe disease activity in IBD.[148-152] Low vitamin D has also been implicated in the pathogenesis of infection with *Clostridioides difficile (C difficile)*, which is much more common in patients with IBD than in the general population.[153] Vitamin D may have anti-inflammatory and anti-proliferative properties.[154] Levels greater than 30 ng/mL or 75 nmol/L are believed to have an anti-inflammatory effect, wherein mRNA production of inflammatory cytokines, such as IL-6 and TNF-α, are inhibited.[155] Therefore, supplementation for patients with insufficient levels (< 30 ng/mL) or deficiency (< 20 ng/mL) is a mainstay of IBD treatment in addition to disease modifying maintenance therapy. Given the ileal absorption of vitamin D via the enterohepatic circulation, hypovitaminosis D may result from ileal disease, decreased oral intake, or decreased sun exposure.

Low vitamin D levels are associated with osteopenia and osteoporosis. This may be more pronounced among patients with significant corticosteroid exposure and/or cigarette smoking and is more frequent among female patients. Therefore, bone mineral density screening with dual-energy X-ray absorptiometry should be routinely performed for female patients and those with a cumulative steroid exposure of more than 3 months in the IBD population with attention to vitamin D and calcium supplementation in at-risk patients.[156] Further attention to prevent osteopenia with vitamin D supplementation in post-menopausal and perimenopausal women is also recommended.

## Zinc

Zinc functions as a superoxide dismutase cofactor and may have indirect antioxidant properties.[157] In experimental animal studies, zinc has been involved with improved redox balance in plasma and colonic tissue, when used in conjunction with vitamin E[157] or an anti-TNF-α drug.[158] Zinc deficiency is a well-described complication of CD in both children[159] and adults.[160] Zinc deficiency has been associated with a worse prognosis among patients with IBD.[161] Therefore, zinc should be supplemented in patients with documented deficiency. However, supplementation may lead to diarrhea, and patients should be counseled on tailoring use to individual symptoms, including reducing use during active IBD flares or during menses if diarrhea is increased. Further human studies are warranted to assess the use of zinc as a CAM.

## Aloe Vera

Aloe vera has been suggested as an herbal supplement that may be useful in the treatment of IBD. It has been purported to have anti-inflammatory properties by inhibition of prostaglandin E2 and IL-2 secretion in the human gut mucosa.[162] Aloe vera was studied in a randomized, double blind, placebo-controlled trial of patients with mild to moderate UC.[163] There were improvements in disease activity and clinical remission in the Aloe vera group, with significantly decreased UC activity index (*P* = .01) and histological score (*P* = .03), which was not observed in the placebo group. No difference was seen between the Aloe vera vs the placebo groups in endoscopic score and biochemical markers. Given the lack of robust clinical endpoints shown to improve with Aloe vera, further clinical trials are warranted to assess its anti-inflammatory effects in IBD. It is important to note that Aloe vera is associated with laxative effects and should be used with consideration of this property.[164] Use within the population of women with constipation as a component of their IBD or following the achievement of remission can be considered.

### Wheatgrass

Wheatgrass in the form of juice has been shown to have anti-inflammatory properties and antioxidant activity.[165] In an experimental study, pigenin, a component of wheatgrass, was found to inactive nuclear factor kappa B by suppression of p65 phosphorylation, resulting in inhibition of IL-1β, IL-8, and TNF.[166] In a clinical randomized, double blind, placebo-controlled trial in UC, wheatgrass users had significantly decreased UC activity index ($P = .03$) and decreased severity of rectal bleeding ($P = .03$) compared to placebo.[167] With a safe side effect profile, wheatgrass should be further studied to assess efficacy in reduction of inflammation in IBD.

## Fatty Acids

### Omega-3 Fatty Acids

Omega-3 fatty acids (FA), found in fish oil, have been widely described as having anti-inflammatory properties. However, the data in the IBD population are contradictory. A preclinical animal study suggests that omega-3 FA may reduce clinical colitis through reduction of colonic pro-inflammatory cytokine synthesis, reduction of myeloid cell recruitment, and promotion of mucosal wound healing.[168] A small clinical trial also observed that fish oil is effective in reducing the rate of relapse in CD.[169] However, in a large randomized controlled trial[170] and in a large epidemiological study,[171] no beneficial protective effect of omega-3 was observed. While further research would be helpful in the clarification of the efficacy of fish oil and omega-3 FA in IBD, the favorable safety profile and possible benefits on lipid profile may justify its use in clinical practice. Women with IBD should discuss supplementation with the clinician and nutrition team prior to its use.

### Butyrate

Butyrate is a short-chain FA, which is a metabolite derived from bacterial fermentation within the colon.[172] Butyrate enemas are known to have possible anti-inflammatory and antioxidant effects in the colon in diversion colitis and active UC.[172-174] However, its effects as a protective agent is controversial. Early clinical trials have shown that topical butyrate or butyrate enema as monotherapy or in conjunction with conventional therapies are effective to treat diversion colitis and acute radiation proctopathy.[172,175,176] A randomized placebo-controlled study of patients with UC in remission only observed a significantly increased colonic mucosal IL-10/IL-12 ratio in the butyrate enema group ($P = .02$).[177] Also, CCL5 levels were increased in the treatment group compared to the placebo group ($P = .03$).[177] All other parameters of inflammation in colonic mucosal biopsy (IL-1β, IL-5, IL-6, IL-10, IL-12, IFN-γ, IL-8, MCP-1, MPO), in fecal marker (calprotectin), as well as in serologic markers (CRP) did not significantly differ between placebo and butyrate, as well as before and after the use of butyrate enema. The oxidative stress parameters measured from colonic mucosal biopsies did not significantly differ between butyrate group and placebo group. Rectal butyrate enemas, thus, had minor effects on inflammation and oxidative stress of UC patients with mild inflammation.[177] More clinical trials are warranted to assess whether butyrate is beneficial as a CAM.

### Evening Primrose

Evening primrose, *Oenothera biennis*, is a fatty oil that is used as an herbal medicine. It contains omega-6 FA, including linoleic acid and gamma-linoleic acid. It has been studied in one early-phase placebo-controlled study in patients with UC.[178,179] The evening primrose group was found to have increased red-cell membrane concentration of dihomogamma-linoleic acid by 40% at 6 months ($P < .05$) whereas placebo patients had reduced levels of dihomogamma-linoleic acid.[179] It also improved stool consistency compared with placebo and it was maintained 3 months after discontinuation of treatment ($P < .05$), but there were no differences between the evening primrose group and placebo groups with regard to disease relapse, stool frequency, rectal bleeding, sigmoidoscopic appearance, or rectal histology.[179] Therefore, it is possible that evening primrose may have mild benefits on UC. Additionally, evening primrose may also have some efficacy in managing premenstrual syndrome, hot flashes, and other ailments relevant to women.[180] Therefore, further controlled clinical studies are necessary to understand the response of women's IBD symptoms to evening primrose oil.

## Therapy for Extraintestinal and Musculoskeletal Manifestations

The most common EIM of CD is joint disease, including inflammatory arthritis, spondyloarthropathies, and ankylosing spondylitis.[117,118,181] However, psoriatic arthritis, osteoarthritis, exercise-induced traumatic arthritis, drug-induced arthritis, autoimmune arthritis, stress fractures, and muscle loss related to steroids and nutritional deficiencies have to be considered.[181] While the list of other EIM observed in IBD is extensive, it is beyond the scope of this chapter. We will briefly discuss management of musculoskeletal manifestations associated with IBD in this section.

## Physical and Psychosocial

Psychosocial aspects of living with IBD include emotional, psychological, and financial burdens. All of these may manifest in women with IBD as stress, anxiety, depression, and sleep disturbance. Sleep disturbance has been widely described in IBD and correlates with disease activity.[182] A prospective population-based study identified that stress was associated as a trigger of symptomatic IBD flares in multivariate logistic regression analysis (adjusted OR = 2.40, 95% CI 1.35 to 4.26), while use of NSAIDs, antibiotics, and infections were not associated with IBD flares.[122] Stress may present as a substantial contributor to the multifactorial causes of IBD. In women, stress needs to be studied with consideration of cyclical variation in hormones (menses, oral contraceptive pill) as a possible confounder. Engaging resources to cope with stress, including attendance in support groups and counseling with social workers and/or mental health professionals may be useful in the IBD population, and further investigation into optimal practices is needed.

### Mind-Body Breathing

Objective studies on breathing, mind, and body complementary alternative approaches are sparse and therefore it is difficult for the practicing clinician to recommend therapies to women with IBD. Of the studies available, a randomized controlled trial studied the effect of breathing through the Qigong method on psychological and physical well-being as well as on biomarkers in IBD patients, 59% of whom were women.[183] This study showed subacute and long-term improvements in psychological symptoms (anxiety, depression, perceived stress, and perceived disability), physical symptoms (bowel symptoms, abdominal pain, and systemic symptoms), QOL (daily function and social function), as well as a transient reduction in CRP and fecal calprotectin.[183] Breathing, involved in yoga and Qigong, may be recommended as a helpful adjunct to medical therapy. Larger scale multicenter trials evaluating the role of stress and intervention strategies in IBD are warranted.

### Antidepressant: Bupropion

Bupropion is a medicine used for atypical depression which has been purported to have antiinflammatory properties. Bupropion has been found to lower levels of TNF and IL-1β in an animal study.[184] The suppression of monoamine oxidase and dopamine by bupropion results in increased intracellular cyclic adenosine monophosphate which inhibits TNF-α synthesis.[184] In human studies, bupropion has been hypothesized to induce clinical remission in CD and lower TNF-α.[185-187] However, no large randomized controlled trials have evaluated bupropion in IBD. As a drug that may be financially affordable with minimal side effects, it is an attractive potential therapy for IBD and large controlled trials are warranted.[187] However, its current use is limited to empiric use based on case reports and preclinical studies.

## Physical Therapy

Physical therapy is an important modality to offset morbidity and/or body composition changes due to IBD.[188] A cross-sectional study of premenopausal patients with IBD, 44% of which were female, revealed low muscle mass in 21% of patients, sarcopenia in 12% of patients, and osteopenia/osteoporosis in 38% of patients.[189] The IBD population may be sarcopenic due to chronic inflammation, sedentary lifestyle, limited mobility, and malnutrition. Malnutrition may be secondary to malabsorption, dietary restriction, surgery, or disordered eating.[19,189,190] Improved nutrition with the involvement of a registered dietitian or clinical nutritionist and guided physical therapy may help with sarcopenia.

Additionally, physical therapy may ameliorate fecal urgency and incontinence, or urinary incontinence experienced after IBD surgeries or during IBD flare.[191,192] A pelvic floor physical therapist can aid in proper instruction of techniques for pelvic floor exercises to improve symptoms.[193] Manual external therapy may also help with pelvic pain in women with IBD. A study on pelvic floor behavioral treatment has observed improved fecal incontinence and constipation in those with IBD diagnoses with previous perianal fistula, pelvic/colorectal surgery, ileoanal pouch, or prior obstetric trauma.[193] Patients with complex pelvic pain should seek pelvic floor specialists to focus on their individual needs, often through a combination of techniques, including stretching, massage, biofeedback, and physical therapy.

## Exercise

Exercise may serve as an adjunctive therapy with possible positive effects on disease, mood, maintenance of muscle mass, and prevention of osteoporosis.[194,195] Exercise may change the gut physiology and research has found that low intensity exercise may reduce transient stool time and decrease the contact time of pathogens with the gastrointestinal mucus layer.[196] This may have beneficial effects such as decreasing risks of colon cancer and confer protection to the gastrointestinal tract.[197] The underlying mechanisms are not well understood and warrant further research.

A study found that CD patients with a higher level of exercise had a decreased likelihood of developing active disease at 6 months.[194,195] However, a recent study of exercise in 227 patients with IBD (with 148 women) revealed that 44% of patients self-reported limitations to exercise due to active IBD.[198] Reasons for limited exercise included fatigue (n = 81), joint pain (n = 37), embarrassment (n = 23), and weakness (n = 1). The disease itself may stand as a barrier to exercise, and recommendations must be individualized based on these limitations and disease activity.

## Yoga

Yoga programs may help reduce gastrointestinal pain, pelvic pain, and improve mood in women with IBD through movement and breathing. A randomized study has shown significantly higher QOL scores (P = .02) and lower disease activity (P = .03) in UC patients taking Hatha yoga than an inactive control group.[199] Another study observed mildly improved anxiety scores (P = .01) and fewer arthralgias (P < .05) in patients with UC, attesting to certain extra-intestinal symptomatic improvements. However, there were no changes observed in patients with CD and no objective immune changes in the potential biomarker eosinophilic cationic protein.[200] A yoga-based lifestyle intervention study, including mind-body therapies, showed no effects of these interventions on inflammatory markers and disease activity.[199] Yoga can be beneficial as a complementary therapy in improving symptoms of IBD in addition to conventional medications; however, more studies are warranted to understand whether it may have direct anti-inflammatory properties.[182]

# Anti-Infective and Microbiome Targeted Therapies
## Microbiome

Probiotics and prebiotics may be used to modulate the intestinal microbiota, although few data exist to support routine probiotic use in IBD. Limited clinical trial data support the use of VSL#3 (now branded as Visbiome) in the adjunctive treatment of mild to moderate UC,[201] treatment of ileal pouchitis,[202] and in the prevention of pouchitis.[203] Several studies have also suggested a benefit for *Escherichia coli* in UC.[204] However, the treatment effects are small and the benefit of probiotic therapies in IBD remains unproven.

Fecal microbiota transplant (FMT) has been shown to be a highly effective therapy in treating *C difficile* and has been studied within the IBD population to treat both *C difficile* and non-*C difficile*–associated inflammation.[205,206] Much work is currently ongoing to elucidate the optimal technique and frequency for performing FMT within the IBD population, but it is not currently an FDA-approved indication.

### Anti-Malarial: Wormwood and Hydroxychloroquine

Wormwood, *Artemisia absinthium*, has been shown to have anti-inflammatory properties. It is originally known for its use as an antimalarial agent, artemisinin, which is extracted from wormwood.[207] This has also been purported to have anticancer effects.[208] In the context of IBD, artemisinin has been found in an animal study to improve colitis by inducing apoptosis of macrophages and dendritic cells, while suppressing IL-12 and TNF-α.[209] A clinical IBD study also has found anti-TNF-α properties of wormwood. In a randomized controlled clinical trial of patients with CD, the effect of wormwood on TNF-α levels was assessed.[210] In the wormwood group, TNF-α levels decreased from a baseline average 24.5 ± 3.5 pg/mL to 8.0 ± 2.5 pg/mL after 6 weeks, whereas the control group only changed from 25.7 ± 4.6 to 21.1 ± 3.2 pg/mL. There were also significant decreases in CDAI scores, accelerated clinical response, and improved mood seen in the wormwood group.

Chloroquine and hydroxychloroquine are anti-malarial drugs that may be used for short-term treatment of mild to moderate UC. They have been shown to display similar efficacy as 5-ASA therapy.[211] Chloroquine and hydroxychloroquine have been shown to be safe during pregnancy and breastfeeding in patients with systemic lupus erythematosus and rheumatoid arthritis.[212,213] In pregnant patients taking chloroquine for chemo suppression of malaria, there were no identified risks of human teratogenicity or fetal adverse effects.[214] In rheumatoid arthritis and systemic lupus erythematosus literature, there were no increased congenital malformations in pregnancies with maternal exposure to anti-malarials daily during the first trimester.[213,215-218] Further human studies are necessary in the context of IBD to survey whether it may be an option for pregnant and lactating women with IBD.

### Parasitic/Anti-Parasitic: Nitazoxanide and Whipworms

Nitazoxanide is an antiparasitic agent that acts peripherally in the gut lumen and may have a role in the management of IBD.[219] However, there is a lack of studies available, with only one study of nitazoxanide use in CD for a concomitant cryptosporidial infection.[220] Randomized controlled trials are needed to discover its properties and effects in IBD treatment.

Whipworms, *Trichuris suis*, may have some beneficial effect in IBD complementary and alternative therapy. This therapy may be administered as ova therapy. These helminths have been found to possibly decrease immune responses in humans colonized with whipworms and may be able to decrease inflammation in the colon.[221-223] Small studies in patients with IBD have seen improved clinical response observed by disease activity scores.[224,225] A randomized clinical trial in patients with UC also showed significant improvement in clinical disease activity in *Trichuris suis* ova therapy than in placebo; however, there were no differences in rate of remission.[226] However, a *Trichuris suis* ova study in patients with CD showed that though the treatment is safe, there were no observed clinically meaningful improvements in gastrointestinal symptoms.[227] More studies are warranted on whipworms and objective measures should be assessed in trials.

### Anti-Bacterial: Rifaximin

Rifaximin may be used in IBD therapy as a gut environment modulator[201] as well as an antibacterial agent.[228] In controlled trials and other studies, rifaximin has been shown to induce remission of CD.[229-231] In an open label study of patients with UC, clinical remission with rifaximin and maintenance mesalazine use was achieved in 76.6% of cases.[232] A double-blind study showed clinical improvement in UC.[233] Therefore, rifaximin may be a useful adjunct medicine for women with IBD.

## Medical Foods

It is important to look toward medical food as an anti-inflammatory and supportive nutritional CAM.[234] Malnutrition is frequent and may be due to malabsorption or restrictive eating in IBD. Modulen, EnteraGam and Vivonex total enteral nutrition may all be effective liquid diets for IBD therapy. Modulen is a liquid enteral nutrition and anti-inflammatory rich in transforming growth factor-beta, which plays a role in immune modulation.[235] It has been found to help in the recovery of weight and earlier disease remission in a pediatric IBD study.[235] Another study showed improvement of clinical remission in patients with CD with use of Modulen, though not clinically significant.[236] Vivonex total enteral nutrition is another medical food that may help with clinical improvement.[237] EnteraGam, serum-derived bovine immunoglobulin/protein isolate, is a medical food formulated for the gut. A retrospective case series showed EnteraGam ameliorated gastrointestinal symptoms in patients not controlled with conventional medicine.[238] A retrospective chart review of patients with IBD also found improved clinical remission.[239] Such medical foods may be used to complement traditional IBD therapies, although further randomized controlled data are needed before widespread use is recommended.

## Other Agents

Frankincense, from the *Boswellia* species, may help treat inflammatory disease through active compound derivatives, boswellic acids. Boswellic acids have been observed to act as non-competitive inhibitors of 5-lipoxygenase, thus blocking leukotriene effects.[240,241] A study of frankincense in patients with UC showed the achievement of clinical remission in 80% of patients, with similar effects to sulfasalazine.[242] Maintenance therapy for CD in a randomized single-center study showed that frankincense was well tolerated and yielded prolonged remission in patients.[243]

Lei gong teng, *Tripterygium wilfordii*, has been shown to be effective in CD therapy. A randomized clinical trial of *Tripterygium* use was comparable to azathioprine use in postoperative recurrence prevention in CD.[244]

Chios mastic gum, *Pistacia lentiscus var. Chia*, was associated with decreased clinical activity and decreased plasma levels of IL-6 and CRP in moderately active patients with CD.[245] Additional TNF-α inhibiting effects were observed in patients with CD treated with mastic.[246] Double-blind placebo-controlled studies are warranted for further evidence of effectiveness in IBD as a CAM.

# Conclusion

Women living with IBD may experience a plethora of overlapping inflammatory and non-inflammatory symptoms. Living with active IBD poses a higher risk of disease complications and progression. Women may be misdiagnosed as having IBS prior to being diagnosed with IBD.[8] We should challenge preexisting diagnoses and use objective measures of disease activity, as well as rule out the potential contribution of non-inflammatory symptoms when evaluating patients with IBD. Women may experience abdominal pain and cramping due to the menstrual cycle, polycystic ovarian syndrome, ovarian cysts, tumors, and other gynecologic processes. Patients should be encouraged to discuss their philosophy about complementary medicine, nutritional supplements, exercise, hydration, and diet. Physicians, care teams, nutritionists, and social workers should be aware of the role of stress, disordered eating, laxatives, and opioid use. The goal for women living with IBD is to maintain clinical remission and mucosal healing with the lowest, safest, most effective dose of anti-inflammatory medications. When conventional therapies fail to obtain remission, women may seek complementary and alternative approaches. As physicians our goal is to personalize and balance conventional and complementary strategies for healing women living with IBD while reversing the natural history of IBD.

# Acknowledgments

This chapter is dedicated to the memory of Jill A. Roberts, founder of The Jill Roberts Center for IBD. Jill was a lifelong, grateful patient and tireless patient advocate.

We extend our gratitude to Dr. Bincy Abraham, Dr. Sunanda Kane, and Dr. Kerri Glassner for the invitation to write this chapter and for their guidance.

We would like to express our appreciation to Dr. Anand Kumar (Weill Cornell Medicine) for his contribution to the background research of this chapter.

---

## KEY POINTS

1. Treating and diagnosing IBD in women should be personalized and focused on recognizing inflammation and overlapping causes of abdominal pain. Women's use of and attitudes toward IBD medications should be identified to emphasize motivational counseling and employ shared decision making for treatment success.

2. Treatment of women with IBD should follow the universal goal of steroid-sparing therapy to obtain IBD remission through use of immune modulators, novel small molecules, and biologic therapy.

3. The physiologic changes of menses, pregnancy, and menopause and diseases often associated with these conditions, such as iron deficiency anemia, VTE, and osteoporosis, should be considered in conjunction with IBD activity for optimal treatment.

4. CAMs may supplement conventional therapies to create a comprehensive IBD treatment regimen. CAMs are versatile and can target different aspects of IBD such as pain management, management of inflammation, psychosocial issues, diet, and nutritional optimization. The usage of CAMs should be implemented only after the medicine is assessed by its ability to reduce inflammatory markers and disease activity in IBD.

---

# References

1.  Crohn BB, Ginzburg L, Oppenheimer GD. Regional ileitis: a pathologic and clinical entity. *JAMA*. 1932;99(16):1323-1329.

2.  Vermeire S, Van Assche G, Rutgeerts P. Classification of inflammatory bowel disease: the old and the new. *Curr Opin Gastroenterol*. 2012;28(4):321-326.

3.  McGovern DP, Kugathasan S, Cho JH. Genetics of inflammatory bowel diseases. *Gastroenterology*. 2015;149(5):1163-1176. e1162.

4.  DeFilippis EM, Longman R, Harbus M, Dannenberg K, Scherl EJ. Crohn's disease: evolution, epigenetics, and the emerging role of microbiome-targeted therapies. *Curr Gastroenterol Rep*. 2016;18(3):13.

5.  Cotton S, Humenay Roberts Y, Tsevat J, et al. Mind–body complementary alternative medicine use and quality of life in adolescents with inflammatory bowel disease. *Inflamm Bowel Dis*. 2010;16(3):501-506.

6.  Jedel S, Hankin V, Voigt RM, Keshavarzian A. Addressing the mind, body, and spirit in a gastrointestinal practice for inflammatory bowel disease patients. *Clin Gastroenterol Hepatol*. 2012;10(3):244-246.

7.  Chouchane L, Mamtani R, Dallol A, Sheikh JI. Personalized medicine: a patient-centered paradigm. In: *BioMed Central*; 2011.

8.  Scherl EJ. Irritable-inflammatory bowel disease: recognizing a new overlap syndrome and an enigma wrapped inside a puzzle. *Gut*. 2002;8:373-374.

9.  Klaus J, Spaniol U, Adler G, Mason RA, Reinshagen M, Christian von Tirpitz C. Small intestinal bacterial over-growth mimicking acute flare as a pitfall in patients with Crohn's disease. *BMC Gastroenterology*. 2009;9(1):61.

10. Lee JM, Lee KM, Chung YY, et al. Clinical significance of the glucose breath test in patients with inflammatory bowel disease. *J Gastroenterol Hepatol*. 2015;30(6):990-994.

11. Pimentel M, Saad RJ, Long MD, Rao SS. ACG clinical guideline: small intestinal bacterial overgrowth. *Am J Gastroenterol*. 2020;115(2):165-178.

12. Ona S, James K, Ananthakrishnan AN, et al. Association between vulvovaginal discomfort and activity of inflam-matory bowel diseases. *Clin Gastroenterol Hepatol*. 2020;18(3):604-611. e601.

13. Yang A, Chen Y, Scherl E, Neugut AI, Bhagat G, Green PH. Inflammatory bowel disease in patients with celiac disease. *Inflamm Bowel Dis*. 2005;11(6):528-532.

14. Jasdanwala S, Babyatsky M. Crohn's disease and acute pancreatitis. a review of literature. *JOP Journal of the Pancreas*. 2015;16(2):136-142.

15. Heikius B, Niemelä S, Lehtola J, Karttunen T, Lähde S. Pancreatic duct abnormalities and pancreatic function in patients with chronic inflammatory bowel disease. *Scand J Gastroenterol*. 1996;31(5):517-523.

16. Heaton K, Read A. Gall stones in patients with disorders of the terminal ileum and disturbed bile salt metabolism. *Br Med J*. 1969;3(5669):494-496.

17. Ramos LR, Sachar DB, DiMaio CJ, Colombel J-F, Torres J. Inflammatory bowel disease and pancreatitis: a review. *J Crohns Colitis*. 2016;10(1):95-104.

18. Couzin-Frankel J. Rethinking anorexia: biology may be more important than culture, new studies reveal. In. *Science*. Vol 368: American Association for the Advancement of Science; 2020:124-127.

19. Satherley R, Howard R, Higgs S. Disordered eating practices in gastrointestinal disorders. *Appetite*. 2015;84:240-250.

20. Barrett JS, Irving P, Shepherd SJ, Muir JG, Gibson PR. Comparison of the prevalence of fructose and lactose malab-sorption across chronic intestinal disorders. *Aliment Pharmacol Ther*. 2009;30(2):165-174.

21. Quezada-Calvillo R, Sim L, Ao Z, et al. Luminal starch substrate "brake" on maltase-glucoamylase activity is located within the glucoamylase subunit. *J Nutr*. 2008;138(4):685-692.

22. Simmer S, Chey WD, Eswaran SL, Ranagan J, Petrucelli S. Is Sucrase-Isomaltase Deficiency an Under-Recognized Cause of IBS-D Symptoms? *Gastroenterology*. 2018;154(6):S-867.

23. Faye A, Metz Y, Hartman B, Crawford CV, Scherl E. Salmonellosis in a patient on Natalizumab for ulcerative colitis and multiple sclerosis. *JSM*. 2016;4(1):1051.

24. Vermeire S, Van Assche G, Rutgeerts P. C-reactive protein as a marker for inflammatory bowel disease. *Inflamm Bowel Dis*. 2004;10(5):661-665.

25. Konikoff MR, Denson LA. Role of fecal calprotectin as a biomarker of intestinal inflammation in inflammatory bowel disease. *Inflamm Bowel Dis*. 2006;12(6):524-534.

26. Rolston VS, Boroujerdi L, Long MD, et al. The influence of hormonal fluctuation on inflammatory bowel disease symptom severity—a cross-sectional cohort study. *Inflamm Bowel Dis*. 2018;24(2):387-393.

27. Bharadwaj S, Kulkarni G, Shen B. Menstrual cycle, sex hormones in female inflammatory bowel disease patients with and without surgery. *J Dig Dis*. 2015;16(5):245-255.

28. Mahadevan U, Sandborn WJ, Li DK, Hakimian S, Kane S, Corley DA. Pregnancy outcomes in women with inflammatory bowel disease: a large community-based study from northern California. *Gastroenterology*. 2007;133(4):1106-1112.

29. Reddy D, Murphy SJ, Kane SV, Present DH, Kornbluth AA. Relapses of inflammatory bowel disease during pregnancy: in-hospital management and birth outcomes. *Am J Gastroenterol.* 2008;103(5):1203-1209.

30. Stephansson O, Larsson H, Pedersen L, et al. Congenital abnormalities and other birth outcomes in children born to women with ulcerative colitis in Denmark and Sweden. *Inflamm Bowel Dis.* 2011;17(3):795-801.

31. de Lima A, Zelinkova Z, Mulders AG, van der Woude CJ. Preconception care reduces relapse of inflammatory bowel disease during pregnancy. *Clin Gastroenterol Hepatol.* 2016;14(9):1285-1292. e1281.

32. Laine L, Kaltenbach T, Barkun A, et al. SCENIC international consensus statement on surveillance and management of dysplasia in inflammatory bowel disease. *Gastroenterology.* 2015;148(3):639-651. e628.

33. Cosnes J, Gower–Rousseau C, Seksik P, Cortot A. Epidemiology and natural history of inflammatory bowel diseases. *Gastroenterology.* 2011;140(6):1785-1794. e1784.

34. Dassopoulos T, Cohen RD, Scherl EJ, Schwartz RM, Kosinski L, Regueiro MD. Ulcerative colitis care pathway. *Gastroenterology.* 2015;149(1):238-245.

35. Bager P, Julsgaard M, Vestergaard T, Christensen LA, Dahlerup JF. Adherence and quality of care in IBD. *Scand J Gastroenterol.* 2016;51(11):1326-1331.

36. Armuzzi A, Riegler G, Furfaro F, et al. Epidemiological features and disease-related concerns of a large cohort of Italian patients with active Crohn's disease. *Dig Liver Dis.* 2019;51(6):804-811.

37. Greenley RN, Kunz JH, Walter J, Hommel KA. Practical strategies for enhancing adherence to treatment regimen in inflammatory bowel disease. *Inflamm Bowel Dis.* 2013;19(7):1534-1545.

38. Campos S, Portela F, Sousa P, Sofia C. Inflammatory bowel disease: adherence to immunomodulators in a biological therapy era. *Eur Gastroenterol Hepatol.* 2016;28(11):1313-1319.

39. Goodhand J, Kamperidis N, Sirwan B, et al. Factors associated with thiopurine non-adherence in patients with inflammatory bowel disease. *Aliment Pharmacol Ther.* 2013;38(9):1097-1108.

40. Siegel CA. Shared decision making in inflammatory bowel disease: helping patients understand the tradeoffs between treatment options. *Gut.* 2012;61(3):459-465.

41. Bernstein M, Graff L, Targownik L, et al. Gastrointestinal symptoms before and during menses in women with IBD. *Aliment Pharmacol Ther.* 2012;36(2):135-144.

42. Zapata LB, Paulen ME, Cansino C, Marchbanks PA, Curtis KM. Contraceptive use among women with inflammatory bowel disease: a systematic review. *Contraception.* 2010;82(1):72-85.

43. Rosenblatt E, Kane S. Sex-specific issues in inflammatory bowel disease. *Gastroenterol Hepatol.* 2015;11(9):592.

44. Preciado-Martínez E, García-Ruíz G, Flores-Espinosa P, et al. Progesterone suppresses the lipopolysaccharide-induced pro-inflammatory response in primary mononuclear cells isolated from human placental blood. *Immunol Invest.* 2018;47(2):181-195.

45. Nguyen GC, Boudreau H, Harris ML, Maxwell CV. Outcomes of obstetric hospitalizations among women with inflammatory bowel disease in the United States. *Clin Gastroenterol Hepatol.* 2009;7(3):329-334.

46. Obstetricians ACo, Gynecologists. Thromboembolism in pregnancy. ACOG practice bulletin. 2011;19.

47. Papa A, Gerardi V, Marzo M, Felice C, Rapaccini GL, Gasbarrini A. Venous thromboembolism in patients with inflammatory bowel disease: focus on prevention and treatment. *World J Gastroenterol.* 2014;20(12):3173.

48. Hansen AT, Erichsen R, Horváth-Puhó E, Sørensen HT. Inflammatory bowel disease and venous thromboembolism during pregnancy and the postpartum period. *J Thromb Haemost.* 2017;15(4):702-708.

49. Safety trial finds risk of blood clots in the lungs and death with higher dose of tofacitinib (Xeljanz, Xeljanz XR) in rheumatoid arthritis patients; FDA to investigate. In: Communication FDS, ed: U.S. Food and Drug Administration; 2019.

50. Dacha S, Devidi M, Osmundson E. Budd-Chiari syndrome in a patient with ulcerative colitis and no inherited coagulopathy. *World J Hepatol.* 2011;3(6):164.

51. Mahadevan U, Kane S. American Gastroenterological Association Institute medical position statement on the use of gastrointestinal medications in pregnancy. *Gastroenterology.* 2006;131(1):278-282.

52. Mahadevan U, Robinson C, Bernasko N, et al. Special report inflammatory bowel disease in pregnancy clinical care pathway: a report from the American Gastroenterological Association IBD Parenthood Project Working Group. 2019;156(5):1508-1524

53. Bell CM, Habal FM. Safety of topical 5-aminosalicylic acid in pregnancy. *Am J Gastroenterol.* 1997;92(12).

54. Lichtenstein GR, Sandborn WJ, Kamm MA, Barrett K, Joseph RE. MMX Mesalamine, a Novel Formulation of 5-ASA, Effectively Induces the Remission of Active Mild-to-Moderate Ulcerative Colitis in Men and Women: 1103. *Am J Gastroenterol.* 2006;101:S432.

55. Blumenstein I, Bock H, Zosel C, et al. Are there gender-related differences in the therapeutic management of patients suffering from inflammatory bowel disease? Subgroup analysis of a prospective multicentre online-based trial. *Z Gastroenterol.* 2009;47(10):1045-1051.

56. Kane SV, Cohen RD, Aikens JE, Hanauer SB. Prevalence of nonadherence with maintenance mesalamine in quiescent ulcerative colitis. *Am J Gastroenterol.* 2001;96(10):2929-2933.

57.  Ali T, Lam D, Bronze MS, Humphrey MB. Osteoporosis in inflammatory bowel disease. *Am J Med.* 2009;122(7):599-604.

58.  Compston J, Judd D, Crawley E, et al. Osteoporosis in patients with inflammatory bowel disease. *Gut.* 1987;28(4):410-415.

59.  Vestergaard P, Rejnmark L, Mosekilde L. Fracture risk associated with different types of oral corticosteroids and effect of termination of corticosteroids on the risk of fractures. *Calcif Tissue Int.* 2008;82(4):249-257.

60.  Schoon EJ, Bollani S, Mills PR, et al. Bone mineral density in relation to efficacy and side effects of budesonide and prednisolone in Crohn's disease. *Clin Gastroenterol Hepatol.* 2005;3(2):113-121.

61.  Quick VM, Byrd-Bredbenner C, Neumark-Sztainer D. Chronic illness and disordered eating: a discussion of the literature. *Adv Nutr.* 2013;4(3):277-286.

62.  Bayle F, Bouvard M. Anorexia nervosa and Crohn's disease dual diagnosis: a case study. *Eur Psychiatry.* 2003;18(8):421-422.

63.  Wabich J, Bellaguarda E, Joyce C, Keefer L, Kinsinger S. Disordered eating, body dissatisfaction, and psychological distress in patients with inflammatory bowel disease (IBD). *J Clin Psychol Med Settings.* 2020:1-8.

64.  Rathbun KM, Singhal M. Addisonian crisis. In: StatPearls [Internet]. StatPearls Publishing; 2019.

65.  Scherl EJ. The "other steroid". In: *Women's Health Advisor.* Vol 8. NY Weill Medical College of Cornell University; 2004:1-7.

66.  Connell WR, Kamm MA, Ritchie J, Lennard-Jones J, Dickson M, Balkwill A. Long-term neoplasia risk after aza-thioprine treatment in inflammatory bowel disease. *Lancet.* 1994;343(8908):1249-1252.

67.  Hutfless S, Fireman B, Kane S, Herrinton L. Screening differences and risk of cervical cancer in inflammatory bowel disease. *Aliment Pharmacol Ther.* 2008;28(5):598-605.

68.  Bhatia J, Bratcher J, Korelitz B, et al. Abnormalities of uterine cervix in women with inflammatory bowel disease. *World J Gastroenterol.* 2006;12(38):6167.

69.  Lees C, Critchley J, Chee N, et al. Lack of association between cervical dysplasia and IBD: a large case–control study. *Inflamm Bowel Dis.* 2009;15(11):1621-1629.

70.  Gómez-García M, Cabello-Tapia MJ, Sánchez-Capilla AD, De Teresa-Galván J, Redondo-Cerezo E. Thiopurines related malignancies in inflammatory bowel disease: local experience in Granada, Spain. *World J Gastroenterol.* 2013;19(30):4877.

71.  Axelrad J, Colombel J, Scherl E, et al. P729 The SAPPHIRE registry: Safety of immunosuppression in a prospec-tive cohort of inflammatory bowel disease patients with a HIstoRy of CancEr. *J Crohns Colitis.* 2020;14(Suppl 1):S585-S587.

72.  Axelrad J, Bernheim O, Colombel J-F, et al. Risk of new or recurrent cancer in patients with inflammatory bowel dis-ease and previous cancer exposed to immunosuppressive and anti-tumor necrosis factor agents. *Clin Gastroenterol Hepatol.* 2016;14(1):58-64.

73.  Mantzaris GJ, Roussos A, Kalantzis C, Koilakou S, Raptis N, Kalantzis N. How adherent to treatment with azathio-prine are patients with Crohn's disease in long-term remission? *Inflamm Bowel Dis.* 2007;13(4):446-450.

74.  Mahadevan U, McConnell RA, Chambers CD. Drug safety and risk of adverse outcomes for pregnant patients with inflammatory bowel disease. *Gastroenterology.* 2017;152(2):451-462. e452.

75.  Tripathi K, Feuerstein JD. New developments in ulcerative colitis: latest evidence on management, treatment, and maintenance. *Drugs Context.* 2019;8:212572.

76.  Verden A, Dimbil M, Kyle R, Overstreet B, Hoffman KB. Analysis of spontaneous postmarket case reports submit-ted to the FDA regarding thromboembolic adverse events and JAK inhibitors. *Drug Saf.* 2018;41(4):357-361.

77.  Sandborn WJ, Panés J, Sands BE, et al. Venous thromboembolic events in the tofacitinib ulcerative colitis clinical development programme. *Aliment Pharmacol Ther.* 2019;50(10):1068-1076.

78.  Sandborn WJ, Peyrin-Biroulet L, Zhang J, et al. Efficacy and safety of etrasimod in a phase 2 randomized trial of patients with ulcerative colitis. *Gastroenterology.* 2020;158(3):550-561.

79.  Vermeire S, Schreiber S, Petryka R, et al. Clinical remission in patients with moderate-to-severe Crohn's disease treated with filgotinib (the FITZROY study): results from a phase 2, double-blind, randomised, placebo-controlled trial. *Lancet.* 2017;389(10066):266-275.

80.  Panaccione R, D'Haens GR, Sandborn WJ, et al. 799–Efficacy of Upadacitinib as an induction therapy for patients with moderately to severely active ulcerative colitis, with or without previous treatment failure of biologic therapy: data from the dose-ranging phase 2B study U-Achieve. *Gastroenterology.* 2019;156(6):S-170.

81.  Panaccione R, Atreya R, Ferrante M, et al. Sa1758-Upadacitinib improves steroid-free clinical and endoscopic end-points in patients with Crohn's disease: data from the celest study. *Gastroenterology.* 2018;154(6):S-384.

82.  Colombel JF, Sandborn WJ, Reinisch W, et al. Infliximab, azathioprine, or combination therapy for Crohn's disease. *N Engl J Med.* 2010;362(15):1383-1395.

83.  Ternant D, Aubourg A, Magdelaine-Beuzelin C, et al. Infliximab pharmacokinetics in inflammatory bowel disease patients. *Ther Drug Monit.* 2008;30(4):523-529.

84. Santos CHMd. Analysis of the factors related to anti-TNF alpha response in the treatment of Crohn's disease. *J Coloproctol.* 2014;34(1):14-18.

85. Scherl EJ, Seidman EG, Wolf DC. Predicting outcomes and tailoring therapy in the diagnosis and treatment of IBD. *Gastroenterol Hepatol.* 2007;3(12 36):1.

86. Laganà B, Zullo A, Scribano ML, et al. Sex differences in response to TNF-inhibiting drugs in patients with spondyloarthropathies or inflammatory bowel diseases. *Front Pharmacol.* 2019;10.

87. Olivera P, Thiriet L, Luc A, Baumann C, Danese S, Peyrin-Biroulet L. Treatment persistence for infliximab versus adalimumab in Crohn's disease: a 14-Year single-center experience. *Inflamm Bowel Dis.* 2017;23(6):976-985.

88. Zelinkova Z, Bultman E, Vogelaar L, Bouziane C, Kuipers EJ, van der Woude CJ. Sex-dimorphic adverse drug reactions to immune suppressive agents in inflammatory bowel disease. *World J Gastroenterol.* 2012;18(47):6967.

89. Tanaka H, Kamata N, Yamada A, et al. Long-term retention of adalimumab treatment and associated prognostic factors for 1189 patients with Crohn's disease. *J Gastroenterol Hepatol.* 2018;33(5):1031-1038.

90. Lördal M, Cars T, Wettermark B. Sa1118 Gender differences of IBD care in the healthcare region of Stockholm. *Gastroenterology.* 2014;146(5):S-204.

91. Mourabet ME, El-Hachem S, Harrison JR, Binion DG. Anti-TNF antibody therapy for inflammatory bowel disease during pregnancy: a clinical review. *Curr Drug Targets.* 2010;11(2):234-241.

92. Osterman MT, Sandborn WJ, Colombel J-F, et al. Increased risk of malignancy with adalimumab combination therapy, compared with monotherapy, for Crohn's disease. *Gastroenterology.* 2014;146(4):941-949. e942.

93. Ghosh S, Goldin E, Gordon FH, et al. Natalizumab for active Crohn's disease. *N Engl J Med.* 2003;348(1):24-32.

94. Feagan BG, Rutgeerts P, Sands BE, et al. Vedolizumab as induction and maintenance therapy for ulcerative colitis. *N Engl J Med.* 2013;369(8):699-710.

95. Sandborn WJ, Feagan BG, Rutgeerts P, et al. Vedolizumab as induction and maintenance therapy for Crohn's disease. *N Engl J Med.* 2013;369(8):711-721.

96. Schneider A-M, Weghuber D, Hetzer B, et al. Vedolizumab use after failure of TNF-α antagonists in children and adolescents with inflammatory bowel disease. *BMC Gastroenterol.* 2018;18(1):140.

97. Sager R, Frei P, Steiner UC, Fink D, Betschart C. Genital dysplasia and immunosuppression: why organ-specific therapy is important. *Inflamm Intest Dis.* 2019;4(4):154-160.

98. Hoffmann P, Krisam J, Wehling C, et al. Ustekinumab:"Real-world" outcomes and potential predictors of nonresponse in treatment-refractory Crohn's disease. *World J Gastroenterol.* 2019;25(31):4481.

99. Park SC, Jeen YT. Anti-integrin therapy for inflammatory bowel disease. *World J Gastroenterol.* 2018;24(17):1868.

100. Blauvelt A, Leonardi CL, Gooderham M, et al. Efficacy and safety of continuous risankizumab therapy vs treatment withdrawal in patients with moderate to severe plaque psoriasis: a phase 3 randomized clinical trial. *JAMA Dermatol.* 2020.

101. Peyrin-Biroulet L, Christopher R, Behan D, Lassen C. Modulation of sphingosine-1-phosphate in inflammatory bowel disease. *Autoimmun Rev.* 2017;16(5):495-503.

102. R Irhimeh M, Cooney J. Management of inflammatory bowel disease using stem cell therapy. *Curr Stem Cell Res Ther.* 2016;11(1):72-77.

103. Cho YB, Park KJ, Yoon SN, et al. Long-term results of adipose-derived stem cell therapy for the treatment of Crohn's fistula. *Stem Cells Transl Med.* 2015;4(5):532-537.

104. Lee WY, Park KJ, Cho YB, et al. Autologous adipose tissue-derived stem cells treatment demonstrated favorable and sustainable therapeutic effect for Crohn's fistula. *Stem Cells.* 2013;31(11):2575-2581.

105. Dietz AB, Dozois EJ, Fletcher JG, et al. Autologous mesenchymal stem cells, applied in a bioabsorbable matrix, for treatment of perianal fistulas in patients with Crohn's disease. *Gastroenterology.* 2017;153(1):59-62. e52.

106. Lightner AL, Dozois EJ, Dietz AB, et al. Matrix-delivered autologous mesenchymal stem cell therapy for refractory rectovaginal Crohn's fistulas. *Inflamm Bowel Dis.* 2020;26(5):670-677.

107. Sanz-Baro R, García-Arranz M, Guadalajara H, de la Quintana P, Herreros MD, García-Olmo D. First-in-human case study: pregnancy in women with Crohn's perianal fistula treated with adipose-derived stem cells: a safety study. *Stem Cells Transl Med.* 2015;4(6):598-602.

108. Ledder O, Turner D. Antibiotics in IBD: still a role in the biological era? *Inflamm Bowel Dis.* 2018;24(8):1676-1688.

109. Cohen D. *Quench: Beat Fatigue, Drop Weight, and Heal Your Body Through the New Science of Optimum Hydration.* Hachette Books; 2019.

110. Burr NE, Smith C, West R, Hull MA, Subramanian V. Increasing prescription of opiates and mortality in patients with inflammatory bowel diseases in England. *Clin Gastroenterol Hepatol.* 2018;16(4):534-541. e536.

111. Hirsch A, Yarur AJ, Dezheng H, et al. Penetrating disease, narcotic use, and loop ostomy are associated with ostomy and IBD-related complications after ostomy surgery in Crohn's disease patients. *J Gastrointest Surg.* 2015;19(10):1852-1861.

112. Lichtenstein GR, Feagan BG, Cohen RD, et al. Serious infection and mortality in patients with Crohn's disease: more than 5 years of follow-up in the TREAT™ registry. *Am J Gastroenterol.* 2012;107(9):1409.

113. Dalal RS, Palchaudhuri S, Snider CK, Lewis JD, Mehta SJ, Lichtenstein GR. Exposure to intravenous opioids is associated with future exposure to opioids in hospitalized patients with inflammatory bowel diseases. *Clin Gastroenterol Hepatol*. 2019.

114. Targownik LE, Nugent Z, Singh H, Bugden S, Bernstein CN. The prevalence and predictors of opioid use in inflammatory bowel disease: a population-based analysis. *Am J Gastroenterol*. 2014;109(10):1613-1620.

115. Hanson KA, Loftus Jr EV, Harmsen WS, Diehl NN, Zinsmeister AR, Sandborn WJ. Clinical features and outcome of patients with inflammatory bowel disease who use narcotics: a case–control study. *Inflamm Bowel Dis*. 2009;15(5):772-777.

116. Felder JB, Korelitz BI, Rajapakse R, Schwarz S, Horatagis AP, Gleim G. Effects of nonsteroidal antiinflammatory drugs on inflammatory bowel disease: a case-control study. *Am J Gastroenterol*. 2000;95(8):1949-1954.

117. O'Neill GP, Ford-Hutchinson AW. Expression of mRNA for cyclooxygenase-1 and cyclooxygenase-2 in human tissues. *FEBS Letters*. 1993;330(2):157-160.

118. Flemstrom G. Stimulation of HCO3-transport in isolated proximal bullfrog duodenum by prostaglandins. *Am J Physiol*. 1980;239(3):G198-G203.

119. Elisa Petrini M, Anna Greco M, Rinaldo Pellicano M. Coxib safety in patients with inflammatory bowel diseases: a meta-analysis. *Pain Physician*. 2015;18:599-607.

120. Takeuchi K, Smale S, Premchand P, et al. Prevalence and mechanism of nonsteroidal anti-inflammatory drug–induced clinical relapse in patients with inflammatory bowel disease. *Clin Gastroenterol Hepatol*. 2006;4(2):196-202.

121. Ananthakrishnan AN, Higuchi LM, Huang ES, et al. Aspirin, nonsteroidal anti-inflammatory drug use, and risk for Crohn disease and ulcerative colitis: a cohort study. *Ann Intern Med*. 2012;156(5):350-359.

122. Bernstein CN, Singh S, Graff LA, Walker JR, Miller N, Cheang M. A prospective population-based study of triggers of symptomatic flares in IBD. *Am J Gastroenterol*. 2010;105(9):1994-2002.

123. Lie MR, van der Giessen J, Fuhler GM, et al. Low dose Naltrexone for induction of remission in inflammatory bowel disease patients. *J Transl Med*. 2018;16(1):55.

124. Lie M, Fuhler G, de Lima A, van der Ent C, van der Woude C. P418 Low dose naltrexone in therapy resistant IBD, a case series. *J Crohns Colitis*. 2014(8):S240.

125. Parker CE, Nguyen TM, Segal D, MacDonald JK, Chande N. Low dose naltrexone for induction of remission in Crohn's disease. *Cochrane Database of Systematic Reviews*. 2018;4(4):CD010410.

126. Katchan V, David P, Shoenfeld Y. Cannabinoids and autoimmune diseases: a systematic review. *Autoimmun Rev*. 2016;15(6):513-528.

127. Massa F, Marsicano G, Hermann H, et al. The endogenous cannabinoid system protects against colonic inflammation. *J Clin Invest*. 2004;113(8):1202-1209.

128. Ahmed W, Katz S. Therapeutic use of cannabis in inflammatory bowel disease. *Gastroenterol Hepatol*. 2016;12(11):668.

129. Naftali T, Schleider LB-L, Dotan I, Lansky EP, Benjaminov FS, Konikoff FM. Cannabis induces a clinical response in patients with Crohn's disease: a prospective placebo-controlled study. *Clin Gastroenterol Hepatol*. 2013;11(10):1276-1280. e1271.

130. Lahat A, Lang A, Ben-Horin S. Impact of cannabis treatment on the quality of life, weight and clinical disease activity in inflammatory bowel disease patients: a pilot prospective study. *Digestion*. 2012;85(1):1-8.

131. Naftali T, Lev LB, Yablecovitch D, Half E, Konikoff FM. Treatment of Crohn's disease with cannabis: an observational study. *Isr Med Assoc J*. 2011;13(8):455-458.

132. Brents LK. Focus: sex and gender health: marijuana, the endocannabinoid system and the female reproductive system. *Yale J Biol Med*. 2016;89(2):175.

133. Yao J, He Q, Liu M, et al. Effects of Δ (9)-tetrahydrocannabinol (THC) on human amniotic epithelial cell proliferation and migration. *Toxicology*. 2018;394:19-26.

134. Almada M, Amaral C, Diniz-da-Costa M, Correia-da-Silva G, Teixeira N, Fonseca B. The endocannabinoid anandamide impairs in vitro decidualization of human cells. *Reproduction*. 2016;152(4):351-361.

135. Swaminath A, Berlin EP, Cheifetz A, et al. The role of cannabis in the management of inflammatory bowel disease: a review of clinical, scientific, and regulatory informationcommissioned by the Crohn's and colitis foundation. *Inflamm Bowel Dis*. 2019;25(3):427-435.

136. Practice CoO. Committee opinion No. 722: marijuana use during pregnancy and lactation. *Obstet Gynecol*. 2017;130(4):e205.

137. Herrmann ES, Weerts EM, Vandrey R. Sex differences in cannabis withdrawal symptoms among treatment-seeking cannabis users. *Exp Clin Psychopharmacol*. 2015;23(6):415.

138. Hanai H, Sugimoto K. Curcumin has bright prospects for the treatment of inflammatory bowel disease. *Curr Pharm Des*. 2009;15(18):2087-2094.

139. Holt P, Katz S, la Therapie Kirshoff R. kurkumin v vnetne črevesne bolezni. *Pilotna študija Dig Dis Sci*. 2005;50(11): 2191.3.

140. Lang A, Salomon N, Wu JC, et al. Curcumin in combination with mesalamine induces remission in patients with mild-to-moderate ulcerative colitis in a randomized controlled trial. *Clin Gastroenterol Hepatol.* 2015;13(8):1444-1449. e1441.

141. Tahan G, Aytac E, Aytekin H, et al. Vitamin E has a dual effect of anti-inflammatory and antioxidant activities in acetic acid–induced ulcerative colitis in rats. *Can J Surg.* 2011;54(5):333.

142. Bostick RM, Potter JD, McKenzie DR, et al. Reduced risk of colon cancer with high intake of vitamin E: the Iowa Women's Health Study. *Cancer Res.* 1993;53(18):4230-4237.

143. Sorice A, Guerriero E, Capone F, Colonna G, Castello G, Costantini S. Ascorbic acid: its role in immune system and chronic inflammation diseases. *Mini Rev Med Chem.* 2014;14(5):444-452.

144. Yan H, Wang H, Zhang X, Li X, Yu J. Ascorbic acid ameliorates oxidative stress and inflammation in dextran sulfate sodium-induced ulcerative colitis in mice. *Int J Clin Exp Med.* 2015;8(11):20245.

145. Aghdassi E, Wendland BE, Steinhart AH, Wolman SL, Jeejeebhoy K, Allard JP. Antioxidant vitamin supplementation in Crohn's disease decreases oxidative stress: a randomized controlled trial. *Am J Gastroenterol.* 2003;98(2):348-353.

146. Linaker B. Scurvy and vitamin C deficiency in Crohn's disease. *Postgraduate medical journal.* 1979;55(639):26-29.

147. Subramanian VS, Sabui S, Subramenium GA, Marchant JS, Said HM. Tumor necrosis factor alpha reduces intestinal vitamin C uptake: a role for NF-κB-mediated signaling. *Am J of Physiol.* 2018;315(2):G241-G248.

148. Ulitsky A, Ananthakrishnan AN, Naik A, et al. Vitamin D deficiency in patients with inflammatory bowel disease: association with disease activity and quality of life. *JPEN J Parenter Enteral Nutr.* 2011;35(3):308-316.

149. Fu Y-TN, Chatur N, Cheong-Lee C, Salh B. Hypovitaminosis D in adults with inflammatory bowel disease: potential role of ethnicity. *Dig Dis Sci.* 2012;57(8):2144-2148.

150. Harries A, Brown R, Heatley R, Williams L, Woodhead S, Rhodes J. Vitamin D status in Crohn's disease: association with nutrition and disease activity. *Gut.* 1985;26(11):1197-1203.

151. Xue LN, Xu KQ, Zhang W, Wang Q, Wu J, Wang XY. Associations between vitamin D receptor polymorphisms and susceptibility to ulcerative colitis and Crohn's disease: A meta-analysis. *Inflamm Bowel Dis.* 2012.

152. Jørgensen SP, Hvas CL, Agnholt J, Christensen LA, Heickendorff L, Dahlerup JF. Active Crohn's disease is associated with low vitamin D levels. *J Crohns Colitis.* 2013;7(10):e407-e413.

153. Ananthakrishnan AN, Cagan A, Gainer VS, et al. Higher plasma vitamin D is associated with reduced risk of Clostridium difficile infection in patients with inflammatory bowel diseases. *Aliment Pharmacol Ther.* 2014;39(10):1136-1142.

154. Raman M, Milestone AN, Walters JR, Hart AL, Ghosh S. Vitamin D and gastrointestinal diseases: inflammatory bowel disease and colorectal cancer. *Therap Adv Gastroenterol.* 2011;4(1):49-62.

155. Zhang Y, Leung DY, Richers BN, et al. Vitamin D inhibits monocyte/macrophage proinflammatory cytokine production by targeting MAPK phosphatase-1. *J Immunol.* 2012;188(5):2127-2135.

156. Farraye FA, Melmed GY, Lichtenstein GR, Kane SV. ACG clinical guideline: preventive care in inflammatory bowel disease. *Am J Gastroenterol.* 2017;112(2):241-258.

157. Bitiren M, Karakilcik AZ, Zerin M, et al. Protective effects of selenium and vitamin E combination on experimental colitis in blood plasma and colon of rats. *Biol Trace Elem Res.* 2010;136(1):87-95.

158. Barollo M, Medici V, D'Incà R, et al. Antioxidative potential of a combined therapy of anti TNFα and Zn acetate in experimental colitis. *World J Gastroenterol.* 2011;17(36):4099.

159. Fritz J, Walia C, Elkadri A, et al. A systematic review of micronutrient deficiencies in pediatric inflammatory bowel disease. *Inflamm Bowel Dis.* 2019;25(3):445-459.

160. Weisshof R, Chermesh I. Micronutrient deficiencies in inflammatory bowel disease. *Curr Opin Clin Nutr Metab Care.* 2015;18(6):576-581.

161. Siva S, Rubin DT, Gulotta G, Wroblewski K, Pekow J. Zinc deficiency is associated with poor clinical outcomes in patients with inflammatory bowel disease. *Inflamm Bowel Dis.* 2017;23(1):152-157.

162. Langmead L, Makins R, Rampton D. Anti-inflammatory effects of aloe vera gel in human colorectal mucosa in vitro. *Aliment Pharmacol Ther.* 2004;19(5):521-527.

163. Langmead L, Feakins R, Goldthorpe S, et al. Randomized, double-blind, placebo-controlled trial of oral aloe vera gel for active ulcerative colitis. *Aliment Pharmacol Ther.* 2004;19(7):739-747.

164. Foster M, Hunter D, Samman S. Evaluation of the nutritional and metabolic effects of Aloe vera. Vol 3: chapter; 2011.

165. Kulkarni SD, Tilak JC, Acharya R, Rajurkar NS, Devasagayam T, Reddy A. Evaluation of the antioxidant activity of wheatgrass (Triticum aestivum L.) as a function of growth under different conditions. *Phytother Res.* 2006;20(3):218-227.

166. Nicholas C, Batra S, Vargo MA, et al. Apigenin blocks lipopolysaccharide-induced lethality in vivo and proinflammatory cytokines expression by inactivating NF-κB through the suppression of p65 phosphorylation. *J Immunol.* 2007;179(10):7121-7127.

167. Ben-Arye E, Goldin E, Wengrower D, Stamper A, Kohn R, Berry E. Wheat grass juice in the treatment of active distal ulcerative colitis: a randomized double-blind placebo-controlled trial. *Scand J Gastroenterol.* 2002;37(4):444-449.

168. Whiting CV, Bland PW, Tarlton JF. Dietary n-3 polyunsaturated fatty acids reduce disease and colonic proinflammatory cytokines in a mouse model of colitis. *Inflamm Bowel Dis.* 2005;11(4):340-349.

169. Belluzzi A, Brignola C, Campieri M, Pera A, Boschi S, Miglioli M. Effect of an enteric-coated fish-oil preparation on relapses in Crohn's disease. *N Engl J Med.* 1996;334(24):1557-1560.

170. Feagan B, Sandborn W, Mittmann U, Ulitsky A. Omega-3 free fatty acids for the maintenance of remission in Crohn disease: the EPIC randomized controlled trials. *Nutr Clin Pract.* 2009;24(1):102.

171. Ananthakrishnan AN, Khalili H, Konijeti GG, et al. Long-term intake of dietary fat and risk of ulcerative colitis and Crohn's disease. *Gut.* 2014;63(5):776-784.

172. Scheppach W, Sommer H, Kirchner T, et al. Effect of butyrate enemas on the colonic mucosa in distal ulcerative colitis. *Gastroenterology.* 1992;103(1):51-56.

173. Rodríguez-Cabezas ME, Galvez J, Lorente MD, et al. Dietary fiber down-regulates colonic tumor necrosis factor α and nitric oxide production in trinitrobenzenesulfonic acid-induced colitic rats. *J Nutr.* 2002;132(11):3263-3271.

174. Lührs H, Gerke T, Müller J, et al. Butyrate inhibits NF-κB activation in lamina propria macrophages of patients with ulcerative colitis. *Scand J Gastroenterol.* 2002;37(4):458-466.

175. Harig JM, Soergel KH, Komorowski RA, Wood CM. Treatment of diversion colitis with short-chain-fatty acid irrigation. *N Engl J Med.* 1989;320(1):23-28.

176. Vernia P, Fracasso P, Casale V, et al. Topical butyrate for acute radiation proctitis: randomised, crossover trial. *Lancet.* 2000;356(9237):1232-1235.

177. Hamer HM, Jonkers DM, Vanhoutvin SA, et al. Effect of butyrate enemas on inflammation and antioxidant status in the colonic mucosa of patients with ulcerative colitis in remission. *Clin Nutr.* 2010;29(6):738-744.

178. Ng S, Lam Y, Tsoi K, Chan F, Sung J, Wu J. Systematic review: the efficacy of herbal therapy in inflammatory bowel disease. *Aliment Pharmacol Ther.* 2013;38(8):854-863.

179. Greenfield S, Green A, Teare J, et al. A randomized controlled study of evening primrose oil and fish oil in ulcerative colitis. *Aliment Pharmacol Ther.* 1993;7(2):159-166.

180. Mahboubi M. Evening primrose (Oenothera biennis) oil in management of female ailments. *J Menopausal Med.* 2019;25(2):74-82.

181. Kane SV, Dubinsky MC. Pocket guide to inflammatory bowel disease. Cambridge University Press; 2005.

182. Qazi T, Farraye FA. Sleep and inflammatory bowel disease: an important bi-directional relationship. *Inflamm Bowel Dis.* 2019;25(5):843-852.

183. Gerberg PL, Jacob VE, Stevens L, et al. The effect of breathing, movement, and meditation on psychological and physical symptoms and inflammatory biomarkers in inflammatory bowel disease: a randomized controlled trial. *Inflamm Bowel Dis.* 2015;21(12):2886-2896.

184. Brustolim D, Ribeiro-dos-Santos R, Kast R, Altschuler E, Soares MBP. A new chapter opens in anti-inflammatory treatments: the antidepressant bupropion lowers production of tumor necrosis factor-alpha and interferon-gamma in mice. *Int Immunopharmacol.* 2006;6(6):903-907.

185. Kast RE, Altschuler EL. Remission of Crohn's disease on bupropion. *Gastroenterology.* 2001;121(5):1260-1261.

186. Kast R, Altschuler E. Bone density loss in Crohn's disease: role of TNF and potential for prevention by bupropion. *Gut.* 2004;53(7):1056-1056.

187. Kane SV, Altschuler EL, Kast RE. Crohn's disease remission on bupropion. *Gastroenterology.* 2003;125(4):1290.

188. Ryan E, McNicholas D, Creavin B, Kelly ME, Walsh T, Beddy D. Sarcopenia and inflammatory bowel disease: a systematic review. *Inflamm Bowel Dis.* 2019;25(1):67-73.

189. Bryant R, Ooi S, Schultz C, et al. Low muscle mass and sarcopenia: common and predictive of osteopenia in inflammatory bowel disease. *Aliment Pharmacol Ther.* 2015;41(9):895-906.

190. DeFilippis E, Webb C, Warren R, Tabani S, Bosworth B, Scherl E. low muscle mass and disordered eating as causes of osteopenia in inflammatory bowel disease. *Aliment Pharmacol Ther.* 2015;41(12):1303-1304.

191. Vollebregt P, van Bodegraven A, Markus-de Kwaadsteniet T, van der Horst D, Felt-Bersma R. Impacts of perianal disease and faecal incontinence on quality of life and employment in 1092 patients with inflammatory bowel disease. *Aliment Pharmacol Ther.* 2018;47(9):1253-1260.

192. Papathanasopoulos AA, Katsanos KH, Tatsioni A, Christodoulou DK, Tsianos EV. Increased fatigability of external anal sphincter in inflammatory bowel disease: significance in fecal urgency and incontinence. *Journal of Crohn's and Colitis.* 2010;4(5):553-560.

193. Khera AJ, Chase JW, Salzberg M, Thompson AJ, Kamm MA. Gut-directed pelvic floor behavioral treatment for fecal incontinence and constipation in patients with inflammatory bowel disease. *Inflamm Bowel Dis.* 2019;25(3):620-626.

194. Bilski J, Mazur-Bialy A, Brzozowski B, et al. Can exercise affect the course of inflammatory bowel disease? experimental and clinical evidence. *Pharmacol Rep.* 2016;68(4):827-836.

195. Moreira LDF, Oliveira MLd, Lirani-Galvão AP, Marin-Mio RV, Santos RNd, Lazaretti-Castro M. Physical exercise and osteoporosis: effects of different types of exercises on bone and physical function of postmenopausal women. *Arq Bras Endocrinol Metabol.* 2014;58(5):514-522.

196. Monda V, Villano I, Messina A, et al. Exercise modifies the gut microbiota with positive health effects. *Oxid Med Cell Longev.* 2017;2017.

197. Peters H, De Vries W, Vanberge-Henegouwen G, Akkermans L. Potential benefits and hazards of physical activity and exercise on the gastrointestinal tract. *Gut.* 2001;48(3):435-439.

198. DeFilippis EM, Tabani S, Warren RU, Christos PJ, Bosworth BP, Scherl EJ. Exercise and self-reported limitations in patients with inflammatory bowel disease. *Dig Dis Sci.* 2016;61(1):215-220.

199. Eckert KG, Abbasi-Neureither I, Köppel M, Huber G. Structured physical activity interventions as a complementary therapy for patients with inflammatory bowel disease–a scoping review and practical implications. *BMC Gastroenterol.* 2019;19(1):115.

200. Sharma P, Poojary G, Dwivedi SN, Deepak KK. Effect of yoga-based intervention in patients with inflammatory bowel disease. *Int J Yoga Ther.* 2015;25(1):101-112.

201. Midha V, Makharia G, Ahuja V, Goswami P. The probiotic preparation, VSL# 3 induces remission in patients with mild-to-moderately active ulcerative colitis. *Clin Gastroenterol Hepatol.* 2009;7(11):1202-1209.

202. Gionchetti P, Rizzello F, Morselli C, et al. High-dose probiotics for the treatment of active pouchitis. *Dis Colon Rectum.* 2007;50(12):2075-2084.

203. Gionchetti P, Rizzello F, Helwig U, et al. Prophylaxis of pouchitis onset with probiotic therapy: a double-blind, placebo-controlled trial. *Gastroenterology.* 2003;124(5):1202-1209.

204. Losurdo G, Iannone A, Contaldo A, Ierardi E, Di Leo A, Principi M. Escherichia coli Nissle 1917 in ulcerative colitis treatment: systematic review and meta-analysis. *J Gastrointestin Liver Dis.* 2015;24(4):499-505.

205. Sokol H, Landman C, Seksik P, et al. Fecal microbiota transplantation to maintain remission in Crohn's disease: a pilot randomized controlled study. *Microbiome.* 2020;8(1):1-14.

206. York A. FMT in the clinic. *Nat Rev Microbiol.* 2019;17(3):127.

207. Tu Y. The discovery of artemisinin (qinghaosu) and gifts from Chinese medicine. *Nat Med.* 2011;17(10):1217-1220.

208. Krishna S, Bustamante L, Haynes RK, Staines HM. Artemisinins: their growing importance in medicine. *Trends Pharmacol Sci.* 2008;29(10):520-527.

209. Sun W, Han X, Wu S, Wu J, Yang C, Li X. Unexpected mechanism of colitis amelioration by artesunate, a natural product from Artemisia annua L. *Inflammopharmacology.* 2019:1-18.

210. Krebs S, Omer TN, Omer B. Wormwood (Artemisia absinthium) suppresses tumour necrosis factor alpha and accelerates healing in patients with Crohn's disease–a controlled clinical trial. *Phytomedicine.* 2010;17(5):305-309.

211. Goenka M, Kochhar R, Tandia B, Mehta S. Chloroquine for mild to moderately active ulcerative colitis: comparison with sulfasalazine. *Am J Gastroenterol.* 1996;91(5):917-921.

212. Borden MB, Parke AL. Antimalarial drugs in systemic lupus erythematosus: use in pregnancy. *Drug safety.* 2001;24(14):1055-1063.

213. Østensen M, Khamashta M, Lockshin M, et al. Anti-inflammatory and immunosuppressive drugs and reproduction. *Arthritis Res Ther.* 2006;8(3):209.

214. Wolfe MS, Cordero JF. Safety of chloroquine in chemosuppression of malaria during pregnancy. *Br Med J (Clin Res Ed).* 1985;290(6480):1466-1467.

215. Dunlop D, Soukop M, McEwan H. Antenatal administration of aminopropylidene diphosphonate. *Ann Rheum Dis.* 1990;49(11):955.

216. Levy M, Buskila D, Gladman DD, Urowitz MB, Koren G. Pregnancy outcome following first trimester exposure to chloroquine. *Am J Perinatol.* 1991;8(03):174-178.

217. Parke A. Antimalarial drugs, systemic lupus erythematosus and pregnancy. *J Rheum.* 1988;15(4):607-610.

218. Costedoat-Chalumeau N, Amoura Z, Duhaut P, et al. Safety of hydroxychloroquine in pregnant patients with connective tissue diseases: a study of one hundred thirty-three cases compared with a control group. *Arthritis Rheum.* 2003;48(11):3207-3211.

219. Hemphill A, Mueller J, Esposito M. Nitazoxanide, a broad-spectrum thiazolide anti-infective agent for the treatment of gastrointestinal infections. *Expert Opin Pharmacother.* 2006;7(7):953-964.

220. Smith S, Shaw J, Nathwani D. Nitazoxanide for cryptosporidial infection in Crohn's disease. *Gut.* 2008;57(8):1179-1180.

221. Elliott DE, Urban Jr JF, Argo CK, Weinstock JV. Does the failure to acquire helminthic parasites predispose to Crohn's disease? *The FASEB Journal.* 2000;14(12):1848-1855.

222. Berg DJ, Davidson N, Kühn R, et al. Enterocolitis and colon cancer in interleukin-10-deficient mice are associated with aberrant cytokine production and CD4 (+) TH1-like responses. *J Clin Invest.* 1996;98(4):1010-1020.

223. Neurath MF, Fuss I, Kelsall BL, Stüber E, Strober W. Antibodies to interleukin 12 abrogate established experimental colitis in mice. *J Exp Med.* 1995;182(5):1281-1290.

224. Summers RW, Elliott D, Urban J, Thompson R, Weinstock J. Trichuris suis therapy in Crohn's disease. *Gut.* 2005;54(1):87-90.

225. Summers RW, Elliott DE, Qadir K, Urban Jr JF, Thompson R, Weinstock JV. Trichuris suis seems to be safe and possibly effective in the treatment of inflammatory bowel disease. *Am J Gastroenterol.* 2003;98(9):2034-2041.

226. Summers RW, Elliott DE, Urban Jr JF, Thompson RA, Weinstock JV. Trichuris suis therapy for active ulcerative colitis: a randomized controlled trial. *Gastroenterology.* 2005;128(4):825-832.

227. Sandborn W, Elliott D, Weinstock J, et al. Randomised clinical trial: the safety and tolerability of T richuris suis ova in patients with Crohn's disease. *Aliment Pharmacol Ther.* 2013;38(3):255-263.

228. Guslandi M. Rifaximin in the treatment of inflammatory bowel disease. *World J Gastroenterol.* 2011;17(42):4643.

229. Shafran I, Johnson LK. An open-label evaluation of rifaximin in the treatment of active Crohn's disease. *Curr Med Res Opin.* 2005;21(8):1165-1169.

230. Sartor R. the potential mechanisms of action of rifaximin in the management of inflammatory bowel diseases. *Aliment Pharmacol Ther.* 2016;43:27-36.

231. Prantera C, Lochs H, Campieri M, et al. Antibiotic treatment of Crohn's disease: results of a multicentre, double blind, randomized, placebo-controlled trial with rifaximin. *Aliment Pharmacol Ther.* 2006;23(8):1117-1125.

232. Guslandi M, Petrone MC, Testoni PA. Rifaximin for active ulcerative colitis. *Inflamm Bowel Dis.* 2006;12(4):335-335.

233. Gionchetti P, Rizzello F, Ferrieri A, et al. Rifaximin in patients with moderate or severe ulcerative colitis refractory to steroid-treatment: a double-blind, placebo-controlled trial. *Dig Dis Sci.* 1999;44(6):1220-1221.

234. Triantafillidis JK, Vagianos C, Papalois AE. The role of enteral nutrition in patients with inflammatory bowel disease: current aspects. *BioMed Res Int.* 2015;2015.

235. Agin M, Yucel A, Gumus M, Yuksekkaya HA, Tumgor G. The effect of enteral nutrition support rich in TGF-β in the treatment of inflammatory bowel disease in Cchildhood. *Medicina.* 2019;55(10):620.

236. Triantafillidis J, Stamataki A, Gikas A, Malgarinos G. Maintenance treatment of Crohn's disease with a polymeric feed rich in TGF-Î². *Ann Gastroenterol.* 2010:113-118.

237. Ciampa BP, Ramos ER, Borum M, Doman DB. The emerging therapeutic role of medical foods for gastrointestinal disorders. *Gastroenterol Hepatol.* 2017;13(2):104.

238. Good L, Panas R. Case series investigating the clinical practice experience of serum-derived bovine immunoglobulin/protein isolate (SBI) in the clinical management of patients with inflammatory bowel disease. *J Gastrointest Dig Syst.* 2015;5(2):268.

239. Shafran I, Burgunder P, Wei D, Young HE, Klein G, Burnett BP. Management of inflammatory bowel disease with oral serum-derived bovine immunoglobulin. *Ther Adv Gastroenterol.* 2015;8(6):331-339.

240. Ammon H. Boswellic acids in chronic inflammatory diseases. *Planta Medica.* 2006;72(12):1100-1116.

241. Hamidpour R, Hamidpour S, Hamidpour M, Shahlari M. Frankincense (Boswellia species): From the selection of traditional applications to the novel phytotherapy for the prevention and treatment of serious diseases. *J Tradit Complement Med.* 2013;3(4):221.

242. Gupta I, Parihar A, Malhotra P, et al. Effects of Boswellia serrata gum resin in patients with ulcerative colitis. *Eur J Med Res.* 1997;2(1):37-43.

243. Sun J, Shen X, Dong J, et al. Tripterygium wilfordii Hook F as maintenance treatment for Crohn's disease. *Am J Med Sci.* 2015;350(5):345-351.

244. Zhu W, Li Y, Gong J, et al. Tripterygium wilfordii Hook. f. versus azathioprine for prevention of postoperative recurrence in patients with Crohn's disease: a randomized clinical trial. *Dig Liver Dis.* 2015;47(1):14-19.

245. Kaliora AC, Stathopoulou MG, Triantafillidis JK, Dedoussis GV, Andrikopoulos NK. Chios mastic treatment of patients with active Crohn's disease. *World J Gastroenterol.* 2007;13(5):748.

246. Kaliora AC, Stathopoulou MG, Triantafillidis JK, Dedoussis GV, Andrikopoulos NK. Alterations in the function of circulating mononuclear cells derived from patients with Crohn's disease treated with mastic. *World J Gastroenterol.* 2007;13(45):6031.

# 6

# Health Maintenance in Women With IBD

Sharmeel K. Wasan, MD | Akriti P. Saxena, MD

## Introduction

Patients with inflammatory bowel disease (IBD) unfortunately do not receive appropriate preventive care at the same rate as the general population, when in fact they are often at increased risk of complications such as infection, malignancy, and developing comorbid conditions such as depression and anxiety. Several of these factors independently lead to adverse outcomes in this vulnerable population.

Historically, primary care physicians (PCPs) were responsible for appropriate health maintenance for patients. However, the management of IBD has become increasingly nuanced in the last decade. Several new agents are now US Food and Drug Administration (FDA)-approved with differing mechanisms of action and in turn, different side effect profiles. Since gastroenterologists are most familiar with these medications and the complexities of preventive health care for patients with IBD, it is important that there be a close working relationship with PCPs to provide this care and recommendations to improve the outcomes of this patient population. Additionally, about half of all IBD patients are women and it is important to note the gender-specific needs of women with IBD such as screening for breast cancer and cervical cancer.

This chapter highlights the necessary vaccinations for patients with IBD and preventive care issues related to skin, breast, cervical, and colon cancer screening, and assessing for bone health, mental health, and smoking.

Abraham BP, Kane SV, Glassner KL, eds.
*Women's Health in IBD: The Spectrum of Care
From Birth to Adulthood* (pp 115-133).
© 2022 Taylor & Francis Group.

# Vaccinations

Preventing opportunistic infections through routine vaccination is recommended for all patients with IBD since most are immunocompromised and many are concurrently malnourished. Gastroenterologists have a unique opportunity to alter the risk profile of patients with IBD early in their disease course. Immunization is generally safe, well tolerated, and has arguably few (if any) disadvantages.

Vaccine uptake in the IBD population remains suboptimal due to lack of awareness, fear regarding safety and adverse events on behalf of both PCPs as well as gastroenterologists and insufficient counseling by providers.[1-3] Counseling rates regarding avoidance of live vaccines in immunosuppressed patients as low as 3.5% to 19% have been reported.[3] Whether the responsibility of vaccination should lie with the gastroenterologist or PCP has been debated. In one study, many gastroenterologists felt that the PCPs should assume responsibility for determining which vaccinations should be given (64%) and actually administer the vaccines as well (83%).[4] To minimize patient suffering due to this ambiguity, however, we encourage gastroenterologists to take charge of health maintenance care as PCPs are not as familiar with managing immunosuppressive medications.

We highlight the additional importance of vaccination early in the course of disease and preferably prior to initiation of immunosuppressive therapy. Several studies have demonstrated that the immune response to vaccine is blunted in patients on immunosuppressive medications[5,6] and particularly in combination therapy. For those on maintenance therapy, conversely, convenience may be prioritized to maximize adherence to vaccination. In one study of pediatric patients on infliximab therapy, the ability to achieve serologic protection from vaccine was not influenced by the timing of their infusion.[7]

In hospitalized patients often in need of an inpatient biologic for rescue therapy, or in outpatients with severe disease, treatment of IBD should take precedence and should not be delayed until after vaccination. Vaccination is not thought to increase the risk of an IBD flare. Greater than 95% of adult patients with IBD who received H1N1 vaccination did not flare when reassessed at 4 weeks.[8]

The vaccination schedule for non-live vaccines is outlined in Table 6-1 and detailed later.

## Influenza Vaccination

Several studies have revealed that patients with IBD are not only more prone to influenza infection but are also at increased risk of complications including requiring hospitalization.[9] The risk is especially heightened for patients on immunosuppressive therapies, particularly corticosteroids, and in such patients the immune response to vaccination may be diminished. Nonetheless, there have been no safety concerns with inactivated vaccines in the IBD population and even partial protection is likely beneficial compared to no protection at all. Therefore, inactivated influenza vaccine should be administered to all patients over age 6 months, as well as household contacts, on an annual basis.

## Pneumococcal Vaccination

The rates of pneumococcal infection in patients with IBD are higher than in those without IBD[10] and even higher in patients on corticosteroids, anti–tumor necrosis factor (TNF) agents[11] or narcotic medications[10] compared with patients who are not exposed to these therapies. In addition, when patients with IBD are admitted to the hospital for pneumonia, their mortality is increased.[12] Furthermore, the risk of invasive pneumococcal pneumonia is increased both before and after the diagnosis of IBD and a study by Kantsø et al suggests that underlying immune dysfunction is a significant driver rather than immunosuppressive therapies alone.[13]

There are 2 pneumococcal vaccines currently available in the United States: the 13-valent pneumococcal conjugate vaccine (PCV13, Prevnar, Pfizer) and the 23-valent pneumococcal

## Table 6-1. Non-Live Vaccines in IBD

| VACCINE | POPULATION | FREQUENCY | COMMENTS |
|---|---|---|---|
| Influenza | All | Annually | Those on immunosuppressive therapies and their household contacts should receive the inactivated vaccine |
| Pneumococcal PCV13 | Patients on or initiating immunosuppression | Once | If PPSV23 is given first, wait for > 1 year to administer this vaccine |
| Pneumococcal PPSV23 | Patients on or initiating immunosuppression | Once, repeat in 5 years and again after age 65 years | If PCV13 is given first, wait for > 8 weeks to administer this vaccine |
| HPV | Ages 9 to 26 years, and using shared decision making for ages 26 to 45 years | 3 dose-series at 0, 2, and 6 months | |
| Tdap | All | See Comments | Tdap booster once at age 11 years (and up to age 64 years), Td every 10 years |
| Hepatitis A | For non-immune patients | Once, 2-dose vaccine | |
| Hepatitis B | For non-immune patients | See Comments | Check hepatitis B core antibody, surface antigen, and surface antibody<br><br>If waning titers, give one booster shot and if unsuccessful, then give the complete vaccination series<br><br>Prophylaxis for patients at risk of HBV reactivations should be considered |

*(continued)*

polysaccharide vaccine (PPSV23, Pneumovax, Merck). Both vaccines are inactivated and target different serotypes. A single administration of PCV13 is recommended for all patients with IBD on immunosuppression, followed by PPSV23 > 8 weeks later. If PPSV23 is given first, then the patient may receive PCV13 > 1 year later. A booster dose of PPSV23 is also recommended 5 years after the original vaccine, and after age 65. As is commonly encountered in clinical practice, patients may receive the pneumococcal vaccines and influenza vaccines during the same visit.

## Human Papillomavirus Vaccine

Human papillomavirus (HPV) infection with strains 16 and 18 is the leading cause of cervical cancer worldwide. Patients with IBD, particularly on azathioprine, are at increased risk for cervical

## Table 6-1 (continued). Non-Live Vaccines in IBD

| VACCINE | POPULATION | FREQUENCY | COMMENTS |
|---|---|---|---|
| Meningococcal vaccine | Healthy adolescents (MenACWY and possibly Men B) and high-risk infants (MenACWY) and high-risk adults (both) | MenACWY (2-dose)<br>MenB-FHbp (3 dose) or MenB-4C (2-dose) | Per ACIP recommendations |
| Herpes zoster vaccine (Shingrix) | Patients > age 50 years | Once, 2-dose series | Inactivated vaccine (Shingrix) recommended even if patient received live attenuated vaccine (Zostavax) or experience shingles previously<br>Although Shingrix is FDA-approved for patients over the age of 50 years, we recommend vaccination in younger immunocompromised patients in clinical practice, cost permitting |

neoplasia. As per ACIP recommendations, HPV vaccine is recommended for children aged 11 or 12 years, and can be given as early as age 9 years. There is emphasis on vaccinating children prior to exposure to maximize efficacy of the vaccine. Between the ages of 26 and 45 years, shared decision making should be used to administer the vaccine selectively in high-risk individuals. Before a patient's 15 birthday, a 2-dose vaccination series at 0 months and at 6 to 12 months is recommended. On or after the 15 birthday, a 3-dose series of the HPV vaccine is recommended at 0, 1 to 2, and 6 months.

## Tdap Vaccine

Tdap is given preferably at age 11 to 12 years as part of a preventive care visit or until age 64 years. To ensure continued protection, a dose of Td or Tdap should be repeated every 10 years, lifelong. Additionally, pregnant women should receive Tdap vaccine during each pregnancy at weeks 27 to 36 (preferably), irrespective of prior immunization. The guidelines in the IBD population mirror that of the general population with respect to the Tdap vaccine.

## Hepatitis A and B Vaccines

Hepatitis A and B vaccination is recommended for all non-immune IBD patients. Hepatitis A IgG indicates immunity against the virus. If non-reactive, hepatitis A vaccination is administered in 2 doses at 0 and 6 months.

Regarding hepatitis B (HBV) infection, it is advisable to check the following panel of tests in all patients with IBD, especially prior to initiation of biologic therapy: HBV surface antibody (HBsAb), HBV surface antigen (HBsAg), and HBV core antibody (anti-HBc).

An isolated HBsAb results from vaccination without prior exposure to HBV. The level of antibody titer that confers immunity is controversial and ranges from 10 IU/L to 100 IU/L. The American College of Gastroenterology (ACG) guidelines from 2017 recommend a single booster vaccination in patients with low titers and to administer the full vaccination series if patients do not respond appropriately to the booster.[14] It is advisable to check titers 1 month post completion of the series and if the response is suboptimal, a double dose can be used. There is a combination Hepatitis A and B vaccine by the name of Twinrix (GlaxoSmithKline) that can also be given. Additionally, a new 2-dose HBV vaccine was approved in 2018: Heplisav-B (HepB-CpG; Dynavax Technologies Corporation).It is only approved for 2 doses administered 4 weeks apart if HepB-CpG is used for both doses. If a vaccine from a different manufacturer is used, then a total of 3 doses should be given. The appropriate HBsAb levels were achieved in 90% to 100% of patients receiving the HepB-CpG compared with 70.5% to 90.2% of patients receiving Engerix-B (GlaxoSmithKline Biologicals) and hence using the HepB-CpG vaccine if available is a reasonable alternative.[15]

It is imperative to consider HBV reactivation in patients with HBsAg or anti-HBc. According to the 2015 American Gastroenterological Association (AGA) guidelines on HBV reactivation, patients treated with anti-TNFs who are anti-HBc–positive (and either HBsAg positive or negative) are considered at moderate risk of HBV reactivation. This is defined as an anticipated incidence of 1% to 10%. Antiviral prophylaxis is recommended for this group (weak recommendation, moderate quality of evidence) and should be continued for 6 months beyond immunosuppressive therapy.[16]

## Meningococcal Vaccine

Recommendations for the meningococcal vaccine in IBD patients with IBD are the same as the general population, per ACIP. Protection from serogroups A, C, W, and Y in healthy adolescents, high-risk infants/children (age 2 months to 10 years) and high-risk adults is available as the MenACWY (Menactra, Menveo, GlaxoSmithKline) vaccine or a polysaccharide (Menomune) vaccine.

There are currently 2 serogroup B vaccines licensed in the United States: MenB-FHbp (Trumenba, Pfizer) and MenB-4C (Bexsero, GlaxoSmithKline). MenB-FHbp is approved as a 3-dose series at 0, 1 to 2, and 6 months but 2 doses are sufficient (at 0 and 6 months) when given to healthy adolescents. MenB-4C is a 2-dose series at 0 and 6 months. The 2 vaccines are not interchangeable and the same vaccine should be used for each dose of the series. The vaccine may be considered in healthy teens (over age 10 but preferably at age 16) and high-risk adults.

## Herpes Zoster Vaccine

Herpes zoster infection has been in the spotlight recently, in part due to the FDA approval of a new inactivated vaccine in 2017—Shignrix (GlaxoSmithKline). The infection is characterized by a rash, caused by reactivation of the varicella zoster virus which lies dormant in the dorsal root ganglia. The risk of herpes zoster infection increases with age and is a significant driver of morbidity and mortality especially when complicated by post-herpetic neuralgia. The incidence of zoster is higher in the IBD population especially for those on immunosuppressive medications and corticosteroids.[17,18] Herpes zoster infection also affects patients with IBD at a younger age.[18] Additionally, there appears to be an increased risk of herpes zoster infection with newer small-molecule IBD therapies such as tofacitinib.[19]

The primary concern with the first-generation vaccine (Zostavax, Merck) is that it is a live attenuated vaccine. As such, it was contraindicated in patients on high-dose immunosuppression. Some of these concerns have been mitigated by the newer recombinant zoster vaccine (Shingrix); which is now recommended for all adults over age 50 years, including those with a prior episode of shingles and those who had received the live vaccine previously. Though the vaccine does not have FDA approval under age 50 years, the vaccine may be offered to younger patients with IBD on immunosuppressive therapies, cost permitting. A recent study demonstrated low rates of IBD flare (1.5%) post-vaccination, and local and systemic adverse reactions similar to the clinical trial data in healthy patients.[20]

## Live Vaccines

In one study, 20% to 30% of gastroenterologists erroneously recommended live vaccines to patients on immunosuppression.[4] In fact, live vaccines are contraindicated in patients either on biologic therapy, tofacitinib, or > 20 mg prednisone daily or who are about to initiate immunosuppressive therapy in the near future. Certain live vaccines can be given to patients on "low-level immunosuppression" comprising of the following therapies and within 3 months of discontinuation: daily corticosteroids for ≥ 14 days (prednisone 20 mg/day or equivalent), alternate day corticosteroid therapy, methotrexate ≤ 0.4 mg/kg/week, 6-mercaptopurine ≤ 1.5 mg/kg/day or azathioprine ≤ 3 mg/kg/day.[22] The live vaccination schedule is summarized in Table 6-2.

## Varicella Vaccine

The vaccine against varicella zoster virus is a live attenuated one, recommended for infants without prior exposure at age 12 to 15 months (2 dose series, 1 month apart). A booster dose is typically repeated at 4 to 6 years. Unfortunately, patient recall of having chickenpox infection is unreliable and therefore, immunity should be documented in 1 of 3 ways: an appropriate vaccination schedule, documentation of infection by a health care provider or the presence of antibody titers. Patients over age 13 years who are not immune should be vaccinated as well. In the IBD population, this is best done at the time of diagnosis as varicella vaccine is contraindicated 1 to 3 months prior to initiation of a biologic agent or other high-dose immunosuppression or with current use of biologic or high-dose immunosuppression.

## Measles, Mumps, and Rubella Vaccine

Measles, mumps, and rubella vaccine (MMR), another live vaccine, is routinely recommended for children aged 12 to 15 months, with the second dose administered at age 4 through 6 years, prior to starting school. For adults over age 18 years, 1 dose is sufficient but 2 doses are recommended for those at higher risk (eg, health care workers, those attending college). As with other lives vaccines, MMR should be avoided within 1 to 3 months of starting immunosuppression and is certainly contraindicated in patients with IBD who are already on these medications.

## Rotavirus Vaccine

There are 2 vaccines currently licensed for use in the United States: RotaTeq (RV5) given at 2, 4, and 6 months of age and Rotarix (RV1) given at 2 and 4 months of age. All doses should be complete by 8 months of age. It is well known that attenuated rotavirus is shed through the stool of infants (more after RV1 compared to RV5) and up to 30 days post-vaccination.[23] ACIP recommends that immunocompromised persons practice good hand hygiene after changing diapers of vaccinated infants whereas the ACG guideline from 2017 recommends that immunocompromised patients avoid handling of diapers altogether for 4 weeks post vaccination.

For infants of mothers on biologic therapy (other than certolizumab, which does not cross the placental barrier) during the third trimester, which is defined as beyond 27 weeks of gestation, live vaccines such as rotavirus should be avoided for the first 6 months of life.[24]

| Table 6-2. Live Vaccines in IBD | | | |
|---|---|---|---|
| **VACCINE** | **POPULATION** | **FREQUENCY** | **COMMENTS** |
| Varicella | For non-immune patients who are not currently on or about to initiate immunosuppression in the next 1 month | Once, 2-dose series | Check titers as recall of chicken pox infection is not reliable |
| Measles, mumps, and rubella | For non-immune patients 6 weeks prior to starting immunosuppressive therapy | Once, 2-dose series | Check titers if vaccination history uncertain |

## Household Contacts

Routine vaccination of household contacts should also be emphasized to immunocompromised patients with IBD.[22] Healthy household contacts should receive MMR, varicella vaccine, and herpes zoster vaccine. Immunocompromised patients with IBD should avoid contact with any members who develop varicella or zoster infection, in addition to patients who develop skin lesions post-vaccination.

## Vaccine Recommendations Among Travelers

There are several vaccines that are infrequently encountered in daily practice but that become relevant when traveling to endemic areas.[25] The live vaccines under consideration include: yellow fever, MMR, oral typhoid, oral polio, intranasal influenza, and tuberculosis Bacillus Calmette-Guerin. As previously discussed, live vaccines are contraindicated in patients on immunosuppression and in select cases, travel should be avoided. Shared decision making between the patient, gastroenterologist, and an infectious disease specialist is highly recommended. Eligibility to receive the yellow fever vaccines should be determined ahead of time in patients traveling to South America and sub-Saharan Africa. Fortunately, there are inactivated vaccines available for influenza, typhoid, and polio and are preferred in the IBD population. Other inactivated vaccines include protection against Japanese encephalitis and rabies.

# Screening for Skin Cancer

Patients with IBD, particularly Crohn's disease (CD), are at increased risk of both melanoma and non-melanoma skin cancer (NMSC) compared to the general population.[26] The effect is likely multi-factorial and related to underlying immune dysfunction in IBD, the use of immunosuppressive medications, and possibly early detection of skin cancer due to more frequent encounters with the health care system.

## Non-Melanoma Skin Cancer

The rise in the incidence of NMSC, the most common malignancy in the United States over the last 3 decades, is associated with significant health care costs and mortality.[27] In patients with IBD, the rise is mostly driven by the use of thiopurines and proportional to the duration of therapy.[26] A meta-analysis quantified the risk to be 2.28 times higher than in patients who do not use thiopurines.[28] Azathioprine and specifically the DNA products of 6-thioguanine are known to increase the photosensitivity of human skin to UVA light.[29] Chronic exposure leads to oxidative stress and the production of free radical species, leading to cutaneous lesions. The risk of NMSC appears to return to baseline after discontinuation of thiopurine therapy (adjusted hazard ratio of 0.7 after stopping therapy compared with unexposed patients).[30]

The use of methotrexate for the treatment of IBD is decreasing with the advent of newer biologic therapies, and therefore, most of the data evaluating the association of methotrexate use and NMSC stems from other autoimmune diseases and solid organ transplant recipients. There is an increased risk of NMSC in psoriasis patients on methotrexate, as well as rheumatoid arthritis (RA) patients on methotrexate and cyclosporine.

During the RA clinical development program, the incidence rate of NMSC for patients on tofacitinib was 0.55 per 100 patient-years,[31] and the higher dose of 10 mg twice daily led to a non-significant increase in NMSC. Newer biologic agents such as vedolizumab and ustekinumab do not appear to increase the rates of NMSC but data are limited.

## Risk of Subsequent Non-Melanoma Skin Cancer After Treatment

Methotrexate use is thought to increase the likelihood of a second NMSC in RA patients, and the risk increases with duration of therapy. Anti-TNF therapy may be associated with an increased risk of a second NMSC especially when used in conjunction with methotrexate. Interestingly, the relative risk of NMSC on thiopurines in IBD was higher than on methotrexate in RA, but thiopurines did not statistically increase the risk of a second NMSC. Due to the known association between thiopurine use and initial NMSC, further studies are needed.

## Melanoma

Similar to the rise in NMSC, the rate of melanoma has increased by 3-fold in the United States over the past 2 decades. IBD is associated with a 37% increase in risk of melanoma.[14] Some data suggest that the use of biologic anti-TNF medication is associated with a risk of melanoma,[26] especially in CD but a recent meta-analysis confirmed that IBD is in fact an independent risk factor.[32] Until more data become available, increased vigilance in patients on immunosuppressive medications would be prudent.

In summary, NMSC is driven by thiopurine use, whereas IBD is an independent risk factor for melanoma. Tofacitinib and methotrexate use (based on data in RA) may also contribute to NMSC, and there may be synergistic effects with combination therapies, but further data are needed. The risk of a subsequent NMSC lesion after treatment of the first in RA patients appears to stem from methotrexate and anti-TNF use in combination.

## Prevention

Primary prevention for skin cancer should include sun avoidance, wearing sun-protective clothing (SPF > 30), the application of broad-spectrum sunscreen against both UVA and UVB, (SPF > 30) and reapplication every 2 hours. Recent data demonstrate that sunscreen decreases both the rates of melanoma and NMSC.[33] Patient should be counseled to avoid tanning beds.

While there are no population-wide screening recommendations for the prevention of skin cancer, patients with IBD especially on immunosuppressive medications are at increased risk. The 2017 ACG guidelines recommend routine screening exams for all patients with IBD, independent of therapy. Skin exams are an integral part of secondary prevention and help to identify lesions at an early stage when the likelihood of treatment success is the highest. In patients with IBD on thiopurines, and particularly over age 50 years, screening specifically for NMSC should be emphasized. Screening patients with CD annually has also been shown to be cost-effective, and led to early detection of about 94% of incident NMSC cases.[34]

# Screening for Breast Cancer

Though breast cancer is the leading cause of cancer-related deaths among women worldwide, there are limited data on the risk of breast cancer in patients with IBD. In a prospective study in Norway, the standardized incidence ratio for breast cancer was significantly increased in both ulcerative colitis (UC) and CD.[35] Whether this is driven by the underlying IBD or immunosuppressive medications is unclear. Interestingly, among women with treated breast cancer and either IBD or RA, one study found that there was no statistically significant increase in the risk of breast cancer recurrence with use of methotrexate or anti-TNF therapy though the thiopurine group needed further study.[36]

Among the screening modalities, mammography has been proven to decrease mortality though society and expert recommendations vary widely. The American College of Radiology recommends annual screening for average-risk women over the age of 40 years[37] whereas the US Preventive Services Task Force recommends screening every 2 years starting at age 50 and shared decision making between age 40 to 50 years.[38] One study found that rates of mammography are < 50% in women with IBD at a screening interval of every 2 years, which was similar to the general population.[39] At this particular center, eligible women received invitation letters for mammograms. Real-world screening rates are likely lower, thus highlighting the importance of reiterating health maintenance recommendations in our patients with IBD.

In accordance with the most conservative guidelines recommending annual mammography for average-risk women over age 40 years, and in light of the increased risk of malignancy with certain immunosuppressive medications, annual mammography for patients with IBD may be reasonable but clear guidelines supporting this practice are lacking.

# Screening for Cervical Cancer

Cervical cancer, characterized by squamous cell carcinoma and adenocarcinoma, is caused by infection and persistence of high-risk HPV. Patients with IBD are at higher risk of cervical cancer compared to the general population[40] as their weakened immune system leads to decreased clearance of HPV.[41] Certainly, the implementation of the HPV vaccine has improved cancer-related incidence and mortality; however, a significant number of women have already been exposed by the time of vaccination. Therefore, annual screening with the Papanicolau (pap) test remains crucial, particularly for women on immunosuppression as recommended by the Centers for Disease Control and Prevention, the American College of Obstetricians and Gynecologists, and the American Cancer Society.

Whether the risk of cervical cancer is driven by the underlying IBD itself is controversial. However, there is growing evidence that patients on immunosuppression carry an increased risk of cervical neoplasia.[40,42] Though most studies included both immunomodulators (6MP, methotrexate) and anti-TNF agents, one study found that only azathioprine but not corticosteroids or anti-TNF therapies contributed to the increased rate of cervical neoplasia.[42] This risk is mirrored in women with other immunodeficiencies (whether innate or acquired) such as women with HIV,[43] systemic lupus erythematosus,[44] and transplant recipients.[45] In fact, some propose that women have annual gynecological examination beyond the cervix due to an increased risk of lower genital lesions including vulvar, vaginal, and anal dysplasia.

Unfortunately, cervical testing rates in women with IBD are suboptimal; one study demonstrated that in patients on immunosuppression, only half received screening during a 15-month period.[46] Factors associated with lower compliance include advanced age, patients on immunosuppression, and those insured by Medicaid—arguably the populations most in need of screening.

## Management of Cellular Abnormalities

Cervical epithelial cell abnormalities can be divided by cell type into squamous cell and glandular cell lesions. According to the updated Bethesda classification from 2014, the former is further classified into atypical squamous cells (ASC) either of undetermined significance (ASC-US) or cannot exclude high-grade squamous intraepithelial lesion (ASC-H), low-grade squamous intraepithelial lesion (LSIL) encompassing HPV, mild dysplasia, cervical intraepithelial neoplasia (CIN-1), or high-grade squamous intraepithelial lesion (HSIL) encompassing moderate and severe dysplasia (CIN-2, CIN-3) and squamous cell carcinoma.

Women aged 25 years and older with ASC-US should undergo either HPV testing immediately (now reflex at most institutions) or repeat cytology in 1 year. If HPV positive, then annual colposcopy is recommended. Women with ASC-H should also undergo colposcopy, and testing for HPV is rarely helpful due to the high rate of prevalence in this population. For women aged 21 to 24 years who carry a lower risk of cervical cancer, colposcopy is only advised if cytologic abnormalities are persistent.

Women over age 30 years with LSIL should undergo both HPV testing and colposcopy, and if the former is negative then repeat co-testing in 1 year is advised. Colposcopy is recommended as the first step for women 25 to 29 years with LSIL.

Since ASC-US, LSIL, HPV 16 or 18 or persistent HPV infection are considered "lesser abnormalities," when these lesions precede CIN-1 then the initial management is conservative with repeat contesting in 1 year. Conversely, when CIN-1 is preceded by ASC-H or HSIL then excision may be pursued earlier in women aged 25 years and older. Prompt treatment is recommended for CIN-2 and CIN-3 due to high risk of progression to cervical cancer and includes excision and ablation.

In general, the management of abnormal cytology in immunocompromised women is similar to immunocompetent women. Nonetheless, the management strategies should ensue in conjunction with a gynecologist.

# Assessing for Bone Health

Osteoporotic fractures are a major cause of morbidity in the general population. Patients with IBD are susceptible to this devastating condition at a younger age due to systemic inflammation, decreased intake of nutrients, malabsorption, and often simultaneous glucocorticoid use.[47] The prevalence of osteoporosis in IBD ranges from 18% to 42%[48] and is as high as 70% in some studies.[49] According to a technical review by the AGA, the overall relative risk of fractures is 40% greater than that in the general population and increases with age.[48] Many studies suggest an increased risk of a hip fracture (> 40%),[49] and increased risk of spine fracture[50] associated with glucocorticoid use. Glucocorticoids are known to impair osteoblasts, reduce intestinal calcium absorption, and increase renal calcium excretion. Conversely, one study showed that the majority of hip fractures in IBD are not in fact attributed to the use of steroids.[51] It is, however, difficult to distinguish corticosteroid use from disease activity in terms of causation of a fracture. IBD may be an independent risk factor for the development of osteoporosis and fractures through the upregulation of inflammatory cytokines resulting in high bone turnover[52] though there is insufficient evidence to draw a definite conclusion at this time. Fractures and reduced BMD are certainly more common in the IBD population as many patients are exposed to glucocorticoids, antibiotics, have poor nutritional status and/or absorption and low sunlight exposure leading to calcium and vitamin D deficiency.

Osteoporosis definitions vary but the underlying pathophysiology entails loss of bone mass with microarchitectural deterioration of bone tissue, resulting in increased fragility.[53] Dual-energy X-ray absorptiometry (DEXA) is the most common imaging modality used to estimate bone mineral density (BMD), which is used as a surrogate to estimate fracture risk. According to the World Health Organization, the presence of a fragility fracture or falling under 2.5 standard deviations of the mean BMD (measured in the lumbar spine or proximal femur) for healthy young adults is diagnostic of osteoporosis.

## Screening Recommendations

Current recommendations for patients with IBD differ in published guidelines by the European Crohn's and Colitis Organisation, the British Society of Gastroenterology, the AGA, and the ACG.[54] While all of the guidelines do recommend a DEXA scan in patients with significant steroid use and/ or recurrent or persistently active IBD, each guideline comments on additional specific risk factors. The British Society of Gastroenterology also recommends including patients over age 70 years, and those with poor nutrition. The European Crohn's and Colitis Organisation recommends screening for patients with long disease duration. Additionally, the AGA alerts practitioners to consider bone density measurements in patients with low trauma fractures, hypogonadism, postmenopausal females or males aged > 50 years.

Acknowledging the low absolute risk of bone fractures, the ACG preventive care guideline recommends following screening practices outlined for the general population and in accordance with the national osteoporosis foundation. Specifically, screening patients with a preexisting fragility fracture, women aged 65 years and men aged 70 years and older, and those with traditional risk factors. In addition to age, traditional risk factors include post-menopausal women, women with hypogonadism or other hormonal imbalances, smokers, and patients with vitamin D or calcium deficiency. Practitioners should have a low threshold to screen patients who have been exposed to glucocorticoids in the past. Additionally, a baseline BMD measurement with DEXA is reasonable for patients starting oral glucocorticoid therapy and certainly for individuals who have received greater than 3 months of steroids at a dose greater than 7.5 mg/day.

The ACG guidelines do not support obtaining baseline BMD measurement for all patients with IBD, or at 1 year after diagnosis as this has not shown to be cost-effective. Additionally, for high-risk patients with conventional risk factors and/or known abnormal BMD, periodic DEXA scans are recommended for patients with UC even post colectomy with ileal pouch-anal anastomosis surgery.

If the initial screen is normal, DEXA may be repeated at a later time. The National Osteoporosis Foundation suggests spacing out screening intervals to every 5 to 10 years if there has been no change in the patient's clinical status or risk factors. For patients who do have osteoporosis, DEXA scan every 2 years is suggested and for patients on treatment for osteoporosis, annual DEXA scans.

## Preventive Measures

Given the association between IBD and the risk of fractures, at-risk patients should be counseled on lifestyle measures such as weight-bearing exercises, smoking cessation, and limiting alcohol intake. Calcium (500 to 1000 mg/day) and vitamin D (800 to 1000 IU/day or higher) should be given to all patients on corticosteroids and in those who have osteopenia.

# Screening for Depression and Anxiety

There is ample anecdotal evidence to suggest that psychological stress exacerbates symptoms in patients with IBD. More recently, there is an increasing breadth of literature to support this. Thus, early recognition is crucial to improve clinical outcomes. A recent study by Lewis at al suggested that the prevalence of depression and anxiety among patients with IBD was on the order of 40% and 30% respectively and that one-third to two-thirds of patients were undiagnosed at the time of screening.[55] One study suggested that male patients and those with a lower education level were at increased risk.[55] Another systematic review confirmed that the prevalence of depression and anxiety is higher in patients with IBD compared to the general population (19% vs 9.6%), and alerts us to the increasing incidence of these disorders even in patients with inactive disease.[56] Other predictors of depressive severity in IBD include aggressive disease, divorced status, disability, and lower socioeconomic status.[57,58]

Regarding disease activity, several studies have demonstrated poorer outcomes in patient with comorbid psychiatric illnesses. In a prospective study of patients with IBD in remission, a higher Beck Depression Inventory score correlated with the number of relapses at 1 year and 18 months.[59] Depression was found to be an independent predictor of active disease in a recent study of patients with active luminal CD on infliximab, with reduced remission rates and shorter time to retreatment.[60] The data are not entirely one-sided; one study showed that perhaps short-term stress but not long-term stress or depression predicted relapse though the hazard risk for short-term stress was only 1.05.[61] IBD-related surgery and hospitalization further increases the risk of developing depression and anxiety, especially in female patients and in patients with CD who have perianal involvement, stoma surgery, patients on immunosuppressants, and those who underwent "early" surgery within 3 years of diagnosis. Therefore, gastroenterologists should pay special attention to screening their patients with IBD for depression by using simple screening questions such as the Patient Health Questionnaire-2.[62] A positive answer to either of the questions should prompt a referral to the patient's PCP or to a psychiatrist for confirmatory testing so that an appropriate treatment plan can be determined.

Fortunately, there are data to support the use of antidepressants in IBD patients. They are proven to be effective,[63] and may reduce the risk of relapse and the use of steroids in one study.[64] The data on whether antidepressants improved adherence to medical therapy for IBD disease activity are conflicting. Cognitive behavioral therapy (CBT) is another promising option. While there is no difference in initial efficacy, relapse or discontinuation rates between CBT and antidepressants, CBT has been shown to be more cost-effective long-term and results in improved quality of life.

The DSM-5 criteria for the diagnosis of major depressive disorder comprises of depressed or irritable mood, or anhedonia for 2 or more weeks with functional impairment and 5 of the following: fatigue, change in sleep, appetite, reduced concentration, motor retardation or agitation, thoughts of death or suicide, guilt, and worthlessness/low self-esteem. The Patient Health Questionnaire-9 is a validated questionnaire based on patient-reported outcomes and is relatively easy to implement and score to screen for depression. The development of several computerized adaptive tests to decrease time to diagnosis and increase precision are now underway.[65] Depression screening should also include screening for mania and substance abuse and assess for seasonal patterns and medical etiologies including alterations in thyroid, vitamin $B_{12}$, vitamin D, sleep apnea, and anemia.

# Screening for Colon Cancer

It is well known that patients with IBD are at increased risk of developing colorectal cancer[66] and that this may occur at a younger age[67] compared to the general population even post colonoscopy.[68] Known risk factors for the development of neoplasia include the presence and severity of both endoscopic and histologic inflammation,[69] extensive disease,[70] younger age at diagnosis,[71] longer duration of disease,[72] family history of colorectal cancer,[73] and concurrent primary sclerosing cholangitis.[74] Since most colorectal cancer arises from dysplasia, surveillance to detect early dysplasia at regular intervals is of paramount importance. Despite probable gender differences, the recommendations for surveillance in women with IBD mirror that of the general population.

The goal of surveillance is to detect and treat colorectal neoplasia, thereby improving mortality. While the data for surveillance colonoscopy stem from retrospective case-control and cohort studies (and not randomized controlled trials), it is considered standard of care and endorsed by several major societies[75,76] from the United States and the United Kingdom. Societies defer in recommendations on when and how frequently to perform surveillance colonoscopy, but several suggest starting 8 years after onset of symptoms and ongoing surveillance in patients who have colonic involvement in greater than one-third of their colon. However, since the development of colorectal cancer is multi-factorial, surveillance should be individualized in each patient as many studies have also shown missed diagnoses when strictly adhering to guidelines[77] and in older patients for instance.[78] There is consensus that patients with primary sclerosing cholangitis undergo annual colonoscopy. For all other patients, societal recommendations for ongoing surveillance differ from 1 to 3 years for the US societies and up to 5 years for the British societies, based on risk factors such as disease activity, anatomy, personal history of dysplasia, and family history.

Prior to the launch of high-definition colonoscopes, the recommendation for surveillance was to use white light endoscopy with random biopsies every 10 cm. New modalities and technologies have improved neoplastic detection in recent years. High-definition colonoscopes allow endoscopists to achieve higher adenoma detection rates than standard scopes.[79] The data on chromoendoscopy (using blue contrast dye to enhance mucosal irregularity) have been conflicting and the use of chromoendoscopy (CE) is currently controversial. The SCENIC guideline recommends CE when using the older, standard colonoscopes but only suggests using CE when high-definition scopes are used. Many subsequent studies have challenged this notion, showing that CE has little benefit over high-definition colonoscopy[80] and that most dysplastic lesions are visible[81] and that targeted biopsies may be superior to random biopsies.[82] Other technologies include the use of narrow-band imaging, panoramic views obtained during colonoscopy, and the use of autofluorescence. Awaiting further data, many practitioners continue to take random biopsies with careful inspection of the mucosa using high-definition scopes.

# Smoking Cessation

The deleterious effects of smoking in all patients include risks of cardiac, respiratory, and oncologic disease. Smoking also negatively affects patients with CD and leads to increased societal costs and decreased health-related quality of life in patients with IBD.[83]

Arguably, the most robust evidence for the development of CD in smokers vs non-smokers stems from a meta-analysis that showed the odds ratio for developing CD among smokers was on the order of 1.76.[84] The data date back several decades. One of the oldest studies to show a 4-fold increased risk of developing CD in smokers was done as early as 1984.[85] Other studies have confirmed this association as evidenced in a study from Oxford that showed that the risk is more than 3-fold in smokers compared with non-smokers.[86] The odds ratios in twin studies similarly ranges from 2.9 to 10 when comparing the twin who smokes to the non-smoking twin.

Smoking in this population also leads to worsening disease activity, increased use of immunosuppressive medications particularly steroids, and IBD-related hospitalizations and surgeries.[87] In a study of 1420 incident cases of CD from 1977 to 2008, current smoking was associated with a change in disease behavior, change in location from ileal disease to colonic or ileocolonic involvement, arthritis, need for steroids, and azathioprine.[88] Conversely, data from the Spanish national IBD registry suggested that smokers with CD were less likely to have colonic involvement, consistent with the known protective effect of smoking in patients with UC.[89] Nonetheless, smokers suffered from early development of both structuring and perianal disease. Smokers are more likely to be on biologic therapy than non-smokers and the tobacco "load" directly correlated with a structuring phenotype.[90] So, in addition to adversely affecting the natural history of CD, tobacco exposure is an independent risk factor for requiring maintenance therapy. Unfortunately, smokers are also less likely to benefit from available therapies. They do not respond as well to infliximab at 4 weeks, and if they do, are more likely to relapse.[91]

As one would surmise, a large meta-analysis and systematic review confirmed that smokers are more likely to flare, need a first and second surgery, and in fact, have a higher probability of flare after surgery.[92] People who smoke also tend to have higher rates of recurrent stricture after endoscopic balloon dilation, and often require a second intervention.[93]

Fortunately, smoking is a modifiable risk factor and more importantly, cessation leads to improved outcomes. Therefore, smoking cessation is an important goal of therapy for patients with CD. Ryan et al showed that patients who quit smoking were less likely to undergo a reoperation for recurrent CD.[94] In a multicenter prospective study, former people who smoke had similar relapse rates to people who don't smoke over a follow up of 4 years.[95] However, only half of people who smoke with CD are in the pre-contemplation phase defined as lack of intent to quit, and in one study, only 11% had quit smoking 6 months later.[96] Education on the perils of smoking is insufficient for quitting as this fails to address the physiologic addiction as well as the social context behind the behavior.[97] Therefore, a multi-targeted approach involving counseling with a nurse, nicotine replacement therapy, and close follow up, for instance, is crucial. In one study, this 3-pronged approach led to smoking cessation in one-half and one-third of patients at 6 and 12 months respectively.[98] An approach combining counseling with nicotine replacement therapy has been shown to be cost-effective [99] and should be offered to all patients with CD who are smokers.

Patients with UC should also be encouraged to stop smoking given the known deleterious effects of tobacco use. However, these patients should also be informed that smoking cessation may be associated with a flare of their colitis and any changes in their symptoms deserves a prompt evaluation.

# Conclusion

Appropriate preventive care can improve outcomes and reduce overall health care costs. Traditionally, the role of the gastroenterologist was to control disease activity and maintain remission while monitoring for the side effects of the medications prescribed for IBD. However, as the therapeutic armamentarium for IBD continues to evolve and the complexity of medications used continues to grow, gastroenterologists as the primary prescribers of these agents are uniquely aware of the nuances of the medications and hence should take ownership over the recommendations for the preventive health care of these patients. Various tools and checklists are available for the practicing gastroenterologist to address these preventive health issues during clinic visits. In addition to routine vaccinations, gastroenterologists should discuss the increased risk of cancer (eg, skin, breast, cervical, colon cancer) with their patients and refer patients to endocrinology (for bone health) and psychiatry (for mental illness) as appropriate.

## KEY POINTS

1. Vaccinating patients with IBD early in their disease course and preferably prior to starting immunosuppressive therapy should be prioritized to minimize the risk of infection.
   - All inactivated vaccines can be given to patients with IBD, regardless of immunosuppression.
   - Live vaccines should not be given to patients with IBD on biologics, tofacitinib, and prednisone > 20 mg daily.
2. The increased risk of both melanoma and NMSC, as well as cervical cancer, may be decreased with routine skin exams and gynecological exams respectively.
3. Patients should be screened for osteoporosis, depression, anxiety, and should be counseled on smoking cessation.
4. Due to the increased risk of colon cancer in patients with IBD, surveillance at an interval of 1 to 3 years is recommended based on disease duration and other risk factors.

# References

1.  Gupta A, Macrae FA, Gibson PR. Vaccination and screening for infections in patients with inflammatory bowel disease: a survey of Australian gastroenterologists. *Intern Med J.* 2011;41(6):462-467. doi:10.1111/j.1445-5994.2009.02114.x

2.  Jung YS, Park JH, Kim HJ, et al. Insufficient knowledge of Korean gastroenterologists regarding the vaccination of patients with inflammatory bowel disease. *Gut Liver.* 2014;8(3):242-247. doi:10.5009/gnl.2014.8.3.242

3.  Wasan SK, Calderwood AH, Long MD, Kappelman MD, Sandler RS, Farraye FA. Immunization rates and vaccine beliefs among patients with inflammatory bowel disease: an opportunity for improvement. *Inflamm Bowel Dis.* 2014;20(2):246-250. doi:10.1097/01.MIB.0000437737.68841.87

4.  Wasan SK, Coukos JA, Farraye FA. Vaccinating the inflammatory bowel disease patient: deficiencies in gastroenterologists knowledge. *Inflamm Bowel Dis.* 2011;17(12):2536-2540. doi:10.1002/ibd.21667

5.  Melmed GY, Agarwal N, Frenck RW, et al. Immunosuppression impairs response to pneumococcal polysaccharide vaccination in patients with inflammatory bowel disease. *Am J Gastroenterol.* 2010;105(1):148-154. doi:10.1038/ajg.2009.523

6.  Nguyen DL, Nguyen ET, Bechtold ML. Effect of immunosuppressive therapies for the treatment of inflammatory bowel disease on response to routine vaccinations: a meta-analysis. *Dig Dis Sci.* 2015;60(8):2446-2453. doi:10.1007/s10620-015-3631-y

7.  deBruyn J, Fonseca K, Ghosh S, et al. Immunogenicity of influenza vaccine for patients with inflammatory bowel disease on maintenance infliximab therapy. *Inflamm Bowel Dis.* 2016;22(3):638-647. doi:10.1097/MIB.0000000000000615

8.  Rahier J-F, Papay P, Salleron J, et al. H1N1 vaccines in a large observational cohort of patients with inflammatory bowel disease treated with immunomodulators and biological therapy. *Gut.* 2011;60(4):456-462. doi:10.1136/gut.2010.233981

9.  Tinsley A, Navabi S, Williams ED, et al. Increased risk of influenza and influenza-related complications among 140,480 patients with inflammatory bowel disease. *Inflamm Bowel Dis.* 2019;25(2):369-376. doi:10.1093/ibd/izy243

10. 1Long MD, Martin C, Sandler RS, Kappelman MD. Increased risk of pneumonia among patients with inflammatory bowel disease. *Am J Gastroenterol.* 2013;108(2):240-248. doi:10.1038/ajg.2012.406

11. Gregory MH, Ciorba MA, Wiitala WL, et al. The Association of Medications and Vaccination with Risk of Pneumonia in Inflammatory Bowel Disease. *Inflamm Bowel Dis.* August 2019. doi:10.1093/ibd/izz189

12. Ananthakrishnan AN, McGinley EL. Infection-related hospitalizations are associated with increased mortality in patients with inflammatory bowel diseases. *J Crohn's Colitis.* 2013;7(2):107-112. doi:10.1016/j.crohns.2012.02.015

13. Kantsø B, Simonsen J, Hoffmann S, Valentiner-Branth P, Petersen AM, Jess T. Inflammatory bowel disease patients are at increased risk of invasive pneumococcal disease: a nationwide Danish cohort study 1977-2013. *Am J Gastroenterol.* 2015;110(11):1582-1587. doi:10.1038/ajg.2015.284

14. Farraye FA, Melmed GY, Lichtenstein GR, Kane S V. ACG clinical guideline: preventive care in inflammatory bowel disease. 2017;112(2):241-258. doi:10.1038/ajg.2016.537

15. Schillie S, Harris A, Link-Gelles R, Romero J, Ward J, Nelson N. Morbidity and mortality weekly report recommendations of the Advisory Committee on Immunization Practices for Use of a Hepatitis B Vaccine with a Novel Adjuvant. https://vaers.hhs.gov. Accessed February 29, 2020.

16. Reddy KR, Beavers KL, Hammond SP, Lim JK, Falck-Ytter YT. American Gastroenterological Association Institute guideline on the prevention and treatment of hepatitis B virus reactivation during immunosuppressive drug therapy. *Gastroenterology*. 2015;148(1):215-219. doi:10.1053/j.gastro.2014.10.039

17. Long MD, Martin C, Sandler RS, Kappelman MD. Increased risk of herpes zoster among 108 604 patients with inflammatory bowel disease. *Aliment Pharmacol Ther*. 2013;37(4):420-429. doi:10.1111/apt.12182

18. Gupta G, Lautenbach E, Lewis JD. Incidence and risk factors for herpes zoster among patients with inflammatory bowel disease. *Clin Gastroenterol Hepatol*. 2006;4(12):1483-1490. doi:10.1016/j.cgh.2006.09.019

19. Winthrop KL, Melmed GY, Vermeire S, et al. Herpes zoster infection in patients with ulcerative colitis receiving tofacitinib. *Inflamm Bowel Dis*. 2018;24(10):2258-2265. doi:10.1093/ibd/izy131

20. Satyam VR, Li PH, Reich J, et al. Safety of recombinant zoster vaccine in patients with inflammatory bowel disease. *Dig Dis Sci*. 2020. doi:10.1007/s10620-019-06016-4

21. Reddy KR, Beavers KL, Hammond SP, Lim JK, Falck-Ytter YT, American Gastroenterological Association Institute. American Gastroenterological Association Institute guideline on the prevention and treatment of hepatitis B virus reactivation during immunosuppressive drug therapy. *Gastroenterology*. 2015;148(1):215-219; quiz e16-7. doi:10.1053/j.gastro.2014.10.039

22. Farraye FA, Melmed GY, Lichtenstein GR, Kane S V. ACG clinical guideline: preventive care in inflammatory bowel disease. *Am J Gastroenterol*. 2017;112(2):241-258. doi:10.1038/ajg.2016.537

23. Prevention of Rotavirus Gastroenteritis Among Infants and Children Recommendations of the Advisory Committee on Immunization Practices. https://www.cdc.gov/mmwr/preview/mmwrhtml/rr5802a1.htm. Accessed February 29, 2020.

24. Mahadevan U, Robinson C, Bernasko N, et al. Inflammatory bowel disease in pregnancy clinical care pathway: a report from the American Gastroenterological Association IBD Parenthood Project Working Group. *Gastroenterology*. 2019;156(5):1508-1524. doi:10.1053/j.gastro.2018.12.022

25. Wasan SK, Baker SE, Skolnik PR, Farraye FA. A practical guide to vaccinating the inflammatory bowel disease patient. *Am J Gastroenterol*. 2010;105(6):1231-1238. doi:10.1038/ajg.2009.733

26. Long MD, Martin CF, Pipkin CA, Herfarth HH, Sandler RS, Kappelman MD. Risk of melanoma and nonmelanoma skin cancer among patients with inflammatory bowel disease. *Gastroenterology*. 2012;143(2):390-399.e1. doi:10.1053/j.gastro.2012.05.004

27. Rogers HW, Weinstock MA, Feldman SR, Coldiron BM. Incidence estimate of nonmelanoma skin cancer (keratinocyte carcinomas) in the us population, 2012. *JAMA Dermatology*. 2015;151(10):1081-1086. doi:10.1001/jamadermatol.2015.1187

28. Ariyaratnam J, Subramanian V. Association between thiopurine use and nonmelanoma skin cancers in patients with inflammatory bowel disease: a meta-analysis. *Am J Gastroenterol*. 2014;109(2):163-169. doi:10.1038/ajg.2013.451

29. Perrett CM, Walker SL, O'Donovan P, et al. Azathioprine treatment photosensitizes human skin to ultraviolet A radiation. *Br J Dermatol*. 2008;159(1):198-204. doi:10.1111/j.1365-2133.2008.08610.x

30. Abbas AM, Almukhtar RM, Loftus E V, Lichtenstein GR, Khan N. Risk of melanoma and non-melanoma skin cancer in ulcerative colitis patients treated with thiopurines: a nationwide retrospective cohort. *Am J Gastroenterol*. 2014;109(11):1781-1793. doi:10.1038/ajg.2014.298

31. Curtis JR, Lee EB, Martin G, et al. Analysis of non-melanoma skin cancer across the tofacitinib rheumatoid arthritis clinical programme. *Clin Exp Rheumatol*. 35(4):614-622. http://www.ncbi.nlm.nih.gov/pubmed/28240592. Accessed January 22, 2020.

32. Singh S, Nagpal SJS, Murad MH, et al. Inflammatory bowel disease is associated with an increased risk of melanoma: a systematic review and meta-analysis. *Clin Gastroenterol Hepatol*. 2014;12(2):210-218. doi:10.1016/j.cgh.2013.04.033

33. Bigby M, Kim CC. A prospective randomized controlled trial indicates that sunscreen use reduced the risk of developing melanoma. *Arch Dermatol*. 2011;147(7):853-854. doi:10.1001/archdermatol.2011.171

34. Okafor PN, Stallwood CG, Nguyen L, et al. Cost-effectiveness of nonmelanoma skin cancer screening in Crohn's disease patients. *Inflamm Bowel Dis*. 2013;19(13):2787-2795. doi:10.1097/01.MIB.0000435850.17263.13

35. Hovde Ø, Høivik ML, Henriksen M, Solberg IC, Småstuen MC, Moum BA. Malignancies in patients with inflammatory bowel disease: results from 20 years of follow-up in the IBSEN study. *J Crohns Colitis*. 2017;11(5):571-577. doi:10.1093/ecco-jcc/jjw193

36. Mamtani R, Clark AS, Scott FI, et al. Association between breast cancer recurrence and immunosuppression in rheumatoid arthritis and inflammatory bowel disease: a cohort study. *Arthritis Rheumatol*. 2016;68(10):2403-2411. doi:10.1002/art.39738

37. Monticciolo DL, Newell MS, Hendrick RE, et al. Breast cancer screening for average-risk women: recommendations from the ACR Commission on Breast Imaging. *J Am Coll Radiol*. 2017;14(9):1137-1143. doi:10.1016/j.jacr.2017.06.001

38. Siu AL. CLINICAL GUIDELINE Screening for Breast Cancer : U.S. Preventive Services Task Force. *Ann Intern Med.* 2016;164(4):279-296. doi:10.7326/M15-2886

39. Singh H, Nugent Z, Demers AA, Bernstein CN. Screening for cervical and breast cancer among women with inflammatory bowel disease: a population-based study. *Inflamm Bowel Dis.* 2011;17(8):1741-1750. doi:10.1002/ibd.21567

40. Allegretti JR, Barnes EL, Cameron A. Are patients with inflammatory bowel disease on chronic immunosuppressive therapy at increased risk of cervical high-grade dysplasia/cancer? a meta-analysis. *Inflamm Bowel Dis.* 2015;21(5):1089-1097. doi:10.1097/MIB.0000000000000338

41. Nguyen ML, Flowers L. Cervical cancer screening in immunocompromised women. *Obstet Gynecol Clin North Am.* 2013;40(2):339-357. doi:10.1016/j.ogc.2013.02.005

42. Rungoe C, Simonsen J, Riis L, Frisch M, Langholz E, Jess T. Inflammatory bowel disease and cervical neoplasia: a population-based nationwide cohort study. *Clin Gastroenterol Hepatol.* 2015;13(4):693-700.e1. doi:10.1016/j.cgh.2014.07.036

43. Ellerbrock T V., Chiasson MA, Bush TJ, et al. Incidence of cervical squamous intraepithelial lesions in HIV-infected women. *J Am Med Assoc.* 2000;283(8):1031-1037. doi:10.1001/jama.283.8.1031

44. Wadström H, Arkema E V., Sjöwall C, Askling J, Simard JF. Cervical neoplasia in systemic lupus erythematosus: a nationwide study. *Rheumatol (United Kingdom).* 2017;56(4):613-619. doi:10.1093/rheumatology/kew459

45. Thimm MA, Rositch AF, VandenBussche C, McDonald L, Garonzik Wang JM, Levinson K. Lower genital tract dysplasia in female solid organ transplant recipients. *Obstet Gynecol.* 2019;134(2):385-394. doi:10.1097/AOG.0000000000003378

46. Long MD, Porter CQ, Sandler RS, Kappelman MD. Suboptimal rates of cervical testing among women with inflammatory bowel disease. *Clin Gastroenterol Hepatol.* 2009;7(5):549-553. doi:10.1016/j.cgh.2008.10.007

47. Chedid VG, Kane S V. Bone Health in patients with inflammatory bowel diseases. *J Clin Densitom.* 2019. doi:10.1016/j.jocd.2019.07.009

48. Bernstein CN, Leslie WD, Leboff MS. AGA technical review on osteoporosis in gastrointestinal diseases. *Gastroenterology.* 2003;124(3):795-841. doi:10.1053/gast.2003.50106

49. Ludvigsson JF, Mahl M, Sachs MC, et al. Fracture risk in patients with inflammatory bowel disease: a nationwide population-based cohort study from 1964 to 2014. *Am J Gastroenterol.* 2019;114(2):291-304. doi:10.14309/ajg.0000000000000062

50. Komaki Y, Komaki F, Micic D, Ido A, Sakuraba A. Risk of fractures in inflammatory bowel diseases: a systematic review and meta-analysis. *J Clin Gastroenterol.* 2019;53(6):441-448. doi:10.1097/MCG.0000000000001031

51. Card T, West J, Hubbard R, Logan RFA. Hip fractures in patients with inflammatory bowel disease and their relationship to corticosteroid use: a population based cohort study. *Gut.* 2004;53(2):251-255. doi:10.1136/gut.2003.026799

52. Targownik LE, Bernstein CN, Leslie WD. Risk factors and management of osteoporosis in inflammatory bowel disease. *Curr Opin Gastroenterol.* 2014;30(2):168-174. doi:10.1097/MOG.0000000000000037

53. Curry SJ, Krist AH, Owens DK, et al. Screening for osteoporosis to prevent fractures us preventive services task force recommendation statement. *JAMA.* 2018;319(24):2521-2531. doi:10.1001/jama.2018.7498

54. Schüle S, Benoit Rossel J-B, Frey D, et al. Prediction of low bone mineral density in patients with inflammatory bowel diseases. *United European Gastroenterol J.* 2016;4(5):669-676. doi:10.1177/2050640616658224

55. Lewis K, Marrie RA, Bernstein CN, et al. The prevalence and risk factors of undiagnosed depression and anxiety disorders among patients with inflammatory bowel disease. *Inflamm Bowel Dis.* 2019;25(10):1674-1680. doi:10.1093/ibd/izz045

56. Mikocka-Walus A, Knowles SR, Keefer L, Graff L. Controversies revisited: a systematic review of the comorbidity of depression and anxiety with inflammatory bowel diseases. *Inflamm Bowel Dis.* 2015;22(3):752-762. doi:10.1097/MIB.0000000000000620

57. Nahon S, Lahmek P, Durance C, et al. Risk factors of anxiety and depression in inflammatory bowel disease. *Inflamm Bowel Dis.* 2012;18(11):2086-2091. doi:10.1002/ibd.22888

58. Bhandari S, Larson ME, Kumar N, Stein D. Association of inflammatory bowel disease (IBD) with depressive symptoms in the United States population and independent predictors of depressive symptoms in an IBD population: a NHANES study. *Gut Liver.* 2017;11(4):512-519. doi:10.5009/gnl16347

59. Mittermaier C, Dejaco C, Waldhoer T, et al. Impact of depressive mood on relapse in patients with inflammatory bowel disease: a prospective 18-month follow-up study. *Psychosom Med.* 66(1):79-84. doi:10.1097/01.psy.0000106907.24881.f2

60. Persoons P, Vermeire S, Demyttenaere K, et al. The impact of major depressive disorder on the short- and long-term outcome of Crohn's disease treatment with infliximab. *Aliment Pharmacol Ther.* 2005;22(2):101-110. doi:10.1111/j.1365-2036.2005.02535.x

61. Langhorst J, Hofstetter A, Wolfe F, Häuser W. Short-Term stress, but not mucosal healing nor depression was predictive for the risk of relapse in patients with ulcerative colitis: a prospective 12-month follow-up study. *Inflamm Bowel Dis.* 2013;19(11):2380-2386. doi:10.1097/MIB.0b013e3182a192ba

62.  Arroll B, Khin N, Kerse N. Screening for depression in primary care with two verbally asked questions: cross sectional study. *BMJ.* 2003;327(7424):1144-1146. doi:10.1136/bmj.327.7424.1144

63.  Mikocka-Walus AA, Turnbull DA, Moulding NT, Wilson IG, Andrews JM, Holtmann GJ. Antidepressants and inflammatory bowel disease: a systematic review. *Clin Pract Epidemiol Ment Heal.* 2006;2. doi:10.1186/1745-0179-2-24

64.  Goodhand JR, Greig FIS, Koodun Y, et al. Do antidepressants influence the disease course in inflammatory bowel disease? a retrospective case-matched observational study. *Inflamm Bowel Dis.* 2012;18(7):1232-1239. doi:10.1002/ibd.21846

65.  Gibbons RD, Weiss DJ, Pilkonis PA, et al. Development of a computerized adaptive test for depression. *Arch Gen Psychiatry.* 2012;69(11):1104-1112. doi:10.1001/archgenpsychiatry.2012.14

66.  Olén O, Erichsen R, Sachs MC, et al. Colorectal cancer in ulcerative colitis: a Scandinavian population-based cohort study. *Lancet.* 2020;395(10218):123-131. doi:10.1016/S0140-6736(19)32545-0

67.  Bogach J, Pond G, Eskicioglu C, Seow H. Age-related survival differences in patients with inflammatory bowel disease-associated colorectal cancer: a population-based cohort study. *Inflamm Bowel Dis.* 2019;25(12):1957-1965. doi:10.1093/ibd/izz088

68.  Stjärngrim J, Ekbom A, Hammar U, Hultcrantz R, Forsberg AM. Rates and characteristics of postcolonoscopy colorectal cancer in the Swedish IBD population: what are the differences from a non-IBD population? *Gut.* 2019;68(9):1588-1596. doi:10.1136/gutjnl-2018-316651

69.  Flores BM, O'Connor A, Moss AC. Impact of mucosal inflammation on risk of colorectal neoplasia in patients with ulcerative colitis: a systematic review and meta-analysis. *Gastrointest Endosc.* 2017. doi:10.1016/j.gie.2017.07.028

70.  Gyde SN, Prior P, Allan RN, et al. Colorectal cancer in ulcerative colitis: a cohort study of primary referrals from three centres. *Gut.* 1988;29(2):206-217. doi:10.1136/gut.29.2.206

71.  Lutgens MWMD, van Oijen MGH, van der Heijden GJMG, Vleggaar FP, Siersema PD, Oldenburg B. Declining risk of colorectal cancer in inflammatory bowel disease: an updated meta-analysis of population-based cohort studies. *Inflamm Bowel Dis.* 2013;19(4):789-799. doi:10.1097/MIB.0b013e31828029c0

72.  Gillen CD, Walmsley RS, Prior P, Andrews HA, Allan RN. Ulcerative colitis and Crohn's disease: a comparison of the colorectal cancer risk in extensive colitis. *Gut.* 1994;35(11):1590-1592. doi:10.1136/gut.35.11.1590

73.  Askling J, Dickman PW, Karlén P, et al. Family history as a risk factor for colorectal cancer in inflammatory bowel disease. *Gastroenterology.* 2001;120(6):1356-1362. doi:10.1053/gast.2001.24052

74.  Ananthakrishnan AN, Cagan A, Gainer VS, et al. Mortality and extraintestinal cancers in patients with primary sclerosing cholangitis and inflammatory bowel disease. *J Crohns Colitis.* 2014;8(9):956-963. doi:10.1016/j.crohns.2014.01.019

75.  Farraye FA, Odze RD, Eaden J, et al. AGA medical position statement on the diagnosis and management of colorectal neoplasia in inflammatory bowel disease. *Gastroenterology.* 2010;138(2):738-745. doi:10.1053/j.gastro.2009.12.037

76.  Lamb CA, Kennedy NA, Raine T, et al. British Society of Gastroenterology consensus guidelines on the management of inflammatory bowel disease in adults. *Gut.* 2019;68:s1-s106. doi:10.1136/gutjnl-2019-318484

77.  Lutgens MWMD, Vleggaar FP, Schipper MEI, et al. High frequency of early colorectal cancer in inflammatory bowel disease. *Gut.* 2008;57(9):1246-1251. doi:10.1136/gut.2007.143453

78.  Baars JE, Kuipers EJ, van Haastert M, Nicolaï JJ, Poen AC, van der Woude CJ. Age at diagnosis of inflammatory bowel disease influences early development of colorectal cancer in inflammatory bowel disease patients: a nationwide, long-term survey. *J Gastroenterol.* 2012;47(12):1308-1322. doi:10.1007/s00535-012-0603-2

79.  Buchner AM, Shahid MW, Heckman MG, et al. High-definition colonoscopy detects colorectal polyps at a higher rate than standard white-light colonoscopy. *Clin Gastroenterol Hepatol.* 2010;8(4):364-370. doi:10.1016/j.cgh.2009.11.009

80.  Li Y, Lopez R, Queener E, Shen B. Adalimumab therapy in Crohn's disease of the ileal pouch. *Inflamm Bowel Dis.* 2012;18(12):2232-2239. doi:10.1002/ibd.22933

81.  Rutter MD, Saunders BP, Wilkinson KH, Kamm MA, Williams CB, Forbes A. Most dysplasia in ulcerative colitis is visible at colonoscopy. *Gastrointest Endosc.* 2004;60(3):334-339. doi:10.1016/s0016-5107(04)01710-9

82.  Van Den Broek FJC, Stokkers PCF, Reitsma JB, et al. Random biopsies taken during colonoscopic surveillance of patients with longstanding ulcerative colitis: Low yield and absence of clinical consequences. *Am J Gastroenterol.* 2014;109(5):715-722. doi:10.1038/ajg.2011.93

83.  Severs M, Mangen MJJ, van der Valk ME, et al. Smoking is associated with higher disease-related costs and lower health-related quality of life in inflammatory bowel disease. *J Crohns Colitis.* 2017;11(3):342-352. doi:10.1093/ecco-jcc/jjw160

84.  Mahid SS, Minor KS, Soto RE, Hornung CA, Galandiuk S. Smoking and inflammatory bowel disease: a meta-analysis. [Erratum appears in Mayo Clin Proc. 2007 Jul;82(7):890]. Mayo Clin Proc. 2006;81(11):1462-1471. http://ovidsp.ovid.com/ovidweb.cgi?T=JS&CSC=Y&NEWS=N&PAGE=fulltext&D=med4&AN=17120402. Accessed January 24, 2020.

85.  Somerville KW, Logan RF, Edmond M, Langman MJ. Smoking and Crohn's disease. *Br Med J (Clin Res Ed).* 1984;289(6450):954-956. doi:10.1136/bmj.289.6450.954

86.  Vessfy M, Jewell D, Smith A, Yeates D, McPhers6N K. Chronic inflammatory bowel disease, cigarette smoking, and use of oral contraceptives: findings in a large cohort study of women of childbearing age. *Br Med J (Clin Res Ed)*. 1986;292(6528):1101-1103. doi:10.1136/bmj.292.6528.1101

87.  Lunney PC, Kariyawasam VC, Wang RR, et al. Smoking prevalence and its influence on disease course and surgery in Crohn's disease and ulcerative colitis. *Aliment Pharmacol Ther*. 2015;42(1):61-70. doi:10.1111/apt.13239

88.  Lakatos PL, Vegh Z, Lovasz BD, et al. Is Current smoking still an important environmental factor in inflammatory bowel diseases? results from a population-based incident cohort. *Inflamm Bowel Dis*. 2013;19(4):1010-1017. doi:10.1097/MIB.0b013e3182802b3e

89.  Nunes T, Etchevers MJ, Domènech E, et al. Smoking does influence disease behaviour and impacts the need for therapy in Crohn's disease in the biologic era. *Aliment Pharmacol Ther*. 2013;38(7):752-760. doi:10.1111/apt.12440

90.  Nunes T, Etchevers MJ, Merino O, et al. Does smoking influence Crohn's disease in the biologic era? the TABACROHN study. *Inflamm Bowel Dis*. 2013;19(1):23-29. doi:10.1002/ibd.22959

91.  Arnott IDR, McNeill G, Satsangi J. An analysis of factors influencing short-term and sustained response to infliximab treatment for Crohn's disease. *Aliment Pharmacol Ther*. 2003;17(12):1451-1457. doi:10.1046/j.1365-2036.2003.01574.x

92.  To N, Gracie DJ, Ford AC. Systematic review with meta-analysis: the adverse effects of tobacco smoking on the natural history of Crohn's disease. *Aliment Pharmacol Ther*. 2016;43(5):549-561. doi:10.1111/apt.13511

93.  Gustavsson A, Magnuson A, Blomberg B, Andersson M, Halfvarson J, Tysk C. Smoking is a risk factor for recurrence of intestinal stricture after endoscopic dilation in Crohn's disease. *Aliment Pharmacol Ther*. 2013;37(4):430-437. doi:10.1111/apt.12176

94.  Ryan WR, Allan RN, Yamamoto T, Keighley MRB. Crohn's disease patients who quit smoking have a reduced risk of reoperation for recurrence. *Am J Surg*. 2004;187(2):219-225. doi:10.1016/j.amjsurg.2003.11.007

95.  Nunes T, Etchevers MJ, García-Sánchez V, et al. Impact of smoking cessation on the clinical course of Crohn's disease under current therapeutic algorithms: a multicenter prospective study. *Am J Gastroenterol*. 2016;111(3):411-419. doi:10.1038/ajg.2015.401

96.  Leung Y, Kaplan GG, Rioux KP, et al. Assessment of variables associated with smoking cessation in Crohn's disease. *Dig Dis Sci*. 2012;57(4):1026-1032. doi:10.1007/s10620-012-2038-2

97.  Kaplan GG. Smoking cessation for Crohn's disease: clearing the haze. *Am J Gastroenterol*. 2016;111(3):420-422. doi:10.1038/ajg.2016.45

98.  Kennelly RP, Subramaniam T, Egan LJ, Joyce MR. Smoking and Crohn's disease: active modification of an independent risk factor (education alone is not enough). *J Crohns Colitis*. 2013;7(8):631-635. doi:10.1016/j.crohns.2012.08.019

99.  Coward S, Heitman SJ, Clement F, et al. Funding a smoking cessation program for Crohn's disease: an economic evaluation. *Am J Gastroenterol*. 2015;110(3):368-377. doi:10.1038/ajg.2014.300

# 7

# Family Planning in Women With IBD

Anita Afzali, MD, MPH | Madalina Butnariu, MD | Kindra Clark-Snustad, DNP, ARNP

## Introduction

Inflammatory bowel diseases (IBD), including Crohn's disease (CD) and ulcerative colitis (UC), are chronic immune-mediated inflammatory diseases commonly diagnosed in the second and third decades of life, during the reproductive years. IBD often requires lifelong treatment, and uncontrolled IBD during conception or pregnancy increases maternal and fetal risks. Given the potential impact of IBD and therapies on family planning, it is important to proactively counsel patients of childbearing age on fertility, contraception, and heredity. While non-operated patients with well-controlled disease have similar fertility as the general population, fertility in patients with IBD is decreased due to voluntary childlessness, active disease, and in patients with a history of ileal pouch-anal anastomosis (IPAA) surgery. CD has also been associated with decreased ovarian reserve. Many contraceptive options exist for people with IBD, but consideration should be given to avoidance of estrogen-containing methods for patients at higher risk of venous thromboembolism (VTE) and depot medroxyprogesterone in patients with known low bone density. Lastly, IBD has a higher rate of heritability if both parents have the disease. This chapter reviews topics relevant to family planning for patients with IBD, including fertility, contraception, and heredity.

Abraham BP, Kane SV, Glassner KL, eds.
*Women's Health in IBD: The Spectrum of Care From Birth to Adulthood* (pp 135-149).
© 2022 Taylor & Francis Group.

# Fertility and Fecundity in IBD

*Fertility* is defined as the ability to conceive children, and *fecundity* refers to the likelihood of pregnancy, considering factors such as age and ovarian reserve. *Sexual health* refers to a state of physical, emotional, mental, and social well-being in relation to sexuality.[1] *Sexuality*, which is defined as the desire for sex and satisfaction with sexual activity, has been found to be lower in patients with IBD.[2] While patients with non-operated, well-controlled UC have similar fertility rates as the general population, overall IBD has been associated with decreased fertility. This is likely due to voluntary childlessness, active UC or CD, history of IPAA, and decreased ovarian reserve in patients with CD.[3] IBD can also negatively impact patients' sexual health, which can lower fecundity and thus impact fertility.

## Patient Concerns

Patients with IBD report concern about the impact of the disease or medical therapies on fertility, the course and outcome of pregnancy, fetal development, mode of delivery, and the safety of lactation. There is also concern that a pregnancy may worsen their disease course, that they may pass on IBD to their child, or that their disease-related symptoms may impair their ability to care for a child.[4] In a survey of 255 patients with IBD, 42.7% reported fear of infertility, concerns about IBD heritability, the risk of congenital abnormalities, and medication teratogenicity.[5] In another patient survey, Walldorf and colleagues reported that females with IBD over the age of 35 had significantly higher rates of childlessness as compared to the general population (36.7% vs 22.9%, odds ratio [OR] 1.9, $P < .001$).[6] A study of 169 patients reported that 14% of females with UC reported voluntary childlessness, compared to 6.2% of the general population ($P = .08$).[7] The relatively high rates of voluntary childlessness among patients with IBD is likely significantly impacted by the psychosocial constraints of chronic disease and may also be due to patients' fear that IBD will negatively impact childbearing. Notably, a prospective study reported that counseling from a health care provider was associated with higher rates of pregnancies and lower rates of voluntary childlessness.[4]

## Sexual Health

The peak prevalence of IBD often occurs in patients' 20s and 30s of age, when forming intimate relationships, body image, and sexuality are of high importance. Unfortunately, IBD can negatively impact sexual health. For example, the disease itself, medications, and surgery can have a profound impact on energy levels, libido, mood, and body image.[2] Symptoms or the fear of symptoms can lead to abstinence, reduced sexual activity, and negative body image, which may impact fertility. Patient surveys suggest that concerns regarding sexual health are common, for example, the European IMPACT study of 4990 patients with IBD reported that 40% of participants felt that their disease prevented them from pursuing intimate relationships.[8,9] Both sexes report that IBD has a negative impact on sexuality; however, women report a greater negative impact as compared to men.[1] While concerns regarding sexual health are commonly reported and of high importance, these concerns are rarely expressed unsolicited and directly by patients to their health care providers.[8]

While IBD is an invisible disease for many patients, surgical scarring, ostomy placement, and weight loss or gain may alter patients' physical appearance. Symptoms, including abdominal pain, diarrhea, fecal incontinence, flatulence, and fistula drainage can affect patients' self-perception and feelings of sexual attractiveness and desire. Symptoms and disease activity can also lead to discomfort during intercourse.[1] In a survey of 347 patients with IBD, 50.2% reported a negative effect on relationships and 66.8% reported impaired body image (74.8% female vs 51.4% males, $P = .0007$). Females reported decreased frequency of sexual activity (66.3% vs 40.5%, $P < .0001$) and decreased libido (67.1% vs 41.9%, $P = .0005$) more often than males. Patients with a history of surgery also reported decreased sexual activity compared to those who had not undergone an operation (50.4%

vs 68.5%, $P = .0113$), and decreased libido (67.4% vs 52.6%, $P = .035$).[10] A longitudinal study of 116 females reported that those with a recent diagnosis of IBD reported sexual dysfunction more frequently than the general population (97% vs 50%).[11] Unfortunately, a high percentage of females with IBD reported sexual dysfunction throughout the 2-year study follow-up despite improvement in disease activity.[11]

Sexual dysfunction in patients with IBD has been associated with the presence of depression.[1] A survey of 169 females and 119 males with IBD reported significantly more impaired sexual function associated with active disease, and disease activity and sexual function were felt to be mediated by depression.[12] A history of surgery has also been associated with sexual dysfunction, with proposed mechanisms including disturbance to the innervation of the genitalia and distortion of the anatomy in the pelvis, which can lead to dyspareunia, decreased lubrication, or decreased vaginal proprioception.[1] Patients with a stoma reported impact on sexual health with regard to appliance leakage, odor, and body image.[2] Despite these concerns, some patients reported improvement in sexual function following surgery, thought to be due to better symptom and disease control.[1]

IBD can also influence body image, and females with IBD report higher rates of dissatisfaction compared to males.[1] Active disease and prednisone treatment can negatively affect body image, as can surgical scars, ostomies, weight and hair loss related to active disease, cutaneous manifestations of IBD, and perianal disease.[1] Additional factors including medication side effects can also contribute to this.[1]

Providers should assess sexual dissatisfaction in patients with IBD, address disease-related issues, and assess for contributing factors, such as depression. Consideration could be given to referral to health care providers specializing in sexual dysfunction.

## Disease Activity

While several studies have reported that fertility rates in non-operated patients with IBD with well-controlled disease are similar to the general population, the presence of active disease has been associated with decreased fertility.

A Danish cohort study of 74,471 pregnancies in women without IBD, 340 pregnancies in women with UC, and 206 with CD compared the time to pregnancy between groups. This study found that women with IBD, especially those with a history of surgery for CD, had a longer time to pregnancy as compared to women without IBD.[13] The adjusted relative risk ratios for time to pregnancy of more than 12 months for those with IBD, UC, and CD were 1.28 (95% confidence interval [CI], 0.99 to 1.65), 1.10 (95% CI, 0.80 to 1.51), and 1.54 (95% CI, 1.03 to 2.30), respectively.[13] For CD patients with a history of surgery, time to pregnancy of more than 12 months was over 2 times greater than for those without IBD (adjusted relative risk 2.54, 95% CI, 1.39 to 4.65).

In patients with UC, several studies have reported no reduction in fertility in patients with well-controlled UC who have not undergone surgery, as compared to those without IBD.[5,6] A systematic review on this topic evaluated 6 studies on fertility in UC. Two small studies reported a reduced fertility rate; however, this was thought to be due to voluntary childlessness. The other 4 studies reported similar fertility rates in females with UC and those without UC.[5]

Patients with CD without a history of surgery have similar or only slightly decreased fertility compared to the general population.[14] In a survey from Scotland, the rate of involuntary infertility in patients with IBD was similar to the general population; however, voluntary childlessness was higher in IBD populations. For example, 36% of patients with CD reported voluntary childlessness, compared to 7% of people in the control population.[14,15] A 2013 systematic review of 11 studies showed that there was a 17% to 44% reduction in fertility in women with CD as compared to controls. Again, the authors felt that this was due to voluntary childlessness.[16]

Studies have attempted to assess fecundity by measuring serum anti-mullerian hormone (AMH) level, which is a reliable indicator of ovarian reserve. A study of 35 patients with CD and 35 age-matched healthy controls showed that patients with CD had significantly lower AMH levels compared to controls (1.02 ± 0.72 vs 1.89 ± 1.80, $P$ = .009), suggesting that patients with CD have decreased ovarian reserve. Further, AMH levels in patients with CD with active disease were significantly lower compared to patients with CD who were in remission (0.33 ± 0.25 vs 1.53 ± 0.49, $P$ = .001). Notably, the authors also described a negative correlation between the CD Activity Index and AMH level (r = -0.718, $P$ < .001).[17]

In 2015, a large cohort study of 9639 females with IBD measured the adjusted fertility rate ratio (AFRR) in women with and without IBD, reporting that the AFRR of women with IBD decreased after diagnosis. In UC, the AFRR was 1.07 (95% CI, 0.99 to 1.16) prior to diagnosis and 0.92 (95% CI, 0.86 to 1.00) after diagnosis. For women with CD, the AFRR was 0.88 (95% CI, 0.81 to 0.97) prior to diagnosis and 0.87 (95% CI, 0.82 to 0.94) after diagnosis.[18] The presence of active endoscopic disease or a history of surgery was found to negatively impact fertility, with a reported AFRR of 0.70 (95% CI, 0.59 to 0.82) following a flare and 0.84 after surgery (95% CI, 0.77 to 0.92). This study reported overall similar fertility in women with a history of pouch and non-pouch surgery.[18] Proposed mechanisms for the negative impact on fertility include decreased sexual activity in patients with active symptoms or associated inflammation in the ovaries and fallopian tubes. Malnutrition, anemia, and depression in the setting of flares are also thought to impact fertility.[14]

## Medical Therapy

Patients report fear that medical therapy may impact their ability to conceive; however, there is no evidence that IBD medications negatively affect female fertility.[14,19] Certain IBD therapies, including methotrexate and thalidomide, are contraindicated during conception and pregnancy given the risk of teratogenicity. Given the limited available human data on the safety of Janus kinase inhibitors in both males and females, avoidance during conception and pregnancy is recommended. In males, sulfasalazine may cause reversible oligospermia, reduced sperm motility, and abnormal sperm morphology. Methotrexate has also been associated with reversible oligospermia.[16]

## Surgery

An estimated 10% to 20% of patients with UC will require surgery in their lifetime,[14,20-22] most commonly with restorative proctocolectomy with IPAA. This surgical technique had been considered superior to other surgical procedures like the ileorectal anastomosis (IRA) given that IPAA aims to remove the entire colon and thus decreases the risk of proctitis, dysplasia, and cancer.[22] IPAA does not appear to impair pregnancy or childbirth; however, IPAA may decrease fecundity due to anatomic changes and fallopian tube scarring due to deep pelvic dissection.[23] A meta-analysis reported infertility rates of 14% for medically treated UC patients and infertility rates of 48% in those who had undergone IPAA.[24] A retrospective study evaluating fecundity reviewed 343 females with UC, documenting the months of unprotected sex leading up to pregnancy or the inability to conceive. From this, they estimated the fecundability ratio (FR) in patients with UC prior to diagnosis, after diagnosis, and after undergoing restorative proctocolectomy with IPAA, reporting that the FR was decreased following colectomy with IPAA (FR 0.20, $P$ < .0001),[23] but not decreased in females with UC prior to diagnosis (FR 1.46, $P$ = .002) or after diagnosis (FR 1.01, $P$ = NS) as compared to healthy females.

A study of females with familial adenomatous polyposis reported that fecundability of females who underwent subtotal colectomy with IRA was not different from the general population, however for those females who underwent proctocolectomy with IPAA, fecundability was decreased to 54% ($P$ = .015).[23,25] IRA may offer an advantage given that it does not involve extensive pelvic dissection; however, it is not an option for patients with IBD with impaired anal sphincter tone, severe perianal or rectal disease, or concern for dysplasia or cancer.[14] Due to the negative impact of IPAA on fertility, some patients with IBD who require surgical treatment for UC may elect for temporary diverting ileostomy or IRA, then may proceed with IPAA after childbearing is complete.[2] More recently, a small retrospective study suggested that a laparoscopic approach to surgery might reduce the risk of infertility. This study reported that 70% of patients who underwent laparoscopic IPAA were able to become pregnant spontaneously, as compared to 39% of those who underwent an open approach.[14,26] A laparoscopic approach to IPAA should be considered if appropriate; however, larger prospective trials are needed to confirm the potential benefit to fertility.

Population studies have reported that 25% of patients with CD will require surgery in their lifetime,[14] and the data are less clear if a history of surgery for CD negatively impacts fertility. A 1986 study of 78 women with CD who had undergone bowel resection reported no difference in the number of live births as compared to the expected live births in the general population.[27] A 1997 retrospective Scottish study of 503 woman with IBD reported that infertility was more frequent in women who had undergone CD surgery compared with those who had not (12% vs 5%).[15] A 2015 cohort study of 1153 patients with UC and CD reported a lower AFRR after any IBD surgery as compared to prior surgery (0.81 vs 0.97).[18] A 2019 Cochrane review including 16 studies reported that the effect of surgery on female infertility was uncertain given the low level of evidence in the included studies.[28] Authors reported that a history of prior surgery was associated with higher rates of miscarriage, use of assisted reproductive therapy, caesarean section delivery, and a low birth-weight infant. The review did not find an association between history of surgery and risk of stillbirth, preterm delivery, or small for gestational age infant.[28] Overall, current data are limited and further studies are needed to understand whether CD-related surgery, particularly limited bowel resection, has a significant impact on fertility.

## Infertility and Assisted Reproduction Technology Treatment

Rates of *infertility*, or the inability to conceive within 1 year of unprotected intercourse, in people with UC are overall similar to the general population. A 2013 systematic review reported that patients with CD have a higher rate of infertility as compared to healthy controls[16]; however, this reduction was thought to be due to voluntary childlessness. For IBD patients with infertility, assisted reproductive technology (ART) treatment including in vitro fertilization, intracytoplasmic sperm injection, and frozen embryo replacement can be successful.[3] Overall, ART for UC patients is successful at similar rates to the general population,[29] including in those patients with a history of IPAA.[30] A Danish cohort study of 381 patients with UC, 158 patients with CD, and 50,321 patients without IBD evaluated the effectiveness of ART to result in a live birth. This study reported that women with UC and women with UC with a history of surgery who underwent ART had a decreased chance of live birth compared to women without IBD, but the result was not statistically significant.[3] Patients with CD and a history of prior surgery were found to have a significantly decreased chance of live birth (OR 0.29, 95% CI, 0.13 to 0.65).[3] Another study evaluated 13,560 women with UC, 711 of whom had undergone restorative proctocolectomy, and reported that patients with a history of IPAA underwent in vitro fertilization more frequently than non-operated UC patients (adjusted hazard ratio 3.2, 95% CI, 2.5 to 4.0), but the odds of live birth following in vitro fertilization were similar between groups.[31] Another study reported that the decreased chance of live birth in patients with UC and CD was likely due to failure to achieve a pregnancy, and not due to issues with fertilization, implantation, or maintenance of the pregnancy.[3,32] A cohort study of 121 women with IBD who underwent ART showed that patients with UC who achieved a live birth were younger ($P = .03$), had shorter duration of disease ($P = .01$), and were more likely to be in remission ($P = .03$). Patients with CD who achieved a live birth were younger ($P < .001$) and had lower body mass index ($P = .02$).[29]

# Family Planning and Contraception in IBD

Patients who conceive in the setting of active IBD have an increased risk of active disease during pregnancy; active disease during pregnancy increases maternal and fetal risks.[33] Furthermore, some IBD therapies including methotrexate and thalidomide are teratogenic and contraindicated pregnancy. Therefore, guidelines recommend that patients aim to achieve remission for at least 3 to 6 months prior to conception to reduce these risks.[34] Proactive family planning for patients with IBD can improve outcomes, and several safe and effective contraceptive options exist.

## Contraceptive Options and IBD Specific Concerns

Options for contraception include progestin-only long-acting hormonal methods (eg, intrauterine devices [IUD] or implants), progestin-only short-acting methods (eg, depot medroxyprogesterone and progesterone only pills), short-acting combined hormonal contraceptives (eg, pills, transdermal patch, or vaginal ring), long-acting non-hormonal method (eg, copper IUD), nonreversible methods (eg, permanent sterilization), and barrier methods (Table 7-1). When selecting a contraceptive method, consideration should be given to patient preference, the effectiveness of the method, and how the contraceptive method could impact patients with IBD.

There are several considerations for choice of contraception in patients with IBD. Given that IBD can negatively affect gastrointestinal absorption, one concern is that a history of bowel resection or severely active disease may cause malabsorption of oral contraceptive pills. Fortunately, studies have suggested that neither colectomy[35,36] nor limited ileal resection[37] significantly change absorption.[38] Given that most oral contraception absorption occurs in the small bowel, this issue is theoretically of greater concern for patients with CD with extensive small bowel involvement or resection. One small study of patients with obesity without IBD with jejunoileal bypass suggested that patients who had undergone surgery had reduced capacity to absorb oral contraception as compared to non-operated controls.[39] Unfortunately, studies in patients with CD who have undergone significant bowel resection or have extensive small bowel disease are lacking.

Another concern is the potential for oral contraception to increase the risk of IBD flares. This does not seem to be the case, as a systematic review on the use of contraceptives in patients with IBD found no increased risk of disease flare in woman with IBD taking combined hormonal contraception.[37]

Concern has also been raised regarding a possible increased risk of VTE in IBD patients on estrogen-containing oral contraception. IBD populations have a 2- to 3-fold increased risk of VTE,[40] and this risk increases to 3- to 8-fold in the setting of active disease.[41] A recent meta-analysis of 33 studies reported that IBD diagnosis was associated with a risk ratio of 1.96 (95% CI, 1.67 to 2.30) for VTE.[42,43] Other studies report that the absolute risk of VTE in IBD patients is 0.1% to 0.5% annually.[42] The increased risk of VTE is thought to be due to an estrogen driven increase in hepatic production of serum globulins involved in the coagulation cascade.[38] Additional risk factors associated with VTE events in patients with IBD include hospitalization, disease that requires corticosteroids, extensive disease, fulminant episodes, and smoking.[44,45]

A 2-fold increased risk of VTE has also been described in healthy females on estrogen-based methods including combination pills, the patch, or the ring,[46,47] but not progestogen-only pills or hormonal releasing intrauterine devices.[38,48] A 2012 meta-analysis did not support an association between VTE and progestin-only contraception.[38,49] There are currently insufficient data to describe the specific risk of VTE in females with IBD using estrogen-based contraception; however, given the theoretical risk, consideration should be given to avoidance of estrogen-containing methods in females with IBD who are at higher risk of VTE.

An additional consideration is the potential influence of IBD medications on VTE risk. A recent interim analysis of an ongoing, post marketing safety study reported that rheumatoid arthritis patients aged 50 years and older with at least one cardiovascular risk factor treated with tofacitinib

## Table 7-1. Contraceptive Methods: Considerations for IBD Patients

| METHODS | | | CONSIDERATIONS |
|---|---|---|---|
| Hormonal | Progestin-only long-acting | IUDs | |
| | | Implants | |
| | Progestin-only short-acting | Depot medroxyprogesterone | Avoid in patients with known low bone density and those at risk |
| | | Progesterone-only pills | |
| | Combined hormonal short-acting | Combined oral contraceptive pills | Avoid in patients at high risk of VTE |
| | | Transdermal patch | |
| | | Vaginal ring | |
| Non-hormonal | Long-acting | Copper IUD | |
| | Non-reversible | Female sterilization (tubal occlusion) | |
| | | Male sterilization (vasectomy) | |
| | Barrier | Male condom | |
| | | Female condom | |
| | | Diaphragm | |
| | Other | Withdrawal | |
| No contraceptive use | | | Patients with active disease have higher risk of complications in the setting of pregnancy |

10 mg twice/day had a higher rate of all-cause mortality, including sudden cardiovascular death, and thrombosis, including pulmonary embolism, deep venous thrombosis, and arterial thrombosis as compared to those treated with tofacitinib 5 mg given twice daily or tumor necrosis factor blockers.[50] The association of VTE risk in patients with UC treated with tofacitinib is less clear and to date has not been found; however, given the concern for increased risk in this population, consideration should be given to avoiding estrogen-containing contraceptives in patients with UC treated with tofacitinib.

In practice, a survey of 1499 females with IBD found that 33.7% (95% CI, 30.6% to 36.9%) of women with CD and 32.6% (95% CI, 28.6% to 36.8%) of those with UC were on hormonal contraception. In this study, hormonal contraception was used as a proxy for estrogen-containing contraceptives. Women with one risk factor for VTE and women with 2 or more risk factors were not significantly less likely to take hormonal contraception as compared to those with no risk factors.[42] This may represent an opportunity for improvement given that while estrogen-containing hormonal contraception is not an absolute contraindication for women with IBD, those patients with additional risk factors for VTE may benefit from alternative contraceptive methods.[42]

Finally, patients with IBD are at increased risk of low bone density. Depot medroxyprogesterone acetate injections have been associated with a negative effect on bone density and therefore considered cautiously as a contraceptive method in the at-risk patient with IBD.[51]

## Preconception Counseling in IBD

Given the increased risk associated with active IBD in the setting of pregnancy, providers should counsel patients on the importance of achieving remission prior to conception. We recommend endoscopic evaluation to confirm remission prior to attempting pregnancy. Additionally, patients with IBD may have misperceptions about the safety of IBD medications during pregnancy, and may discontinue or decrease their medications once they conceive, which increases the risk of IBD flare. Patients should be counseled on the importance of continuing effective, low-risk medications during pregnancy to decrease disease-related risks. Patients should discontinue methotrexate and likely avoid tofacitinib in pregnancy.

For these reasons, proactive preconception counseling for patients with IBD by their gastroenterology provider is essential, and can optimize disease control during conception and throughout pregnancy. Not all patients may be aware of the implications of IBD on family planning and pregnancy; therefore, health care providers should proactively discuss this issue with all patients of childbearing potential. For example, preconception counseling could be provided near the time of diagnosis, and then revisited when the patient reaches the age of childbearing potential and when they have an interest in potential pregnancy. This will help patients to be better informed about concerns about disease, medications, and heritability, and will also allow for optimization of disease control and medical therapy prior to pregnancy. Furthermore, education on family planning may modify some patients' decision to have children or proceed with voluntary childlessness. All patients with IBD who are considering pregnancy should also have a consultation with a high-risk obstetrician/maternal fetal medicine provider to discuss routine management during pregnancy, the safety of medical therapy, and a potential management plan in case of disease flare during pregnancy.

# Heritability in IBD

*Heritability* is defined as the proportion of phenotypic variance that can be attributed to genetic variance.[52] As discussed earlier, voluntary childlessness is more common among women with IBD. An important concern is the potential to pass the disease to offspring.[6] In a recent survey, this concern was expressed in 67.8% of women with IBD.[4,52]

## Familial Risk of IBD

There is an increased risk of IBD among family members of patients with IBD. One Danish population-based cohort study completed between 1977 and 2011 (N = 8,295,773; 200 million person-years) reported that the incidence relative risk (IRR) of CD was significantly increased among CD patients' relatives, particularly in first-degree (IRR, 7.77; 95% CI, 7.05 to 8.56) or second-degree relatives (IRR, 2.44; 95% CI, 2.01 to 2.96), and less so in third-degree relatives (IRR, 1.88; 95% CI, 1.30 to 2.71). In UC, the risk was increased among first-degree relatives (IRR, 4.08; 95% CI, 3.81 to 4.38), and less among second-degree (IRR, 1.85; 95% CI, 1.60 to 2.13) or third-degree relatives (IRR, 1.51; 95% CI, 1.07 to 2.12). The study concluded that the risk of developing CD among offspring was 2.7% and 1.6% for UC.[53]

Patients with Ashkenazi Jewish heritage have a high prevalence of IBD and heritability in this population appears higher than in other groups. A recent United Kingdom study revealed that 40% of patients with Ashkenazi Jewish heritage and IBD also had a family history of IBD, with 25%

having at least one affected first-degree relative, suggesting a higher familial aggregation among the Ashkenazi Jewish population.[54]

To determine the risk of IBD in offspring born to women with IBD, researchers evaluated data from the Danish Medical Birth Registry, a nationwide register-based cohort study, including all live births in Denmark between 1989 and 2013. This included 9238 children born to women with IBD (exposed) and 1,371,407 born to women without IBD (unexposed). The median follow-up period was 9.7 years for exposed and 13.8 years for unexposed children. In children exposed to maternal UC, the hazard risk of IBD in the offspring was 4.63 (95% CI, 3.49 to 6.16). In children exposed to a mother with CD, the risk of IBD in the offspring was 7.70 (95% CI, 5.66 to 10.47).[55] While the study had the strength of a national registry, the follow-up period was limited, and therefore the long-term risk was not evaluated.

Although the risk of developing IBD in offspring of mothers with IBD is relatively low, the risk increases significantly when both parents have IBD. Several small studies of families in which both parents have IBD identified the risk to be between 28% and 36%.[56-58]

## Genetic Considerations in IBD

Genetics play an important role in IBD pathogenesis, and familial clustering of IBD has been documented since the beginning of the 20th century.[60] More recently, genome-wide association studies have identified more than 200 single-nucleotide polymorphisms associated with IBD.[53] Healthy individuals can carry the IBD risk alleles without developing IBD, thus proving that genetics play only a partial role in the heritability of IBD. At this time, no available genetic tests can predict if offspring will develop IBD.

The first genetic locus described in IBD was NOD2. NOD2 is a receptor found on gut epithelial cells, monocytes, macrophages, and lamina propria lymphocytes that recognizes and binds to muramyl dipeptide and increases the transcription of inflammatory cytokines.[59] Other loci are genes involved in the autophagy pathway, interleukin (IL)10, IL-12, and IL-23 genes. Some of the loci are common to all ethnicities and others are specific to certain populations.

Twin studies provide further insight into the role of genetics in IBD. The first twin study in IBD identified 80 pairs of twins with IBD out of 25,000 pairs of twins from the Swedish twin registry. The proband concordance rate among monozygotic twins was 58.3% for CD and 6.3% for UC, suggesting that heredity is stronger in CD than in UC. Of note, monozygotic twins with CD were more likely to be people who smoke than monozygotic twins with UC.[60] Another twin study from Denmark evaluated 103 twin pairs in which at least one twin had IBD. Again, the proband concordance was higher in monozygotic twins with CD (58.3%) vs UC (18.3%). Among the dizygotic twins the rates were 0% for CD and 4.5% for UC.[61]

## Anticipation

It is described in the literature that the presence of IBD in offspring appears at an earlier age and is more severe. This phenomenon is named *anticipation*. In a study of 160 families from Northern France and Belgium in which 2 or more first-degree relatives had IBD, 57 parent-first affected child pairs were identified. In 84% of the cases, children were younger than their parents at diagnosis, with a median age difference of 16 years ($P < .0001$). However, this difference was not present in 12 parent-child pairs with an early age at diagnosis for the parents.[62]

Ballester and colleagues performed a retrospective single center of 1211 patients and found that 14.2% had relatives with IBD. Median age at diagnosis was lower in the familial group (32 vs 29 years old; $P = .07$). There was a higher proportion of extraintestinal manifestations: peripheral arthropathy (OR = 2.3, $P = .015$) and erythema nodosum (OR = 7.6, $P = .001$) in patients with familial UC and higher treatment requirements: immunomodulators (OR = 1.8, $P = .029$); biologics

(OR = 1.9, $P$ = .011); and surgery (OR = 1.7, $P$ = .044) in patients with familial CD. These findings strengthen the hypothesis that familial IBD is associated with earlier onset and may present with more severe disease.[63]

## Very-Early-Onset IBD

Very-early-onset IBD (VEO-IBD) refers to the diagnosis of IBD in children less than 6 years old, while patients diagnosed at less than 2 years old are considered to have infantile IBD. Patients with VEO-IBD are nearly twice as likely to have a family history of IBD as compared to those with later-onset IBD.[64] In patients with VEO-IBD, causative monogenic variants are more frequently found and mostly reflect primary immune deficiencies. There are different categories including general immune dysregulation, phagocytic defects, hyper- and autoinflammatory conditions, and epithelial barrier dysfunction, all with different modes of inheritance. However, despite higher prevalence of genetic disorders, more than 70% to 80% of cases have no specifically identified causal genetic etiology.[65] This points toward the robust role of the environment in the etiology of even VEO-IBD.

## Environmental Factors and Microbiome

Although genetics play an important role in IBD pathogenesis, the lack of 100% concordance in twin studies suggests an environmental or microbiome influence. There are multiple risk factors implicated in the pathogenesis of IBD such as smoking, diet, medications (eg, antibiotics, nonsteroidal anti-inflammatory drugs), geography, and stress.

It is generally considered that the gut microbiome is introduced in the newborn at birth and equilibrates in the first few years. The composition of the microbiome is influenced by environmental factors including medications (especially antibiotics), diet, smoking, and pollution. There are specific changes seen in the microbiome of patients with IBD such as an increase in *Proteobacteria* and *Actinobacteria* and decreased amounts of *Bacteroidetes* and *Firmicutes*.[59] Although these changes are recognized, there is no causation described since active inflammation can itself alter the microbiome. For infants, the mode of delivery has been described to influence the colonization of the gut microbiome; therefore, consideration has been given to the potential impact of the mode of delivery on the development of IBD. However, a systematic review and meta-analysis from 2014 did not report a difference in the risk of IBD in offspring birthed vaginally vs via caesarean section.[66] The infant gut microbiome is also impacted by breastmilk. Low quality evidence suggests possible reduced risk of eczema and allergic rhinitis in breastfed infants,[67] and other studies have suggested that breastfed individuals had lower risk of asthma exacerbations compared to those who were not breastfed.[68] However, evidence regarding the association between breastfeeding and IBD is lacking.

# Conclusion

IBD is associated with decreased fertility in the setting of active disease, history non-laparoscopic open surgery IPAA, and in CD, due to decreased ovarian reserve. Non-operative patients with well-controlled disease have similar fertility rates as the general population. Proactive family planning is important given that certain IBD medications should be avoided in pregnancy and conceiving in the setting of active disease is associated with increase maternal and fetal risks. Many effective contraceptive options exist for family planning and patients with IBD should consider avoiding estrogen-containing contraception if possible. Lastly, IBD is an inheritable disease, with higher rates of heritability if both parents are affected by IBD (Table 7-2).

## Table 7-2. Summary of Recommendations Regarding Family Planning, Fertility, Infertility, Contraception, and Heredity in IBD

| TOPIC | CONSIDERATIONS FOR PATIENTS WITH IBD | RECOMMENDATIONS FOR IBD CARE |
|---|---|---|
| Family planning | Active IBD during conception or pregnancy increases maternal and fetal risks<br>Medications<br>• Most IBD medications are low risk in pregnancy<br>• Methotrexate and thalidomide are teratogenic<br>• Limited safety data exist on Janus kinase inhibitors | Recommend proactive pre-conception counseling<br>Recommend highly effective birth control to aid in family planning<br>If pregnancy is desired, recommend consultation with high-risk obstetrician/maternal fetal medicine<br>Recommend achieving remission for 3 to 6 months prior to conception<br>Continue safe, effective therapy during pregnancy to maintain disease control<br>Discontinue methotrexate, thalidomide, and Janus kinase inhibitors 3 to 6 months prior to conception |
| Fertility | Non-operated patients with well-controlled IBD have similar fertility as the general population<br>Fertility may be decreased due to voluntary childlessness, active disease, and following IPAA<br>Crohn's disease is associated with decreased ovarian reserve | Recommend counseling patients on fertility and family planning<br>While fertility may be decreased in the setting of active disease or following IPAA, pregnancy may occur at any time and highly effective birth control is recommended to aid in family planning |
| Infertility | In general, infertility rates are similar to healthy populations<br>In patients with UC, ART treatments are successful at similar rates as the general population<br>In patients with CD and a history of surgery, ART may be less effective compared to the general population | Patients with infertility who desire pregnancy should be referred to an infertility specialist for consideration of ART |

*(continued)*

## Table 7-2 (continued). Summary of Recommendations Regarding Family Planning, Fertility, Infertility, Contraception, and Heredity in IBD

| TOPIC | CONSIDERATIONS FOR PATIENTS WITH IBD | RECOMMENDATIONS FOR IBD CARE |
|---|---|---|
| Contraception | Most contraceptives are safe and effective in patients with IBD<br><br>Estrogen-containing oral contraceptives are associated with an increased risk of VTE<br><br>Depot medroxyprogesterone is associated with a negative effect on bone density | IUDs are safe and highly effective<br><br>Avoid estrogen-containing methods for patients at high risk of VTE<br><br>Avoid depot medroxyprogesterone in patients with low bone density and those at high risk |
| Heredity | Genome-wide association studies identify > 200 single-nucleotide polymorphisms associated with IBD<br><br>There is not 100% concordance of IBD in twin studies; therefore, environment plays a role in pathogenesis<br><br>~12% of IBD patients have a family history of IBD<br><br>The prevalence of CD in offspring of first-degree relatives with IBD ranges from 0.35% to 4.5%, and in UC ranges from 0.3% to 2.7%<br><br>In offspring of both parents with IBD, the risk of developing IBD is between 28% and 36%<br><br>Currently no available genetic tests can predict if offspring will develop IBD | Providers should counsel patient on the heritability of IBD |

## KEY POINTS

1. Patients with well-controlled IBD without a history of surgery have similar fertility as the general population. Fertility is decreased due to voluntary childlessness, active disease, and history of IPAA surgery.

2. Providers should proactively counsel patients on the importance of achieving remission prior to conception to reduce disease-related risks.

3. Many contraceptive options exist. Avoid estrogen-containing contraception for IBD patients at higher risk of VTE and depot medroxyprogesterone in patients with low bone density.

4. IBD is heritable with higher rates if both parents have the disease.

# References

1.  Feagins LA, Kane SV. Caring for women with inflammatory bowel disease. *Gastroenterol Clin North Am.* 2016;45(2):303-315.

2.  Nee J, Feuerstein JD. Optimizing the care and health of women with inflammatory bowel disease. *Gastroenterol Res Pract.* 2015;2015:435820.

3.  Friedman S, Larsen PV, Fedder J, Nørgård BM. The efficacy of assisted reproduction in women with inflammatory bowel disease and the impact of surgery-a nationwide cohort study. *Inflamm Bowel Dis.* 2017;23(2):208-217.

4.  Ellul P, Zammita SC, Katsanos KH, et al. Perception of reproductive health in women with inflammatory bowel disease. *J Crohns Colitis.* 2016;10(8):886-891.

5.  Mountifield R, Bampton P, Prosser R, Muller K, Andrews JM. et al. Fear and fertility in inflammatory bowel disease: a mismatch of perception and reality affects family planning decisions. *Inflamm Bowel Dis.* 2009;15(5):720-725.

6.  Walldorf J, Brunne S, Gittinger FS, Michl P. Family planning in inflammatory bowel disease: childlessness and disease-related concerns among female patients. *Eur J Gastroenterol Hepatol.* 2018;30(3):310-315.

7.  Marri, SR, Ahn C, Buchman AL. Voluntary childlessness is increased in women with inflammatory bowel disease. *Inflamm Bowel Dis.* 2007;13(5):591-599.

8.  Leenhardt R, Rivière P, Papazian P, et al. Sexual health and fertility for individuals with inflammatory bowel disease. *World J Gastroenterol.* 2019;25(36):5423-5433.

9.  Ghosh S, Mitchell R. Impact of inflammatory bowel disease on quality of life: results of the European Federation of Crohn's and Ulcerative Colitis Associations (EFCCA) patient survey. *J Crohns Colitis.* 2007;1(1):10-20.

10. Muller KR, Prosser R, Bampton P, Mountifield R, Andrews JM. Female gender and surgery impair relationships, body image, and sexuality in inflammatory bowel disease: patient perceptions. *Inflamm Bowel Dis.* 2010;16(4):657-663.

11. Shmidt E, Suárez-Fariñas M, Mallette M, et al. A longitudinal study of sexual function in women with newly diagnosed inflammatory bowel disease. *Inflamm Bowel Dis.* 2019;25(7):1262-1270.

12. Bel LG, Vollebregt AM, Van der Meulen-de Jong AE. Sexual dysfunctions in men and women with inflammatory bowel disease: the influence of IBD-related clinical factors and depression on sexual function. *J Sex Med.* 2015;12(7):1557-1567.

13. Friedman S, Nielsen J, Nøhr EA, Jølving LR, Nørgård BM. Comparison of time to pregnancy in women with and without inflammatory bowel diseases. *Clin Gastroenterol Hepatol.* 2020;18(7):1537-1544.e1.

14. Martin J, Kane SV, and LA Feagins. Fertility and contraception in women with inflammatory bowel disease. *Gastroenterol Hepatol (N Y).* 2016;12(2):101-109.

15. Hudson M, Flett G, Sinclair TS, Brunt PW, Templeton A, Mowat NA. Fertility and pregnancy in inflammatory bowel disease. *Int J Gynaecol Obstet.* 1997;58(2):229-237.

16. Tavernier N, Fumery M, Peyrin-Biroulet L, Colombel JF, Gower-Rousseau C. Systematic review: fertility in non-surgically treated inflammatory bowel disease. *Aliment Pharmacol Ther.* 2013;38(8):847-853.

17. Şenateş E, Çolak Y, Erdem ED, et al. Serum anti-Mullerian hormone levels are lower in reproductive-age women with Crohn's disease compared to healthy control women. *J Crohns Colitis.* 2013;7(2):e29-34.

18. Ban L, Tata LJ, Humes DJ, Fiaschi L, Card T. Decreased fertility rates in 9639 women diagnosed with inflammatory bowel disease: a United Kingdom population-based cohort study. *Aliment Pharmacol Ther.* 2015;42(7):855-866.

19. van der Woude CJ, Ardizzone S, Bengtson MB, et al. The second European evidenced-based consensus on reproduction and pregnancy in inflammatory bowel disease. *J Crohns Colitis.* 2015;9(2):107-124.

20. Bernstein CN, Ng SC, Lakatos PL, Moum B, Loftus EV Jr, Epidemiology and Natural History Task Force of the International Organization of the Study of Inflammatory Bowel Disease. A review of mortality and surgery in ulcerative colitis: milestones of the seriousness of the disease. *Inflamm Bowel Dis.* 2013;19(9):2001-2010.

21. Niewiadomski O, Studd C, Hair C, et al. Prospective population-based cohort of inflammatory bowel disease in the biologics era: Disease course and predictors of severity. *J Gastroenterol Hepatol.* 2015;30(9):1346-1353.

22. Faye AS, Oh A, Kumble LD, et al. Fertility impact of initial operation type for female ulcerative colitis patients. *Inflamm Bowel Dis.* 2020;26(9):1368-1376.

23. Ording Olsen K, Juul S, Berndtsson I, Oresland T, Laurberg S. Ulcerative colitis: female fecundity before diagnosis, during disease, and after surgery compared with a population sample. *Gastroenterology.* 2002;122(1):15-19.

24. Waljee A, Waljee J, Morris AM, Higgins PD. Threefold increased risk of infertility: a meta-analysis of infertility after ileal pouch anal anastomosis in ulcerative colitis. *Gut.* 2006;55(11):1575-1580.

25. Olsen KO, Juul S, Bülow S, et al. Female fecundity before and after operation for familial adenomatous polyposis. *Br J Surg.* 2003;90(2):227-231.

26. Bartels SA, D'Hoore A, Cuesta MA, Bensdorp AJ, Lucas C, Bemelman WA. Significantly increased pregnancy rates after laparoscopic restorative proctocolectomy: a cross-sectional study. *Ann Surg.* 2012;256(6):1045-1048.

27. Lindhagen T, Bohe M, Ekelund G, Valentin L. Fertility and outcome of pregnancy in patients operated on for Crohn's disease. *Int J Colorectal Dis.* 1986;1(1):25-27.

28. Lee S, Crowe M, Seow CH, et al. The impact of surgical therapies for inflammatory bowel disease on female fertility. Cochrane Database Syst Rev, 2019;7:Cd012711.

29. Oza SS, Pabby V, Dodge LE, et al. In vitro fertilization in women with inflammatory bowel disease is as successful as in women from the general infertility population. *Clin Gastroenterol Hepatol.* 2015;13(9):1641-1646.e3.

30. Pabby V, Oza SS, Dodge LE, et al. In vitro fertilization is successful in women with ulcerative colitis and ileal pouch anal anastomosis. *Am J Gastroenterol.* 2015;110(6):792-797.

31. Pachler FR, Toft G, Bisgaard T, Laurberg S. Use and success of in vitro fertilisation following restorative proctocolectomy and ileal pouch-anal anastomosis. A nationwide 17-year cohort study. *J Crohns Colitis.* 2019;13(10):1283-1286.

32. Friedman S, Larsen PV, Fedder J, Nørgård BM. The reduced chance of a live birth in women with IBD receiving assisted reproduction is due to a failure to achieve a clinical pregnancy. *Gut.* 2017;66(3):556-558.

33. Abhyankar A, Ham M, Moss AC. Meta-analysis: the impact of disease activity at conception on disease activity during pregnancy in patients with inflammatory bowel disease. *Aliment Pharmacol Ther.* 2013;38(5):460-466.

34. Mahadevan U, Robinson C, Bernasko N, et al. Inflammatory bowel disease in pregnancy clinical care pathway: a report from the American Gastroenterological Association IBD Parenthood Project Working Group. *Inflamm Bowel Dis.* 2019;25(4):627-641.

35. Grimmer SF, Back DJ, Orme ML, Cowie A, Gilmore I, Tjia J. The bioavailability of ethinyloestradiol and levonorgestrel in patients with an ileostomy. *Contraception.* 1986;33(1):51-59.

36. Nilsson LO, Victor A, Kral JG, Johansson ED, Kock NG. Absorption of an oral contraceptive gestagen in ulcerative colitis before and after proctocolectomy and construction of a continent ileostomy. *Contraception.* 1985;31(2):195-204.

37. Zapata LB, Paulen ME, Cansino C, Marchbanks PA, Curtis KM. Contraceptive use among women with inflammatory bowel disease: a systematic review. *Contraception.* 2010;82(1):72-85.

38. Limdi JK, Farraye J, Cannon R, Woodhams E, Farraye FA. Contraception, venous thromboembolism, and inflammatory bowel disease: what clinicians (and patients) should know. *Inflamm Bowel Dis.* 2019;25(10):1603-1612.

39. Victor A, Odlind V, Kral JG. Oral contraceptive absorption and sex hormone binding globulins in obese women: effects of jejunoileal bypass. *Gastroenterol Clin North Am.* 1987;16(3):483-491.

40. Bernstein CN, Blanchard JF, Houston DS, Wajda A. The incidence of deep venous thrombosis and pulmonary embolism among patients with inflammatory bowel disease: a population-based cohort study. *Thromb Haemost.* 2001;85(3):430-434.

41. Grainge MJ, West J, Card TR. Venous thromboembolism during active disease and remission in inflammatory bowel disease: a cohort study. *Lancet.* 2010;375(9715):657-663.

42. Cotton CC, Baird D, Sandler RS, Long MD. Hormonal contraception use is common among patients with inflammatory bowel diseases and an elevated risk of deep vein thrombosis. *Inflamm Bowel Dis.* 2016;22(7):1631-1638.

43. Fumery M, Xiaocang C, Dauchet L, Gower-Rousseau C, Peyrin-Biroulet L, Colombel JF. Thromboembolic events and cardiovascular mortality in inflammatory bowel diseases: a meta-analysis of observational studies. *J Crohns Colitis.* 2014;8(6):469-479.

44. Isene R, Bernklev T, Høie O, et al. Thromboembolism in inflammatory bowel disease: results from a prospective, population-based European inception cohort. *Scand J Gastroenterol.* 2014;49(7):820-825.

45. Vegh Z, Golovics PA, Lovasz BD, et al. Low incidence of venous thromboembolism in inflammatory bowel diseases: prevalence and predictors from a population-based inception cohort. *Scand J Gastroenterol.* 2015;50(3):306-311.

46. Wilks JF. Hormonal birth control and pregnancy: a comparative analysis of thromboembolic risk. *Ann Pharmacother.* 2003;37(6):912-916.

47. Dinger JC, Heinemann LA, Kuhl-Habich D. The safety of a drospirenone-containing oral contraceptive: final results from the European Active Surveillance Study on oral contraceptives based on 142,475 women-years of observation. *Contraception.* 2007;75(5):344-354.

48. Lidegaard O, Nielsen LH, Skovlund CW, Skjeldestad FE, Løkkegaard E. Risk of venous thromboembolism from use of oral contraceptives containing different progestogens and oestrogen doses: Danish cohort study, 2001-9. *BMJ.* 2011;343:d6423.

49. Mantha S, Karp R, Raghavan V, Terrin N, Bauer KA, Zwicker JI. Assessing the risk of venous thromboembolic events in women taking progestin-only contraception: a meta-analysis. *BMJ.* 2012;345:e4944.

50. Communication FDS. Safety trial finds risk of blood clots in the lungs and death with higher dose of tofacitinib (Xeljanz, Xeljanz XR) in rheumatoid arthritis patients; FDA to investigate. 2019: fda.gov.

51. Sridhar A, Cwiak CA, Kaunitz AM, Allen RH. Contraceptive considerations for women with gastrointestinal disorders. *Dig Dis Sci.* 2017;62(1):54-63.

52. Gordon H, Trier Moller F, Andersen V, Harbord M. Heritability in inflammatory bowel disease: from the first twin study to genome-wide association studies. *Inflamm Bowel Dis.* 2015;21(6):1428-1434.

53. Turpin W, Goethel A, Bedrani L, Croitoru Mdcm K. Determinants of IBD heritability: genes, bugs, and more. *Inflamm Bowel Dis.* 2018;24(6):1133-1148.

54. Schiff ER, Frampton M, Semplici F, et al. A new look at familial risk of inflammatory bowel disease in the Ashkenazi Jewish population. *Dig Dis Sci.* 2018;63(11):3049-3057.

55. Jolving LR, Nielsen J, Beck-Nielsen SS, et al. The association between maternal chronic inflammatory bowel disease and long-term health outcomes in children-a nationwide cohort study. *Inflamm Bowel Dis.* 2017;23(8):1440-1446.

56. Laharie D, Debeugny S, Peeters M, et al. Inflammatory bowel disease in spouses and their offspring. *Gastroenterology.* 2001;120(4):816-819.

57. Comes MC, Gower-Rousseau C, Colombel JF, et al. Inflammatory bowel disease in married couples: 10 cases in Nord Pas de Calais region of France and Liege county of Belgium. *Gut.* 1994;35(9):1316-1318.

58. Bennett RA, Rubin PH, Present DH. Frequency of inflammatory bowel disease in offspring of couples both presenting with inflammatory bowel disease. *Gastroenterology.* 1991;100(6):1638-1643.

59. Kuhnen A. Genetic and environmental considerations for inflammatory bowel disease. *Surg Clin North Am.* 2019;99(6):1197-1207.

60. Tysk C, Lindberg E, Järnerot G, Flodérus-Myrhed B. Ulcerative colitis and Crohn's disease in an unselected population of monozygotic and dizygotic twins. A study of heritability and the influence of smoking. *Gut.* 1988;29(7):990-996.

61. Orholm M, Binder V, Sørensen TI, Rasmussen LP, Kyvik KO. Concordance of inflammatory bowel disease among Danish twins. Results of a nationwide study. *Scand J Gastroenterol.* 2000;35(10):1075-1081.

62. Grandbastien B, Peeters M, Franchimont D, et al. Anticipation in familial Crohn's disease. *Gut.* 1998;42(2):170-174.

63. Ballester MP, Martí D, Tosca J, et al. Disease severity and treatment requirements in familial inflammatory bowel disease. *Int J Colorectal Dis.* 2017;32(8):1197-1205.

64. Paul T, Birnbaum A, Pal DK, et al. Distinct phenotype of early childhood inflammatory bowel disease. *J Clin Gastroenterol.* 2006;40(7):583-586.

65. Ouahed J, Spencer E, Kotlarz D, et al. Very early onset inflammatory bowel disease: a clinical approach with a focus on the role of genetics and underlying immune deficiencies. *Inflamm Bowel Dis.* 2020;26(6):820-842.

66. Bruce A, Black M, Bhattacharya S. Mode of delivery and risk of inflammatory bowel disease in the offspring: systematic review and meta-analysis of observational studies. *Inflamm Bowel Dis.* 2014;20(7):1217-1226.

67. Lodge CJ, Dharmage SC. Breastfeeding and perinatal exposure, and the risk of asthma and allergies. *Curr Opin Allergy Clin Immunol.* 2016;16(3):231-236.

68. Ahmadizar F, Vijverberg SJH, Arets HGM, et al. Breastfeeding is associated with a decreased risk of childhood asthma exacerbations later in life. *Pediatr Allergy Immunol.* 2017;28(7):649-654.

# 8

# Pregnancy and Delivery in the IBD Patient

Jill K. J. Gaidos, MD | Katrina H. Naik, MD

## Introduction

Many patients are under the age of 35 years when they are first diagnosed with inflammatory bowel disease (IBD), which is considered the peak childbearing years for females. Naturally, many women with IBD turn to their gastroenterologist with questions regarding how IBD and its therapies will affect them and their developing baby during pregnancy. Previous studies have shown high rates of voluntary childlessness in the IBD population due to these concerns.[1] The aim of this chapter is to provide the most updated evidence on the effect of IBD on pregnancy, the impact of pregnancy on IBD, review the safety of our current IBD medications for use throughout pregnancy, recommendations on the mode of delivery for special populations of IBD patients, review the management of IBD flares during pregnancy, and discuss the importance of preconception counseling for women with IBD. Fertility in IBD and medication safety during lactation will be covered in other chapters.

## Effect of IBD on Pregnancy

Women with IBD who are considering pregnancy or are already pregnant should be counseled that they may be at an increased risk for fetal and obstetric complications (Table 8-1) compared to the general population. In 2007, a meta-analysis of 12 studies including 3907 pregnancies in women with IBD compared to 320,531 pregnancies in women without IBD found that women with IBD were at a significantly increased risk for adverse fetal outcomes.[2] In the sensitivity analysis limited to only higher quality studies, women with IBD were more likely to have premature birth (odds ratio

Abraham BP, Kane SV, Glassner KL, eds.
*Women's Health in IBD: The Spectrum of Care
From Birth to Adulthood* (pp 151-176).
© 2022 Taylor & Francis Group.

## Table 8-1. Definitions of Adverse Outcomes

| ADVERSE CONCEPTION OUTCOMES | |
| --- | --- |
| *SPONTANEOUS ABORTION* | Spontaneous delivery of a nonviable fetus, usually prior to 20 weeks' gestation |
| *ABORTION FOR UNKNOWN REASON* | Delivery of unclear reasons of a nonviable fetus |
| **ADVERSE OBSTETRIC OUTCOMES** | |
| *CAESAREAN DELIVERY* | Delivery by intra-abdominal incision |
| *PRELABOR CAESAREAN* | Delivery by intra-abdominal incision prior to labor onset |
| *PRETERM BIRTH* | Birth of an infant prior to 37 weeks' gestation |
| *INDUCED PRETERM DELIVERY* | Labor induction when the indicated benefit outweighs the risk of delivery prior to 37 weeks, when fetal lung development is incomplete |
| *VENOUS THROMBOEMBOLISM* | Blood clot formation in deep veins |
| *ANTEPARTUM HEMORRHAGE* | Life-threatening vaginal bleeding after 20 to 24 weeks' gestation |
| *GESTATIONAL DIABETES* | New maternal hyperglycemia at any point in pregnancy |
| *MATERNAL HYPERTENSION* | New elevations in blood pressure > 140/90 mm Hg on at least 2 measurements at least 4 hours apart after 20 weeks' gestation, without proteinuria |
| *PREECLAMPSIA* | New elevations in blood pressure > 140/90 mm Hg on at least 2 measurements at least 4 hours apart after 20 weeks' gestation, with proteinuria or other signs and symptoms of significant end-organ damage |

*(continued)*

[OR] 1.74, 95% confidence interval [CI] 1.14 to 2.65, $P = .01$) and small for gestational age (SGA) infants (OR 1.96, 95% CI 1.01 to 3.81, $P = .05$). There was no increased risk of stillbirth or congenital anomalies.[2] A more recent meta-analysis of 23 studies including 15,007 pregnancies in women with IBD compared to 4,614,271 pregnancies in healthy controls found an increased odds of preterm delivery (OR 1.85, 95% CI 1.67 to 2.05, I2 = 31%) and an increase in the pooled odds for stillbirth (OR 1.57, 95% CI 1.03 to 2.38, I2 = 30%). Though the data suggested that women with IBD have an increased odds of SGA (OR 1.36, 95% CI 1.16 to 1.60, I2 = 56%) and major congenital anomalies (OR 1.29, 95% CI 1.05 to 1.58, I2 = 46%), these studies had significant heterogeneity suggestive of publication bias.[3]

Results from pregnancy registry studies also support an increased risk for preterm birth in both Crohn's disease (CD) and ulcerative colitis (UC). A large pregnancy registry including 2637 primiparous women with UC and 868,942 primiparous women without UC in Denmark and Sweden found an increased odds of preterm birth before 37 weeks (prevalence odds ratio [pOR] 1.77, 95% CI 1.54 to 2.05), preterm birth before 32 weeks (pOR 1.41, 95% CI 1.02 to 1.96), SGA (pOR 1.27, 95% CI 1.05 to 1.54), and neonatal death (pOR 1.93, 95% CI 1.04 to 3.60), but no increased risk for congenital anomalies.[4] Using these same registries to look at pregnancy and fetal outcomes in

## Table 8-1 (continued). Definitions of Adverse Outcomes

| ADVERSE FETAL OUTCOMES | |
| --- | --- |
| PREMATURITY | Birth at or before 37 weeks' gestation |
| LOW BIRTH WEIGHT | Weighing less than 2500 g at birth, regardless of gestational age |
| CONGENITAL ANOMALIES | Structural or functional abnormality that has been present since birth |
| • Major | Structural and functional defects in development of the cardiac, nervous, musculoskeletal, digestive, respiratory, or genitourinary system; chromosomal abnormalities, limb deformities, facial deformities including orofacial cleft, ear, eye, neck, abdominal wall, asplenia, situs inversus, severe skin disorders |
| • Minor | Only structural changes without significant impact on function or neonatal health |
| STILLBIRTH | Delivery of a deceased fetus at least 28 weeks' gestation after dying in the womb |
| NEONATAL DEATH | Death of a 28-week-old or less infant |
| SMALL FOR GESTATIONAL AGE | Fetus or infant with less weight gain than is expected for an average fetus or infant at the same weeks' gestation, usually under the 10th percentile |
| INTRAUTERINE GROWTH RESTRICTION | Fetus with slower rate of weight gain than is expected for an average fetus at the same weeks' gestation |

primiparous women with CD, including 2377 women with CD and 869,202 women without CD, also showed an increased risk for preterm birth before 37 weeks (pOR 1.76, 95% CI 1.51 to 2.05) and preterm birth before 32 weeks (pOR 1.86, 95% CI 1.38 to 2.52) with no increased odds for stillbirth or congenital malformation.[5]

Population-based studies have also shown a small increase in adverse outcomes, particularly preterm birth and low birth weight (LBW), among women with IBD. A population-based study from the United States, which compared pregnancy outcomes between 461 pregnant women with IBD matched with 493 pregnant healthy controls, found that pregnancies in women with IBD were less likely to result in a live birth (60% vs 68%, $P = .01$), were more likely to have an adverse conception outcome (23% vs 17%, $P = .03$) and more likely to have a complication in pregnancy (25% vs 16%, $P < .01$).[6] When each of these broad categories (ie, "adverse conception outcome") was broken down into the specific types of adverse events, the differences between the IBD cohort and the non-IBD cohort were no longer significant. Further, this study did not find any increased risk of adverse pregnancy outcomes, adverse newborn outcomes or congenital anomalies.[6] Complications were not associated with the severity of IBD disease activity; however, this population was noted to have higher health access, fewer comorbidities, and overall low disease activity.[6] Another population-based cohort study from Sweden included 3053 singleton births to women with IBD compared to 470,110 singleton births to women without IBD and found an increased odds of preterm birth in women with UC (adjusted odds ratio [aOR] 1.78, 95% CI 1.49 to 2.13) and CD (aOR 1.65, 95% CI 1.33 to 2.06), LBW in women with UC (aOR 1.64, 95% CI 1.31 to 2.04) and CD (aOR 1.86, 95% CI 1.46 to 2.38), and stillbirth among patients with CD (aOR 2.93, 95% CI 1.57 to 5.47).[7] A third population-based study from the United Kingdom looking specifically at congenital anomalies included 1703 children born to women with IBD compared to 384,811 children born to women without IBD and found the risk for any major congenital anomaly in women with IBD was 2.7% compared to 2.8% in the non-IBD cohort (aOR 0.98, 95% CI 0.73 to 1.31).[8] A retrospective study looking at pregnancy and fetal outcomes in 97 pregnancies in women prior to a diagnosis of IBD and 70 pregnancies in the same cohort of women after their diagnosis of IBD and found that pre-term birth (P = .008) and LBW (P = .048) were more common after the IBD diagnosis, but there was no increased risk for congenital anomalies.[9]

Studies have consistently shown that disease activity at conception is the most important predictor for adverse pregnancy and neonatal outcomes. The previously described population-based cohort study using a Swedish health registry also showed that the risks for adverse outcomes increased further in the setting of a disease flare during pregnancy.[7] In this cohort, the risk for preterm birth nearly doubled with active UC (aOR 2.72, 95% CI 2.12 to 3.40) and active CD (aOR 2.66, 95% CI 1.89 to 3.74), as did the risk for LBW in active UC (aOR 2.10, 95% CI 1.51 to 2.90) compared to nearly triple the risk in active CD (aOR 3.30, 95% CI 2.29 to 4.74). The risk of stillbirth also doubled in active CD (aOR 4.48, 95% CI 1.67 to 11.90).[7] In contrast, the European Crohn's Colitis Organisation (ECCO) group case-control study of outcomes from 332 pregnant women with IBD who were age and parity-matched to 332 pregnant women without IBD showed that the presence of active UC was associated with a higher risk for LBW (defined as < 3200 g; P = .04).[10] These results underscore the importance of having quiescent disease prior to conception and throughout pregnancy for healthy pregnancy and fetal outcomes.

Similarly, the risk of other adverse pregnancy outcomes, including uterine bleeding and venous thromboembolism (VTE), may also be increased in women with IBD. One population-based study using administrative health records from England including 1969 singleton pregnancies in women with IBD compared to 362,394 singleton pregnancies in women without IBD and found that women with CD had an increased risk of postpartum hemorrhage (OR 1.27, 95% CI 1.04 to 1.55), but not in the UC cohort.[11] Another population-based cohort study using Swedish health registry data including 1996 pregnant patients with IBD compared to 10,773 pregnant women without IBD and found that women with CD had a higher risk of antepartum hemorrhage compared to controls without IBD (aOR 1.66, 95% CI 1.12 to 2.45), with this risk most pronounced in those with inactive disease (aOR 1.79, 95% CI 1.07 to 3.01).[12] This study also showed an almost 4-fold increased odds of VTE in women with UC (aOR 3.78, 95% CI 1.52 to 9.38) with a 25-fold increase in the odds in the setting of active UC (aOR 25.0, 95% CI 2.49 to 250). The risk for VTE was not found to be increased among women with CD.[12] A recent meta-analysis of 5 studies, including 17,636 pregnant women with IBD and 11,251,778 pregnant healthy controls, found that women with IBD had a significantly increased risk of VTE during pregnancy (pooled risk ratio [RR] 2.13, 95% CI 1.66 to 2.73) and in the postpartum period (RR 2.61, 95% CI 1.84 to 3.69).[13] Comparing UC to CD, the risk of VTE was increased among the cohort of women with UC during pregnancy (RR 2.24, 95% CI 1.6 to 3.11) and in the postpartum period (RR 2.85, 95% CI 1.79 to 4.52).[13] With few studies showing an increased risk of bleeding during pregnancy but growing data to support the increased risk for VTE in pregnancy and the postpartum period, recent clinical care guidelines recommend the use of medical VTE pro-phylaxis for hospitalized pregnant women with IBD in conjunction with her obstetrical care.[14-16]

# Effect of Pregnancy on IBD

The results from studies on the impact of pregnancy on IBD disease activity are inconsistent. Older studies have shown that pregnant women with UC or CD had the same rate of flares as their non-pregnant counterparts.[17,18] However, a recent prospective cohort study including 209 pregnant women with IBD (92 CD, 117 UC) found no difference in the rate of flares for pregnant compared to non-pregnant women with CD; however, women with quiescent UC at conception are more likely to relapse during pregnancy (RR 2.19, 95% CI 1.25 to 3.97, $P$ = .004) and within 6 months postpartum (RR 6.22, 95% CI 2.05 to 79.3, $P$ = .0004) compared to non-pregnant women with UC.[19] In contrast, other studies have suggested improvement in the IBD course following pregnancy. A retrospective cohort study from Europe including 580 pregnancies (403 before and 177 after the diagnosis of IBD) found that the rate of disease flares decreased in the years after the pregnancy in both women with UC (0.34 vs 0.18 flares/year, $P$ = .008) and CD (0.76 vs 0.12 flares/year, $P$ = .004).[20]

Women with active disease at conception are more likely to experience disease flares during pregnancy. In a meta-analysis of 14 studies, including 1130 pregnant women with UC and 590 pregnant women with CD, women with active disease at the time of conception were more likely to continue to have active disease throughout pregnancy.[21] Specifically, 55% of the women with UC who had active disease at conception continued to have active disease during pregnancy compared to 36% of women with UC who were in remission at conception and developed active disease during pregnancy (RR 2.0, 95% CI 1.5 to 3, $P$ < .001). Similarly, 46% of the women with CD who had active disease at conception continued to have active disease during pregnancy compared to disease flares in 23% of the women with CD who were in remission at conception who developed a disease flare (RR 2.0, 95% CI 1.2 to 3.4, $P$ = .006).[21] In a survey of 324 pregnant IBD patients, 70% of women had no change or an improvement in their disease activity during pregnancy while 30% experienced a worsening of disease.[22] Importantly, those with quiescent disease had a milder disease course throughout pregnancy compared to those with moderate or severe disease at conception ($P$ < .001). This study also showed that active disease at delivery resulted in worsening disease postpartum. Only 13% of women with quiescence or mild disease at delivery experienced a relapse postpartum compared to 53% of those with active disease at delivery ($P$ < .001).[22]

Disease activity during pregnancy adversely impacts pregnancy and fetal outcomes.[9,11,17-20] Active UC during pregnancy has been associated with an increased risk for premature rupture of membranes (aOR 2.82, 95% CI 1.87 to 4.26), preterm birth (aOR 2.72, 95% CI 2.12 to 3.48), and LBW (aOR 2.10, 95% CI 1.51 to 2.90).[7] Active CD during pregnancy is associated with an increased risk for premature rupture of membranes (aOR 2.74, 95% CI 1.53 to 4.92), preterm birth (aOR 2.66, 95% CI 1.89 to 3.74), LBW (aOR 3.30, 95% CI 2.29 to 4.74), SGA (aOR 2.75, 95% CI 1.72 to 4.38), and stillbirth (aOR 4.48, 95% CI 1.67 to 11.9).[7] Another retrospective health registry study showed a 2-fold increased risk for preterm birth among women with active CD during pregnancy compared to women with quiescent CD.[23] These results strongly support the importance of achieving disease remission prior to conception on a steroid-free regimen that is safe to continue throughout pregnancy.[15,16]

A subset of women with IBD require surgical treatment prior to pregnancy. The presence of an ostomy during pregnancy may lead to possible stomal complications as the pregnancy progresses. Due to the increase in abdominal size with the growing fetus, the stoma may become displaced, stenosed, prolapsed, or retracted.[24] These alterations can be mitigated by working with a nutritionist or dietitian to ensure adequate but not excessive weight gain. Further, ongoing care with a colorectal surgeon and/or ostomy nurse can be helpful to address any active stomal issues.

# Safety of IBD Medications in Pregnancy

In 2014, the US Food and Drug Administration (FDA) updated the drug labeling requirements to include summaries of the current evidence for drug safety in pregnancy such as findings from animal studies and human studies and any evidence to assess the safety for use while breastfeeding. All newly approved medications are required to use these new standards established by the Pregnancy and Lactation Labeling Rule[25]; however, not all previously approved drugs have been relabeled to the new standards. Furthermore, because pregnant women, lactating women, and newborns are excluded from most clinical drug trials, evidence for drug safety in preconception and peripartum is limited to early exposure in clinical trial participants who become pregnant, then are required to discontinue the medication, or based on post-marketing data. At best, drug safety in pregnancy is defined by the FDA as, "not known to be embryocidal, teratogenic, or fetotoxic, as well as indicating that the drug is safe for the woman herself."[26] The Pregnancy and Lactation Labeling Rule also requires a subsection of drug labels to include information about fertility, contraception recommendations, and the need for pregnancy testing when indicated for patients of reproductive potential. The aim of this section is to review the safety of commonly used medications in the management of patients with IBD for use during pregnancy (Table 8-2).

## Aminosalicylates

Aminosalicylates (including sulfasalazine and 5-aminosalicylates [5-ASA]: balsalazide, mesalamine, olsalazine) have limited evidence for use in CD; however, continued aminosalicylate therapy is recommended for patients with mild to moderate UC.[27] Two recent meta-analyses have demonstrated no increased risk for LBW, stillbirth, preterm delivery, or spontaneous abortion (SA) with the continued use of aminosalicylates during pregnancy.[2,28] In terms of the mode of administration of the medication, there does not appear to be any difference in the risk for the mother or the fetus when aminosalicylates are used orally or topically, though rectal application may be impractical for the pregnant patient.[16]

Some 5-ASA formulations, including Mesasal, contain phthalates in the tablet coating to promote delayed release of the active ingredient, mesalamine, in the gut. Animal studies have demonstrated an association with dibutyl phthalate (DBP) and male urogenital defects and external skeletal defects, and human studies have shown a possible link between di-(2-ethyl-hexyl) phalate (DEHP) and neurodevelopmental problems. It should be noted that these animal exposures were 190 times higher than therapeutic doses used in humans.[29] Given the above evidence, Mesasal is no longer available in the United States[30] but may still be available in other countries.[31] Women currently taking a DBP-containing 5-ASA who are considering pregnancy should be counseled on these risks and recommended to switch to one of the many other effective 5-ASA brands that do not contain DBP. Furthermore, women with IBD should not be initiated on a DBP-containing 5-ASA during pregnancy.[16]

Although there has been a proposed risk for congenital anomalies associated with sulfasalazine use due to the ability of the sulfa moiety to cross the placenta,[32] recent studies have not supported this increased risk. Because sulfasalazine inhibits folate-metabolizing enzymes, guidelines recommend the addition of 2 mg folic acid supplementation daily to prevent neural tube defects during pregnancy.[14,15] Overall, given the good evidence for efficacy and safety of aminosalicylates, continued aminosalicylate therapy throughout pregnancy is recommended.[14-16]

## Antibiotics

Several situations may arise during pregnancy that warrant the use of antibiotics. These include acute or recurrent pouchitis, *Clostridioides difficile* (*C difficile*) colitis, and active perianal disease. This section discusses the safety of commonly used antibiotics to treat these possible complications.

### Quinolones

Ciprofloxacin is one of the commonly used antibiotics in IBD management. The use of ciprofloxacin during pregnancy was previously controversial due to an association with transient arthropathy in animal models; however, this has only rarely been demonstrated in humans. A recent meta-analysis of 10 studies including 2821 pregnant women exposed to fluoroquinolones during the first trimester compared to 159,592 controls found no associated increase in major or minor congenital defects, premature birth, or LBW.[33] A second meta-analysis including 13 studies assessed for congenital malformations as well as other adverse fetal or pregnancy outcomes following exposure

## Table 8-2. Safety of Medications for IBD in Pregnancy

| MEDICATIONS | SAFETY IN PREGNANCY |
| --- | --- |
| *AMINOSALICYLATES* | |
| 5-aminosalicylates (balsalazide, osalazine, mesalamines) | Safe for use during pregnancy<br>Avoid formulation containing phthalates (no longer available in the United States) |
| Sulfasalazine | Safe for use during pregnancy<br>Supplement with 2 mg folic acid daily |
| *ANTIBIOTICS* | |
| Quinolones (ciprofloxacin) | Safe to use for short durations for pouchitis or perianal disease |
| Metronidazole | Safe for use for short courses for pouchitis or perianal disease |
| Vancomycin | Safe for use for short courses for *Clostridioides difficile* colitis |
| *CORTICOSTEROIDS* | |
| Prednisone | Safe for use in short courses, not for long-term use |
| Budesonide | Safe for use in short courses, not for long-term use |
| *IMMUNOMODULATORS* | |
| Methotrexate | Not safe in pregnancy<br>Discontinue at least 3 months prior to conception |
| Azathioprine/6-mercaptopurine | Safe to continue for maintenance therapy<br>Avoid starting during pregnancy due to long onset of action and possible risk of adverse side effect<br>Consider discontinuation of the thiopurine prior to conception if in a durable remission in combination with an anti-TNF based on the individual clinical history and disease severity |
| *CALCINEURIN-INHIBITORS* | |
| Cyclosporine | Limited data in pregnancy, appears safe for use as rescue therapy for a severe ulcerative colitis flare |
| Tacrolimus | Limited data in pregnancy, appears safe for use as rescue therapy for a severe ulcerative colitis flare<br>Insufficient data to recommend for routine use in pregnancy |

*(continued)*

## Table 8-2 (continued). Safety of Medications for IBD in Pregnancy

| MEDICATIONS | SAFETY IN PREGNANCY |
|---|---|
| *SMALL MOLECULE AGENTS* | |
| Tofacitinib | Limited safety data in pregnancy, should discontinue at least 1 week prior to conception if other treatment options are available |
| *ANTI-TUMOR NECROSIS FACTOR AGENTS* | |
| Infliximab | Safe for use during pregnancy |
| Adalimumab | Consider obtaining serum trough drug levels at conception and dose adjusting as needed |
| Golimumab | Infants with in-utero exposure to all except certolizumab pegol should avoid live vaccines for the first 6 months of life |
| Certolizumab pegol | |
| *ANTI-INTEGRIN AGENTS* | |
| Natalizumab | Safe for use during pregnancy |
| | Not recommended in any patients with prior exposure to JC virus |
| | Infants with in-utero exposure should avoid live vaccines for the first 6 months of life |
| Vedolizumab | Safe for use during pregnancy |
| | Infants with in-utero exposure should avoid live vaccines for the first 6 months of life |
| *ANTI-IL 12/23* | |
| Ustekinumab | Safe for use during pregnancy |
| | Infants with in-utero exposure should avoid live vaccines for the first 6 months of life |
| *OTHER MEDICATIONS* | |
| Bisphosphonates | Not safe for use during pregnancy, should be discontinued |
| Antidiarrheals (loperamide, diphenoxylate) | Limited safety data for use in pregnancy, some evidence of an increased risk of congenital anomalies |
| | Avoid or limit use during pregnancy when possible |

to fluoroquinolones and found no increase in fetal malformations (pooled OR 1.08, 95% CI 0.96 to 1.21), preterm birth (pooled OR 0.97, 95% CI 0.75 to 1.24), miscarriage (pooled OR 1.78, 95% CI 0.93 to 3.38), or stillbirth (pooled OR 1.11, 95% CI 0.34 to 3.6).[34] Looking specifically at exposure in the first trimester, a meta-analysis of 12 studies found no increased risk for congenital malformation (pooled OR 0.89, 95% CI 0.72 to 1.09, I2 =0%), preterm birth (OR=1.10, 95% CI 0.83 to 1.48, I2 =41%) LBW (OR=1.29, 95% CI 0.54 to 3.12, I2 =67%), or stillbirth (OR=1.32, 95% CI 0.33 to 5.34, I2 =16%).[35] Most experts recommend avoiding ciprofloxacin use during pregnancy when possible, as amoxicillin/clavulanate may be a safer alternative in combination with metronidazole for coverage of infections due to either gram-negative rods or anaerobes, such as in the treatment of perianal or intra-abdominal abscesses and fistulizing disease. In the setting of pouchitis or perianal disease, however, current guidelines recommend treating pregnant women in the same manner as non-pregnant women, with a short course of ciprofloxacin and metronidazole.[14-16]

### Metronidazole

Metronidazole crosses the placental barrier.[32] Though a few older case reports have suggested a possible association with oral cleft malformations with first-trimester metronidazole treatment,[36,37] a large cohort study comparing 1387 women exposed to metronidazole during the first trimester of pregnancy to 1387 women unexposed in pregnancy found no increased risk of congenital malformations (OR 1.2, 95% CI 0.90 to 1.60).[38] Further, a subsequent meta-analysis of 7 studies including 1336 women exposed to metronidazole in the first trimester also found no increased risk for congenital malformations (OR 0.93, 95% CI 0.73 to 1.18).[39] Based on the current evidence, short courses of metronidazole appear to be safe for use during pregnancy when appropriate to treat an active infection.[14-16]

### Vancomycin

Pregnancy and IBD are conditions associated with an increased risk for *C difficile* infection (CDI). Studies have shown that pregnant women are at a higher risk for CDI particularly around the time of labor, especially in the setting of cesarean delivery.[40] The Infectious Disease Society of America recommends vancomycin or fidaxomicin for treatment of an initial CDI,[41] though there are no current recommendations for treatment specifically in the pregnant patient. Intravenous vancomycin crosses the placenta and has been detected in amniotic fluid and infant serum, however to date there is no evidence for teratogenicity.[42,43] It is unknown if oral vancomycin crosses the placenta, but, as the bioavailability of oral vancomycin is less than 10%, it is very unlikely.[43] If needed for the treatment of an active infection, the current evidence suggests that the use of vancomycin during pregnancy is safe.

## Corticosteroids

Corticosteroid use during pregnancy has previously been associated with a 3-fold increase in orofacial cleft deformities[44]; however, more recent studies have not supported this finding. A Danish study of more than 51,973 pregnancies with corticosteroid exposure during prenatal development found no increased risk of cleft lip and/or cleft palate.[45] Several case reports have suggested that long-term, moderate- to high-dose corticosteroid use throughout pregnancy, particularly in the third trimester, may suppress fetal adrenal hormone production, resulting in neonatal adrenal insufficiency.[46,47] A subsequent case report consisting of 16 cases of in utero exposure to prednisolone (mean dose of 29.7 ± 16.1 mg/day for a mean duration of 18.4 ± 15.4 weeks), however, found no evidence for an increase in neonatal adrenal insufficiency in the infants.[48] The Pregnancy in Inflammatory Bowel Disease and Neonatal Outcomes (PIANO) registry including over 900 women who received either oral or intravenous corticosteroids at any point in pregnancy resulted in an increased odds of gestational diabetes (OR 2.8, 95% CI 1.30 to 6.00) and LBW (OR 1.2, 95% CI 0.60 to 2.50) but no congenital anomalies.[49] One small series of 8 patients with CD treated with budesonide did not show any increased risk for adverse pregnancy outcomes.[50]

As previously discussed, women with IBD who are of childbearing age should be counseled on the importance of having quiescent disease on a steroid-free long-term treatment regimen prior to conception due to the negative impact of active disease on pregnancy and fetal outcomes. The current recommendation is for patients be in remission for at least 3 months prior to pregnancy. If treatment with steroids is needed, they can safely be used at the lowest dose possible for the shortest duration needed while current medications are being optimized or a new treatment regimen is implemented.[14-16]

# Immunomodulators

## Methotrexate

Methotrexate inhibits the enzymes that convert folic acid into its active form for DNA synthesis and is a well-known abortifacient and teratogen. Its use early in pregnancy has been associated with cardiovascular and orofacial congenital abnormalities, though this risk was partially mediated by folate supplementation.[51] Based on the existing evidence, the use of methotrexate is contraindicated in pregnancy.[14-16] Methotrexate elimination varies widely from patient to patient with positive levels detected in the red blood cells of patients anywhere between 2 to 32 weeks after medication discontinuation.[52] For those planning to conceive, women are recommended to discontinue methotrexate at least 3 months prior to conception to allow sufficient time for drug elimination and to pursue an alternative therapy, ensuring sustained remission is achieved prior to conception.[14-16] Otherwise, any woman in her childbearing years who is being treated with methotrexate should be strongly encouraged to also use a reliable form of birth control, in addition to folate supplementation. If an unplanned pregnancy is detected, experts recommend immediate discontinuation of methotrexate, continued folate supplementation, and referral to an obstetrician, though termination is not strictly mandated.[14,16]

## Azathioprine/6-Mercaptopurine

Thiopurine therapy in pregnancy was previously controversial; however, there is now good evidence to support continued use in pregnancy. The active metabolite of both AZA and 6MP, 6-thioguanine (6-TGN), crosses the placenta and can be detected in neonates following intrauterine exposure.[53] Studies in animal models suggest teratogenic potential, resulting in neonatal hepatoxicity and myelosuppression; however both prospective and retrospective studies in humans have not consistently supported these findings. A meta-analysis of 5 studies including 3045 pregnancies exposed to thiopurines found an increased odds of preterm birth (OR 1.67, 95% CI 1.26 to 2.20), but no increase for LBW or congenital anomalies.[54] A subsequent cohort study using Swedish health registry data also found an increased odds for preterm birth among women treated with thiopurines during pregnancy in the setting of both stable disease (aOR 2.41, 95% CI 1.05 to 5.51) and active disease (aOR 4.90, 95% CI 2.76 to 8.69).[7] In contrast, a recent, multicenter retrospective study including 187 pregnancies exposed to thiopurines did not find any increase in adverse pregnancy or neonatal outcomes compared to unexposed pregnancies or pregnancies exposed to anti-TNF agents.[55] In terms of long-term consequences, a small prospective study including 30 children with intrauterine thiopurine exposure compared to unexposed children found no difference in development, risk of infection, or immunodeficiency.[56]

Pregnancy alters the metabolism of thiopurines with a decrease in 6-TGN and an increase in the other AZA metabolite, 6-methylmercaptopurine, throughout pregnancy with a return to preconception levels after delivery.[57] For this reason, there may be a role for therapeutic drug monitoring (TDM) to optimize thiopurine therapy in the setting of active disease among pregnant IBD patients.[16]

Thiopurine initiation in pregnancy is not recommended due to the side effect profile and the length of time required to achieve a therapeutic effect.[58] Thiopurine therapy for maintenance of remission is recommended to be continued throughout pregnancy.[14-16] Infants exposed to thiopurines in utero may be at a higher risk for anemia at birth, which should be closely monitored with consideration for checking hemoglobin levels on a case-by-case basis.[14,16]

# Calcineurin-Inhibitors

## Cyclosporine

In the treatment of IBD, cyclosporine is typically used for severe acute UC that is unresponsive to steroids or infliximab.[59] A meta-analysis of the use of cyclosporine during pregnancy in a post-transplant population demonstrated no increased risk for congenital malformations.[60] A small case-control study and a retrospective study on the treatment of flares in pregnant IBD patients, including treatment with intravenous cyclosporine, did not show any increase in adverse outcomes among the cohort exposed to cyclosporine; however, the narrow therapeutic window and the associated toxicities of this drug limit its use to specialized centers.[61,62]

## Tacrolimus

Tacrolimus, a calcineurin-inhibitor, is also most commonly used for steroid-refractory severe UC and fistulizing CD; however, much of what is known about its safety profile in pregnancy is derived from transplant research. One study including 100 pregnancies with exposure to tacrolimus found the incidence of congenital malformations to be comparable to other cohorts of transplant recipients.[63] There are a few case reports that have demonstrated no adverse obstetric or neonatal complications with tacrolimus used as monotherapy[64] or in combination with granulocyte apheresis[65] to treat refractory UC during pregnancy; however, larger studies are indicated before this can be recommended for routine use.

# Small Molecule Agents

## Tofacitinib

Tofacitinib is a Janus kinase inhibitor that was approved by the FDA for the treatment of UC in 2018. As a result, the safety profile of this drug in pregnant patients with IBD is largely unknown. As tofacitinib is a small molecule, it is presumed to cross the placenta, though concentrations in the newborn are not known. Animal studies have demonstrated teratogenic potential though this was seen at doses over 10 times higher than the therapeutic dose used in humans.[66] In one small study of 47 pregnant patients with rheumatoid arthritis or psoriasis, including 33 treated with tofacitinib monotherapy, there was no increased risk of congenital malformations, fetal death, or SA with tofacitinib use compared to the general population.[67] A recent review of the safety data from the Tofacitinib Development Program, including 11 pregnancies in women with UC who were exposed to tofacitinib at the time of conception or during pregnancy, showed no difference in fetal or neonatal deaths, SA, or congenital malformations.[66] Given the scarcity of data with this new therapy, experts recommend discontinuation of tofacitinib at least 1 week prior to conception or discontinued immediately in the event of an unplanned pregnancy, if another treatment option is available to maintain remission throughout pregnancy.[15]

# Anti-Tumor Necrosis Factor Inhibitors

Anti–tumor necrosis factor (anti-TNF) inhibitors are monoclonal antibodies. Of all the antibodies in the human humoral system, only immunoglobulin G (IgG) can cross the placenta. There are several IgG subtypes. Of these, the IgG1 subtype is most easily transported via the Fc receptor-mediated active transport, which is required for transcellular placental transfer due to their large size at 160 kDA. This process most effectively takes place in the second and third trimesters, after organogenesis.[68] The IgG1 antibodies currently approved for IBD management are infliximab (IFX), adalimumab (ADA), and golimumab (GOL). Certolizumab pegol (CZP) is a Fab fragment which binds IgG4 but lacks the Fc component required for active transport, so it crosses the placenta by passive diffusion only.[32] To evaluate the degree of fetal exposure conferred by maternal use in pregnancy, cord blood drug levels of anti-TNF medications obtained at birth showed a medial level of IFX that was 160% of maternal levels and median cord level of ADA was 153% maternal levels, while the median cord level of CZP was 3.9% maternal levels with IFX and ADA detectable until 6 months of age.[69]

Over the past few years, several biosimilars to anti-TNF medications have been approved by the FDA; however, only biosimilars to infliximab are commercially available in the United States. A biosimilar is a biological product that is highly similar, but not identical, to a biologic product already approved for use.[70] Because of their similarity in structure, the safety of using biosimilar anti-TNF medications is thought to be equivalent for all the anti-TNF medications.

The anti-TNF class of medications are known to be immunosuppressive, which initially led to concerns regarding the safety of their use during pregnancy. First, was the initial concern about the impact of intrauterine exposure on the developing fetus. Then, there were questions about a possible increased short-term risk for infections in the newborn due to exposure to an immunosuppressive therapy. Further, there was the concern that intrauterine exposure would impact the immune development of the fetus, leading to a long-term increased risk for infections or malignancy. To date, all these areas of concern have been studied with no evidence of increased risks for adverse fetal or neonatal outcomes following intrauterine exposure to anti-TNF medications.

## Maternal and Pregnancy Outcomes

As the role of TNF in human pregnancy is not well understood, the effects of anti-TNF therapy on the child or the mother have been a subject of much interest. Preclinical animal studies of anti-TNF therapy at doses over 100 times higher than the therapeutic doses in humans, however, have not been associated with any teratogenic effects.[68] Much of what is known about the safety of biologics stem from large meta-analyses (including over 1000 pregnancies) and pregnancy registries. A multicenter European retrospective cohort study evaluated outcomes of 841 pregnancies in women with IBD (388 exposed to anti-TNF medications and 453 women without anti-TNF exposure) and found an increase in maternal infections in the TNF exposed cohort (4.1% vs 0.9%, $P = .002$) but no increase in other pregnancy complications.[71] The authors also reported an overall increase in neonatal complications (19% in the TNF exposed cohort vs 10.5% in the unexposed cohort, $P < .01$), with an increase in neonatal intensive care unit admission (7% in the TNF exposed cohort vs 3.1% in the unexposed cohort, $P < .01$) and for LBW (9.8% in the TNF exposed vs 5% in the unexposed, $P > .01$).[71] Of note, the cohort of pregnant women treated with anti-TNF medications had a higher proportion of CD, prior surgery, tobacco use, and 25% were also being treated with thiopurines.[71] A large retrospective administrative database study also showed an increased risk for maternal infections with anti-TNF exposure during pregnancy (aOR 1.31, 95% CI 1.16 to 1.47).[72]

Studies from the large PIANO registry have also shown the safety of anti-TNF use during pregnancy, including no increased risk of SA, intrauterine growth retardation, congenital anomaly, preterm birth, or neonatal intensive care unit admissions associated with in utero anti-TNF exposure, even in the third trimester.[73,74] A recent meta-analysis of 1242 pregnancies with exposure to anti-TNF therapies compared to disease-matched controls found no increased risk of any adverse pregnancy outcomes including preterm birth, LBW, or congenital anomalies.[75]

Looking specifically at the safety of ADA use in pregnancy, the Organization of Teratology Information Specialists prospective cohort study evaluated the outcomes of 602 pregnancies (257 with CD or rheumatoid arthritis [RA] who received ADA, 120 unexposed with CD or RA and 225 without CD or RA) and found that women in the ADA exposed cohort were more likely to have preterm delivery compared to the healthy, unexposed cohort (adjusted hazard ratio [aHR] 2.59, 95% CI 1.22 to 5.50) but not compared to the unexposed CD or RA cohort (aHR 0.82, 95% CI 0.66 to 7.20).[76] No increased risk was found in preterm delivery, SA, LBW, or congenital anomalies. In a worldwide, prospective, post-marketing pharmaceutical analysis of 1137 pregnancies with maternal CZP therapy for CD and rheumatic diseases, rates of fetal loss, congenital malformations, and maternal complications, including diabetes and preeclampsia, were similar to that of the general population in the United States and Europe.[77] GOL is one of the newer anti-TNF therapies to receive FDA approval for the treatment of moderate to severe UC. As a result of how recently this drug was approved, it is the most infrequently prescribed anti-TNF inhibitor in pregnancy.[78] Safety data are therefore quite limited; however, GOL is presumed safe based on large studies of all anti-TNF therapies that have included GOL.[71,72,79,80] One retrospective study including 20 pregnancies in women with IBD who were treated with biosimilar IFX showed no increased risk for adverse pregnancy or fetal outcomes,[81] suggesting a shared safety profile.

## Neonatal Outcomes

Due to the increased active transport of anti-TNF therapies in the second and third trimester, there have been concerns regarding the impact on fetal immune development and the risk of infections. One of the initial studies from the PIANO registry, including 102 women with anti-TNF exposure during pregnancy and 59 women on combination anti-TNF and immunomodulator therapy, found an increased risk for infections at 12 months of age in the cohort exposed to combination therapy compared to the unexposed cohort (RR 1.50, 95% CI 1.08 to 2.09), not compared to the anti-TNF monotherapy cohort, but no differences in height, weight, or developmental milestones in any cohort (when adjusted for maternal disease activity) at 4, 9, and 12 months of age.[73] The multicenter European TEDDY retrospective cohort study found no difference in the risk of infection between the 388 children exposed to TNF and 453 unexposed children for a mean follow-up period of 4 years.[71] On multivariate analysis, after adjusting for LBW, preterm birth was the only risk factor associated with an increased risk for severe infections (hazard risk 2.5, 95% CI 1.5 to 4.3).[71] A prospective, multicenter study including 72 children exposed to anti-TNF in utero and 69 unexposed children found no differences in infection rates, a diagnosis of allergies, growth, or psychomotor development for up to 3 years of follow-up.[79] Looking specifically at the concerns for developmental delays, a subsequent study from the PIANO registry found that, when controlling for preterm birth, infants with intrauterine exposure to immunomodulator and/or biologic therapy did not exhibit any developmental delay compared to unexposed infants when followed for up to 4 years of age.[82]

Response to vaccinations has also been a concern following exposure to anti-TNFs during fetal development. A prospective cohort study showed that the serologic response to live and non-live vaccines was equal or better in infants with intrauterine anti-TNF exposure compared to unexposed controls.[79] In addition, data from the PIANO registry also demonstrated that infants exposed to biologics in utero developed adequate humoral immunity to routine vaccinations with no difference in the IFX cord blood levels between those who responded and those who did not.[84]

As IFX and ADA can be detected for up to 6 months in infants with intrauterine exposure,[69] these infants should not receive live vaccines for the first 6 months or until drug levels are undetectable.[15,16] In the United States the only live vaccine given in the first year is rotavirus, however Bacillus Calmette-Guerin (BCG) is given in infants outside of the United States. There has been one report of a fatal disseminated infection following BCG vaccination of an infant with detectable serum IFX levels[83]; however, another report of BCG exposure in IFX exposed infants resulted in axillar lymphadenopathy and large local skin reactions but not death.[79] Further, exposure to rotavirus in anti-TNF exposed infants has been reported to result in mild reactions[84]; however, given the risk for a more severe reaction in the newborn, avoidance of live vaccines is recommended. Those exposed to CZP only, however, may receive live vaccines on schedule as CZP is found in much lower concentrations due to passive transport across the placenta.[85]

In older guidelines, the recommendations were to stop these medications in the second trimester in women in clinical remission to lower the drug concentration in the fetus at the time of birth.[16] Data from the PIANO registry showed that exposure to anti-TNF medications during the third trimester of pregnancy did not increase the risk of preterm birth, infant infections (up to 12 months of age), or the risk of disease activity for the first 4 months postpartum.[74] Further, a recent large retrospective study using the French national health system database found no difference in the overall infection rate between children exposed to anti-TNF in the third trimester compared to children who were unexposed (43.7% in the exposed cohort vs 45.9% unexposed cohort, aOR 0.89, 95% CI 0.76 to 1.05, $P = .242$).[72] Importantly, there were significantly more IBD relapses in women who stopped anti-TNF therapy before 24 weeks of gestation (45.8%) compared to women who continued anti-TNF therapy after 24 weeks (30.6%, $P = .005$). After adjusting for disease severity, IBD type, age, and concomitant thiopurine use, this increased risk of flare persisted on multivariate analysis (aOR 1.98, 95% CI 1.25 to 3.15). Given more recent studies showing the safety of this class of medications throughout pregnancy, and the increased risk of a complication with discontinuing these medications, the current recommendation is to continue these medications throughout pregnancy.[79] If possible, prescribers can adjust the dosing schedule to achieve the lowest drug concentration at the time of delivery, but dosing should not be interrupted for more than 1 to 2 weeks. For CZP, the dosing intervals do not need to be altered.

## Combination Therapy

Recent studies have suggested an increased risk for infections in infants with intrauterine exposure to the combination of anti-TNF and thiopurine medications. Safety reports have not shown any increased risk for adverse maternal or fetal outcomes with the use of combination anti-TNF and thiopurine therapies.[86] However, data from the PIANO registry showed an increased risk for infections at 12 months of age in the infants with prior in-utero exposure to combination therapy compared to an unexposed cohort (RR 1.50, 95% CI 1.08 to 2.09).[73] Another prospective study including 80 pregnant women with IBD found that infants exposed to anti-TNF therapy and thiopurines were 2.7 times more likely to develop an infection in the first year of life compared to those exposed to anti-TNF monotherapy (RR 2.7, 95% CI 1.09 to 6.78, $P = .02$).[87] In a recent European multicenter study of 841 children, including 99 children with intrauterine exposure to combination therapy, there was no increased prevalence of severe infections between the children exposed to combination therapy compared to those exposed to anti-TNF monotherapy (12% vs 11%, $P > .05$) with a median follow-up period of 4 years.[71] Given the increased risk of infections in infants following exposure to combination therapy, the current recommendations are to consider discontinuing the thiopurine during preconception planning to ensure sustained remission on monotherapy. However, this needs to be decided on an individual basis depending on the patient's severity of disease and indication for using combination therapy prior to pregnancy.[15,16]

## Therapeutic Drug Monitoring

Current guidelines support the use of TDM for patients with signs and symptoms of active inflammation to help guide the next steps in their medication management.[88] However, there may also be a role for TDM as part of preconception planning or early in pregnancy. A prospective study including 15 pregnant women on stable doses of IFX and 10 pregnant women on stable doses of ADA assessed maternal drug concentrations in each trimester and showed that the IFX concentration increases throughout pregnancy, even after adjusting for albumin, body mass index and C-reactive protein, while the ADA concentration remained stable.[89] This increased IFX level is thought to be due to decreased IFX clearance as pregnancy progresses.[90] These levels normalize to pre-pregnancy levels at delivery,[89] and the normal dosing schedule can then be resumed based on pre-pregnancy body weight.[15]

# Anti-Integrin Agents

## Natalizumab

Natalizumab (NAT) is a monoclonal IgG4 antibody that crosses the placenta through active transport.[91] NAT specifically inhibits the α-subunit on the α4β1 and α4β7 integrin-adhesion molecules, which mediate the process by which leukocytes are targeted toward tissue in the first steps of the inflammatory cascade.[92,93] Importantly, α4 integrin is involved in fertilization, implantation, and placental and cardiac development, raising concerns for a potential risk of teratogenicity or congenital malformation.[94] In terms of maternal risk, NAT crosses the blood-brain barrier and is known to lead to progressive multifocal encephalopathy in patients with prior exposure to the John Cunningham (JC) virus, which can be fatal. Testing for prior exposure to the JC virus is required prior to starting NAT, and routine testing is required for all patients being treated with NAT with drug discontinuation if JC virus antibody is positive.

Animal studies have not shown any abortifacient or teratogenic effects of NAT; however, there were associated changes in hematopoiesis and leukocyte trafficking in some exposed fetuses.[95] Similarly, a case series including 13 pregnancies in 12 women with multiple sclerosis who were exposed to NAT during the third trimester reported hematologic abnormalities in 10 of the 13 newborns, including anemia or thrombocytopenia, which all resolved at 4 months.[96] A prospective observational study including 101 women with multiple sclerosis who were exposed to NAT during the first trimester compared to disease matched controls and healthy controls found no increased rates of congenital malformations, preterm birth, or LBW between the groups.[97] Higher rates of miscarriage ($P = .002$) and lower birth weights, but not < 2500 g ($P = .001$), were seen in the exposed and disease-matched cohorts compared to the healthy controls, but there was no significant difference in the exposed and disease matched groups, suggesting these findings are related to the underlying disease and not due to NAT exposure.[97] Further, 9 patients exposed to NAT in the third trimester were included in the PIANO registry and were found to have no increased risk for preterm birth or an increase in newborn infections.[74] Given the overall evidence suggesting the safety of use during pregnancy, the current recommendations are for continued use of NAT during pregnancy to maintain disease remission with dose adjusting to allow for the lowest dose concentration at the time of delivery, when possible.[15]

### Vedolizumab

Vedolizumab (VDZ) was only recently approved for the treatment of moderate to severe CD and UC, therefore, data for the efficacy and safety of use in pregnancy remain limited. VDZ inhibits only integrins containing α4β7, which is expressed by T cells to promote pro-inflammatory cell migration into gastrointestinal tissues. In this way, the action of VDZ is specific to the gut, and thus avoids the risk of maternal development of progressive multifocal encephalopathy seen with NAT use.[91-93] Similar to other IgG1 antibodies, VDZ has a high affinity for the Fc receptor and is actively transported across the placenta, with placental transfer steadily increasing throughout pregnancy.[68] In an analysis of the clinical trial data for VDZ including 23 pregnant IBD patients there were no new safety concerns identified following use in pregnancy.[98] A multicenter retrospective case-control study from Europe compared pregnancy and neonatal outcomes in women with IBD exposed to VDZ (n = 79 pregnancies) to women with IBD exposed to anti-TNF therapy (n = 186 pregnancies) and women without exposure to biologics (n = 184) and found no increased risk of SA, prematurity, SGA, LBW, or congenital anomalies between the cohorts.[99] Further, there was no difference in neonatal infections or malignancies in the first year of life between the groups. In an early analysis of the ongoing Organization of Teratology Information Specialists pregnancy registry including 28 patients with IBD who received VDZ in the first trimester of pregnancy or later found no increased risk of congenital malformations compared to disease-matched and healthy control cohorts.[100]

Looking at serum drug concentrations, a recent assessment of patients enrolled in the PIANO registry compared drug levels in maternal and cord blood in 4 mother/infant pairs exposed to VDZ and found that concentrations of VDZ were lower in the infant than the mother by approximately 50%. Furthermore, the timing of the last dose of VDZ prior to delivery was not associated with any increased risk in neonatal infections.[101] In summary, evidence from current studies support the safety of continued use of VDZ throughout pregnancy. As with other biologic agents, adjusting the timing of the last dose to allow for the lowest fetal drug concentration is recommended, if possible, and live vaccines should be avoided in infants with exposure to VDZ in utero for the first 6 months of life.[15]

## Anti-Interleukin 12/23 Medications

Ustekinumab (UST) is an IgG1κ monoclonal antibody that prevents pro-inflammatory T-cell recruitment by binding to the p40 subunit of both IL-12 and IL-23 and is one of the newest drugs approved for treatment of moderate to severe CD and UC. As UST is an IgG1 antibody, it crosses the placenta via active transport throughout pregnancy but to the greatest extent in the second and third trimesters, after organogenesis.[68] There is no evidence of teratogenicity in animal studies[102] but studies in humans are limited. Review of the company safety database including outcomes for 206 pregnancies with exposure to UST showed rates of SA and congenital anomalies similar to the general population in the United States.[103] Analysis of 24 pregnancies that occurred during the CD Clinical Development Program for UST also found no significant increases in LBW or preterm birth regardless of the duration of UST exposure during pregnancy.[104] Two case reports of women with CD treated with UST until 30 and 33 weeks of pregnancy reported that cord blood concentrations of UST were significantly higher (2-fold higher in 1 report) than maternal serum levels at delivery though both pregnancies resulted in healthy newborns.[105,106] One of the infants was followed up after 1 year and had no associated developmental delay or an increase in infections.[105] There remains a paucity of data on the safety of UST in pregnancy, however, based on the current literature there does not appear to be any safety concerns for use during pregnancy. The current recommendation is to continue UST throughout pregnancy with the timing of the last dose adjusted to allow for the lowest fetal drug concentration, if possible, and avoid giving live vaccines to infants with intrauterine exposure to UST for the first 6 months of life.[15]

## Other Commonly Used Medications

### Bisphosphonates

Osteoporosis is a common complication seen in patients with IBD, with an estimated prevalence of 14% to 42%.[107] The etiology of osteoporosis is likely multifactorial with risk factors including nutritional deficiencies, in the setting of poor intake or malabsorption, chronic systemic inflammation, and corticosteroid exposure. Bisphosphonates decrease bone turnover, therefore preserving bone mass, and are often prescribed for the treatment for osteoporosis. Animal studies have demonstrated the transfer of bisphosphonates across the placenta as well as storage in the fetal skeleton. Though these studies evaluated exposures to doses 10 times higher than the therapeutic dose in humans, the exposures resulted in severe alterations in fetal growth or outright fetal loss.[108] Case reports have suggested a possible link between bisphosphonate use in pregnancy and neonatal electrolyte derangements (eg, transient hypocalcemia) and LBW.[109] A recent systematic review was only able to identify reports of 40 pregnancies with exposure to bisphosphonates and no serious pregnancy or fetal adverse effects were reported.[110] Due to the adverse outcomes in animal studies and limited reports of safety in humans, bisphosphonates should be avoided in pregnancy.[111] If long-term use is indicated for female IBD patients, it is recommended they follow closely with an endocrinologist and consider discontinuing therapy during pregnancy.[111]

### Antidiarrheal Medications

Antidiarrheal medications (eg, loperamide, diphenoxylate) are frequently used as adjuvant treatment for ongoing symptoms, not due to inflammation, in IBD patients. Patients with IBD can also have symptoms of irritable bowel syndrome, including diarrhea in the absence of active intestinal inflammation.[111] A multicenter, prospective study on the use of loperamide during pregnancy, including during the first trimester, did not show any increased incidence of adverse pregnancy or fetal outcomes compared to a matched cohort of women without loperamide use.[112] Another study using the Swedish Birth Registry to assess for an increase in congenital malformations following first trimester exposure to loperamide and found an increase in the odds of any congenital malformation (OR = 1.43, 95% CI 1.04 to 1.96), with an increased risk for hypospadias (RR = 3.2, 95% CI 1.3 to 6.6).[113] Overall, these authors concluded that the use of loperamide during pregnancy may be associated with an increased risk of malformation. For diphenoxylate, animal studies have not shown any evidence of teratogenicity[114]; however, there are no studies of its use in humans during pregnancy. Given the potential for congenital malformations with the use of loperamide and no evidence to support the safety of use of diphenoxylate and atropine during pregnancy, these medications should be avoided, if possible. Safer options to consider for the treatment of non-inflammatory diarrhea include the use of bile acid binding agents or fiber supplementation.

# Mode of Delivery

The mode of delivery (ie, vaginal or caesarean section [c-section]) is typically a decision made between the patient and her obstetrician based on obstetric factors. However, c-section delivery occurs much more commonly among women with IBD. In a cohort of 543 women with IBD including 403 pregnancies prior to the diagnosis of IBD and 177 after the diagnosis of IBD, the use of c-section delivery occurred 3 times more often after the diagnosis of IBD (28.7% vs 8.1%).[115] A large meta-analysis also found that women with IBD were more likely to have a caesarean delivery (pOR 1.5, 95% CI 1.26 to 1.79).[2] A prospective cohort study including 179 births in women with IBD found that c-section deliveries were more common in women with IBD (30% vs 21% in healthy controls, RR 1.6, 95% CI 1.2 to 2.6, $P = .02$); however, there was not a higher incidence of emergency c-sections in the IBD cohort compared to healthy controls (35% vs 40%, $P = .08$).[116]

One possible reason women and their physicians are electing for c-sections is an inability to predict which patients will experience complications during a vaginal delivery, such as perianal trauma or the need for an episiotomy, as trauma to the perianal region, particularly injury to the anal sphincters, should be avoided when possible in women with IBD to maintain continence, which significantly impacts quality of life.[117] Most experts agree that delivery by elective c-section is clearly indicated for women with IBD with active perianal or rectal disease and should be highly considered in those with an ileal pouch.[15] However, in a retrospective cohort study including 369 births in women with IBD found that women with CD were more likely to have a caesarean delivery if they had a prior c-section (aOR 22.2, 95% CI 6.16 to 80.2) or a history of perianal disease (aOR 13.6, 95% CI 3.87 to 47.5), although only 42% of the women with prior perianal disease had active disease during pregnancy. For women with UC, c-section delivery was more likely in women with a history of colectomy (aOR 5.08, 95% CI 1.95 to 13.20).[118]

Fistulizing perianal disease develops in approximately 25% of patients with CD.[119] Active perianal disease is characterized by anorectal fistulas or abscesses, anal fissures, anal stenosis, and rectovaginal fistulas. Despite the use of c-section delivery for women with prior perianal disease, a systematic review of 18 studies demonstrated no increase in new onset or recurrence of perianal disease with vaginal delivery compared to caesarean delivery.[120] However, in the setting of active perianal disease, 67% developed worsening disease following vaginal delivery. Using a large health database, women with CD without perianal involvement were found to have the same risk of fourth-degree lacerations after vaginal delivery as women without CD (1.4% vs 1.3%). However, perianal disease was found to significantly increase the risk of severe lacerations following vaginal delivery (12.3%, $P < .001$).[121] Due to the use of administrative data, the presence of active perianal disease could not be determined. Screening for active perianal disease should occur in patients who are symptomatic, have a history of perianal disease, or at the time of rectovaginal culture for group B streptococcus which is obtained between weeks 35 to 37 of pregnancy.[15] The current delivery recommendation for all women with active rectal or perianal disease is elective caesarean.[14-16]

Total colectomy with an ileal pouch-anal anastomoses (IPAA) is a frequently used surgical treatment for patients with UC. There is a higher risk for infertility following an IPAA,[122] however, once pregnant, women with an IPAA commonly have normal pregnancies that result in healthy babies.[123] Studies have shown an increase in bowel frequency and incontinence in the later stages of pregnancy,[124] likely due to rising pelvic floor pressure. One study showed a higher incidence of anterior sphincter damage and lower mean squeeze anal pressure following vaginal delivery compared to cesarean delivery; however, these changes did not impact pouch function.[125] Other studies have also shown a return of pouch function immediately postpartum,[126] no difference in pouch function after vaginal delivery compared to c-section delivery (mean follow-up of 2.4 years)[124] or compared to women who have never been pregnant (mean follow-up of 13 years).[123] For many women with and without IBD, vaginal delivery has been shown to increase the risk of anal sphincter injury and pudendal nerve injury,[127] both of which can further impair pouch function.[125] Due to the potential risk for anal sphincter damage during vaginal delivery, delivery by cesarean section should be considered for women with a prior IPAA.[14-16]

# Management of a Flare in Pregnancy

A pregnant patient with IBD and symptoms suggestive of active inflammation should undergo an evaluation similar to the non-pregnant IBD patient. Prior to making any medication changes, it is pertinent to ensure that her symptoms are due to active inflammation. Risk factors for disease flares in pregnancy and postpartum include active inflammation at conception, discontinuation of medical therapy, and postpartum resumption of smoking[128]; however evaluation for any new medications (including over the counter medications) or infectious etiologies such as viral infections or C difficile should also be considered. As part of the laboratory evaluation for a flare, it is important to note that normal laboratory changes during pregnancy include a decrease in albumin and hemoglobin and an increase in inflammatory markers.[15] If imaging is required to assess for areas of active inflammation, ultrasound and magnetic resonance imaging are preferred due to the absence of radiation exposure risk to the fetus compared to x-ray or computed tomography. Gadolinium is considered a potential teratogen and should be avoided until after the first trimester when organogenesis is complete.[128,129] Hospitalized patients with IBD should be treated with anticoagulation for prophylaxis of venothromboembolism,[130] including in pregnant patients.[15] Endoscopy is safe during pregnancy and lower endoscopy appears to be safe during all trimesters of pregnancy.[131,132] It is highly recommended to have a preprocedural consultation with an obstetrician, have a strong indication for the procedure, minimize procedure time, and use the lowest doses of sedation medication possible to minimize the risk to the fetus. Positioning the patient in the left lateral position, as typically used for endoscopy, prevents compression of major blood vessels and resultant maternal hypotension and placental hypoperfusion. When obtaining informed consent, maternal and fetal risks of the procedure and sedation should be discussed including the risk for emergent delivery.[133]

Medical treatment for an IBD flare in pregnancy, in most cases, can be treated similarly to flares in the non-pregnant patients. A short course of corticosteroids may be enough to regain a symptomatic remission while determining if a dose adjustment of the current treatment or if a change in treatment is needed. Steroids should not be continued long term for maintenance, even in pregnancy. Methotrexate is contraindicated and thiopurines should not be started in pregnancy due to the long onset of action and the adverse side effect profile. Anti-TNF medications can be safely started in pregnancy if needed for control of active IBD following negative screening for hepatitis B and tuberculosis exposure. Small studies have shown the safety of using cyclosporine for acute severe UC in pregnancy,[61] however due to the narrow therapeutic window for this medication, use should be under the guidance of an experienced provider.

Surgery may be indicated during pregnancy for several reasons, such as obstruction, hemorrhage, perforation, or ongoing active inflammation.[14] Surgery appears to be relatively safe in any trimester; however, some small series have suggested SA following first trimester surgeries and preterm birth following surgery in the third trimester.[134] In summary, evaluation, and treatment of an IBD flare is similar between pregnant and non-pregnant patients.

# Preconception Counseling

Every female patient with IBD between the ages of 15 and 40 years should receive preconception counseling. Preconception counseling should include a medication review, an assessment for active inflammation, a review of preventative health maintenance, and a discussion about tobacco, alcohol, and recreational drug use.[15] The medication review should include a detailed review of the patient's current medication regimen to ensure she can safely continue the medications throughout pregnancy as well as a detailed discussion with the patient on the safety and importance of continuing those medications throughout pregnancy to try to keep her IBD in remission. Discontinuation of maintenance therapy is associated with a > 20% higher rate of relapse compared with those who continue their medications,[6] therefore, medication adherence must be strongly encouraged throughout pregnancy. If the patient is on methotrexate, this should be discontinued and a new treatment regimen started at least 3 months prior to conception. If the patient is on tofacitinib, and another treatment regimen is available, then the tofacitinib should be discontinued at least 1 week prior to conception. If she is taking sulfasalazine, the folate supplement should be increased to 2 mg daily.

As part of preconception counseling, the patient should be assessed for signs and/or symptoms of active inflammation based on patient reported symptoms and objective criteria, such as inflammatory markers, fecal calprotectin, and/or endoscopy if not recently completed. If she continues to have active inflammation, dose optimization or a change in treatment to a medication that is safe to continue throughout pregnancy should be made. Ideally, the patient should be in clinical and endoscopic remission for at least 3 months prior to conception on a steroid-free maintenance medication regimen. If the patient is in remission, a thorough review of health maintenance recommendations based on the patient's age, medication regimen, and other risk factors should be completed with any pending preventative care updated prior to conception. Further, patients should be informed of the importance of smoking and alcohol cessation as well as abstinence from recreational drug use during pregnancy on fetal development. Women with CD who are trying to become or are already pregnant should be counseled that smoking increases the risk for LBW, SA, and stillbirth[135] and is associated with more severe disease activity,[136] whereas cessation is associated with disease improvement.[137]

When caring for pregnant women with IBD, physicians may consider referring them to a nutritionist to optimize nutritional status. If nutritional support is not available, part of the preconception evaluation should include screening for deficiencies in vitamin $B_{12}$, vitamin D, and iron as many patients with IBD, particularly those with ileal disease, are nutritionally deficient.[15,128,138] If deficiencies are found, supplementation should be prescribed. Regardless of folic acid levels, supplementation with 2 mg of folate daily is recommended for patients with ileal disease, on a low-residue diet, or therapies that inhibit enzymes of folate metabolism.[139] Adequate weight gain is another important factor in optimizing pregnancy outcomes. Women with IBD are at an increased risk for inadequate weight gain in pregnancy even with quiescent disease.[140] Moreover, when compared to non-IBD controls matched for inadequate weight gain, mothers with IBD were twice as likely to deliver SGA infants.[140] Poor weight gain in pregnancy among mothers with IBD has also been associated with preterm births and LBW infants.[141] Weight gain should therefore be regularly monitored throughout the pregnancy.

Preconception education is extremely important for women with IBD. Many patients, as well as providers, are unaware of the safety of IBD medication during pregnancy. In one survey of 145 women with IBD, 24% of the respondents felt that tolerating symptoms of a flare is more important than medical therapy while 36% felt that all IBD medications are harmful to unborn children.[142] Pregnant women who have received preconception counseling, however, have been found to have an increased adherence to folate (aOR 3.15, 95% CI 2.47 to 4.03),[143,144] multivitamin supplementation (aOR 4.40, 95% CI 4.00 to 4.70), alcohol cessation (aOR 1.30, 95% CI 1.20 to 1.50),[145] and tobacco cessation ($P$ = .0013).[144] Further, preconception counseling is significantly associated with lower disease activity regardless of smoking status, duration of disease, or disease activity at conception (OR 0.441, 95% CI 0.232 to 0.838).[144] Preconception counseling, specifically providing patients with updated information regarding the safety of their IBD medications and the importance of maintaining a steroid-free remission throughout pregnancy, has been shown to improve pregnancy and fetal outcomes.[144] Given the improved pregnancy and fetal outcomes after preconception counseling, current guidelines recommend that women of childbearing age with IBD should receive counseling prior to conception.[14-16]

# Postpartum

Women with IBD are at an increased risk for a disease flare in the postpartum period for several reasons. Many discontinue their medications to breastfeed despite strong evidence that the benefits of continuing IBD medications far outweigh the risk of exposure to the neonate.[136] Other reasons include resumption of cigarette smoking, hormonal fluctuations, and loss of the disinhibiting anti-inflammatory cytokines of pregnancy.[136,146] To prevent a flare, maintenance therapy that was at any point discontinued in pregnancy should be resumed within 24 hours of a vaginal delivery or within 48 hours of a caesarean delivery if there is no evidence of infection using the pre-pregnancy weight.[15] Exceptions to this rule are methotrexate, which is contraindicated with breastfeeding, and tofacitinib, which is not known to be safe in either pregnancy or breastfeeding.[146,147]

# Conclusion

Most women with IBD have healthy pregnancies and deliver healthy babies; however, studies suggest a higher incidence of preterm birth and LBW among women with IBD. Women with UC, however, are more likely to experience an exacerbation of their disease, particularly early in pregnancy and in the postpartum period. Disease remission prior to conception is the most important factor for a healthy pregnancy and healthy newborn. Methotrexate and tofacitinib should be discontinued prior to pregnancy, but other IBD therapies can be safely continued throughout pregnancy. A c-section delivery is recommended for women with active perianal or rectal disease at the time of delivery and should be considered for women with an ileal pouch due to the risk for perianal injury and the potential impact on fecal incontinence. A suspected flare in a pregnant IBD patient should be evaluated and treated similarly to non-pregnant IBD patients; however, imaging should be restricted to ultrasounds at any time or MRI after the first trimester. It is paramount that providers who care for women with IBD during their childbearing years implement preconception counseling so that patients are up to date on their preventive care; they are aware of the importance of active remission prior to conception; their medication regimen is reviewed for safety; and they receive the most updated information about the safety of continuing their medications, which improves compliance and improves pregnancy and fetal outcomes.

## KEY POINTS

1. Most women with IBD have healthy pregnancies, but there is a higher risk of having a preterm birth or LBW infant.

2. Methotrexate and tofacitinib should be discontinued prior to pregnancy, but other IBD medications can be safely continued.

3. Disease remission prior to conception is the most important factor for a healthy pregnancy and healthy newborn.

4. Delivery via c-section is recommended for women with active perianal or rectal disease and should be considered for women with an ileal pouch. Otherwise, vaginal delivery is recommended.

# References

1. Mountifield R, Bampton P, Prosser R, et al. Fear and fertility in inflammatory bowel disease: a mismatch of perception and reality affects family planning decisions. *Inflamm Bowel Dis.* 2009;15:720-725.

2. Cornish J, Tan E, Teare J, et al. A meta-analysis on the influence of inflammatory bowel disease on pregnancy. *Gut.* 2007;56(6):830-837.

3. O'Toole A, Nwanne O, Tomlinson T. Inflammatory bowel disease increases risk of adverse pregnancy outcomes: a meta-analysis. *Dig Dis Sci.* 2015;60(9):2750-2761.

4. Stephansson O, Larsson H, Pedersen L, et al. Congenital abnormalities and other birth outcomes in children born to women with ulcerative colitis in Denmark and Sweden. *Inflamm Bowel Dis.* 2011;17(3):795-801.

5. Stephansson O, Larsson H, Pedersen L, et al. Crohn's disease is a risk factor for preterm birth. *Clin Gastroenterol Hepatol.* 2010;8(6):509-515.

6. Mahadevan U, Sandborn WJ, Li D, et al. Pregnancy outcomes in women with inflammatory bowel disease: a large community-based study from northern California. *Gastroenterology.* 2007;133(4):1106-1112.

7. Bröms G, Granath F, Linder M, et al. Birth outcomes in women with inflammatory bowel disease: effects of disease activity and drug exposure. *Inflamm Bowel Dis.* 2014;20(6):1091-1098.

8. Ban L, Tata LJ, Fiaschi L, Card T. Limited risks of major congenital anomalies in children of mothers with IBD and effects of medications. *Gastroenterology.* 2014;146(1):76-84.

9. Molnár T, Farkas K, Nagy F, et al. Pregnancy outcome in patients with inflammatory bowel disease according to the activity of disease and the medical treatment: a case-control study. *Scand J Gastroenterol.* 2010;45:11:1302-1306.

10. Bortoli A, Pedersen N, Duricova D, et al. Pregnancy outcome in inflammatory bowel disease: prospective European case-control ECCO-EpiCom study, 2003–2006. *Aliment Pharm Ther.* 2011;34(7):724-734.

11. Abdul Sultan A, West J, Ban L, et al. Adverse pregnancy outcomes among women with inflammatory bowel disease: a population-based study from England. *Inflamm Bowel Dis.* 2016;22(7):1621-1630.

12. Bröms G, Granath F, Linder M, et al. Complications from inflammatory bowel disease during pregnancy and delivery. *Clin Gastroenterol Hepatol.* 2012;10(11):1246-1252.

13. Kim YH, Pfaller B, Marson A, et al. The risk of venous thromboembolism in women with inflammatory bowel disease during pregnancy and the postpartum period. *Medicine (Baltimore).* 2019;98(38):e17309.

14. van der Woude CJ, Ardizzone S, Bengtson MB, et al. The second European evidenced-based consensus on reproduction and pregnancy in inflammatory bowel disease. *J Crohns Colitis.* 2015;9(2):107-124.

15. Mahadevan U, Robinson C, Bernasko N, et al. Inflammatory bowel disease in pregnancy clinical care pathway: a report From the American Gastroenterological Association IBD Parenthood Project Working Group. *Gastroenterology.* 2019;156(5):1508-1524.

16. Nguyen GC, Seow CH, Maxwell C, et al. The Toronto consensus statements for the management of inflammatory bowel disease in pregnancy. *Gastroenterology.* 2016;150(3):734-757.e1.

17. Nielsen O, Andreasson B, Bondesen S, et al. Pregnancy in Crohn's disease. *Scan J Gastroenterol.* 1984;19(6):724-732.

18. Nielsen OH, Andreasson B, Bondesen S, et al. Pregnancy in ulcerative colitis. *Scan J Gastroenterol.* 1983;18(6):735-742.

19. Pedersen N, Bortoli B, Duricova D, et al. The course of inflammatory bowel disease during pregnancy and postpartum: a prospective European ECCO-Epicom study of 209 pregnant women. *Aliment Pharm Ther.* 2013;38:501-512.

20. Riis L, Vind I, Politi P, et al. Does pregnancy change the disease course? A study in a European cohort of patients with inflammatory bowel disease. *Am J Gastroenterol.* 2006;101(7):1539-1545.

21. Abhyankar A, Ham M, Moss AC. Meta-analysis: the impact of disease activity at conception on disease activity during pregnancy in patients with inflammatory bowel disease. *Aliment Pharm Ther.* 2013;38(5):460-466.

22. Mogadam M, Korelitz BI, Ahmed SW, et al. The course of inflammatory bowel disease during pregnancy and postpartum. *Am J Gastroenterol.* 1981;75(4):265-269.

23. Nørgård B, Hundborg HH, Jacobsen BA, et al. Disease activity in pregnant women with Crohn's disease and birth outcomes: a regional Danish cohort study. *Am J Gastroenterol.* 2007;102(9):1947-1954.

24. Aukamp V, Sredl D. Collaborative care management for a pregnant woman with an ostomy. *Complement Ther Nurs Midwifery.* 2004;10(1):5-12.

25. Food and Drug Administration. Content and format of labeling for human description drug and biological products; requirements for pregnancy and lactation labeling (Federal Register Web Site). Available at: https://www.fda.gov/regulatory-information/search-fda-guidance-documents/labeling-human-prescription-drug-and-biological-products-implementing-plr-content-and-format.

26. Brucker MC, King TL. The 2015 US Food and Drug Administration pregnancy and lactation labeling rule. *Journal of Midwifery & Women's Health.* 2017;62(3):308-316.

27. Rubin D, Ananthakrishnan A, Siegel C, et al. ACG clinical guideline ulcerative colitis in adults. *Am J Gastroenterol.* 2019;114(3):384-413.

28. Rahimi R, Nikfar S, Rezaie A, Abdollahi M. Pregnancy outcome in women with inflammatory bowel disease following exposure to 5-aminosalicylic acid drugs: a meta-analysis. *Reproductive Toxicology.* 2008;25(2):271-275.

29. Gallinger ZR, Nguyen GC. Presence of phthalates in gastrointestinal medications: is there a hidden danger? *World J Gastroenterol.* 2013;19(41):7042-7047.

30. Drugs A to Z: Mesasal, Drugs.com (available at https://www.drugs.com/cons/mesasal-rectal.html).

31. International: Mesasal, Drugs.com (available at https://www.drugs.com/international/mesasal.html).

32. Damas OM, Deshpande AR, Avalos DJ, Abreu MT. Treating inflammatory bowel disease in pregnancy: the issues we face today. *J Crohns Colitis.* 2015;9(10):928-936.

33. Acar S, Keskin-Arslan E, Erol-Coskun H, et al. Pregnancy outcomes following quinolone and fluoroquinolone exposure during pregnancy: a systematic review and meta-analysis. *Reprod Toxicol.* 2019;85:65-74.

34. Yefet E, Schwartz N, Chazan B, et al. The safety of quinolones and fluoroquinolones in pregnancy: a meta-analysis. *BJOG.* 2018;125(9):1069-1076.

35. Ziv A, Masarwa R, Perlman A, et al. Pregnancy outcomes following exposure to quinolone antibiotics—a systematic-review and meta-analysis. *Pharm Res.* 2018;35(5):109.

36. Schwebke JR. Metronidazole: utilization in the obstetric and gynecologic patient. *J Sex Transm Dis.* 1995;22(6):370-376.

37. Cantú JM, García-Cruz D. Midline facial defect as a teratogenic effect of metronidazole. *Birth Defects Orig Artic Ser.* 1982;18(3 Pt A):85-88.

38. Piper JMD, Mitchel EFM, Ray WA. Prenatal use of metronidazole and birth defects: no association. *Obstetrics & Gynecology.* 1993;82(3):348-352.

39. Burtin P, Taddio A, Ariburnu O, Einarson TR, Koren G. Safety of metronidazole in pregnancy: a meta-analysis. *Am J Obstet Gynecol.* 1995;172(2 Pt 1):525-529.

40. Cózar-Llistó A, Ramos-Martinez A, Cobo J. *Clostridium difficile* infection in special high-risk populations. *Infect Dis Ther.* 2016;5(3):253-269.

41. McDonald LC, Gerding DN, Johnson S, et al. Clinical practice guidelines for *Clostridium difficile* infection in adults and children: 2017 update by the Infectious Diseases Society of America (IDSA) and Society for Healthcare Epidemiology of America (SHEA). *Clin Infect Dis.* 2018;66(7):e1-e48.

42. Bourget P, Fernandez H, Delouis C, Ribou F. Transplacental passage of vancomycin during the second trimester of pregnancy. *Obstet Gynecol.* 1991;78(5):908-910.

43. Patel S, Preuss CV, Bernice F. Vancomycin. [Updated 2020 Feb 28]. In: StatPearls [Intranet]. Treasure Island (FL): StatPearls Publishing; 2020 Jan. Available from: https://www.ncbi.nlm.nih.gov/books/NBK459263/, accessed 3/19/20.

44. Park-Wyllie L, Mazzotta P, Pastuszak A, et al. Birth defects after maternal exposure to corticosteroids: prospective cohort study and meta-analysis of epidemiological studies. *Teratology.* 2000;62(6):385-392.

45. Hviid A, Mølgaard-Nielsen D. Corticosteroid use during pregnancy and risk of orofacial clefts. *CMAJ.* 2011;183(7):796-804.

46. Homar V, Grosek S, Battelino T. High-dose methylprednisolone in a pregnant woman with Crohn's disease and adrenal suppression in her newborn. *Neonatology Basel.* 2008;94(4):306-309.

47. Saulnier PJ, Piguel X, Perault-Pochat MC, et al. Hypoglycaemic seizure and neonatal acute adrenal insufficiency after maternal exposure to prednisone during pregnancy: a case report. *Eur J Pediatr.* 2010;169(6):763-765.

48. de Vetten L, van Stuijvenberg M, Kema IP, Bocca G. Maternal use of prednisolone is unlikely to be associated with neonatal adrenal suppression-a single-center study of 16 cases. *Eur J Pediatr.* 2017;176(8):1131-1136.

49. Lin K, Martin CF, Dassopoulos T, et al. Pregnancy outcomes amongst mothers with inflammatory bowel disease exposed to systemic corticosteroids: results of the PIANO registry. *Gastroenterology*. 2014;146(5):S-1.

50. Beaulieu DB, Ananthakrishnan AN, Issa M, et al. Budesonide induction and maintenance therapy for Crohn's disease during pregnancy. *Inflamm Bowel Dis*. 2009;15:25-28.

51. Hernández-Díaz S, Werler MM, Walker AM, Mitchell AA. Folic acid antagonists during pregnancy and the risk of Birth Defects. *NEJM*. 2000;343(22):1608-1614.

52. Dalrymple JM, Stamp LK, O'Donnell JL, et al. Pharmacokinetics of oral methotrexate in patients with rheumatoid arthritis. *Arthritis Rheum*. 2008;58(11):3299-3308.

53. de Boer NKH, Jarbandhan SVA, de Graaf P, et al. Azathioprine use during pregnancy: unexpected intrauterine exposure to metabolites. *Am J Gastroenterol*. 2006;101(6):1390-1392.

54. Akbari M, Shah S, Velayos FS, Mahadevan U, Cheifetz AS. Systematic review and meta-analysis on the effects of thiopurines on birth outcomes from female and male patients with inflammatory bowel disease. *Inflamm Bowel Dis*. 2013;19(1):15-22.

55. Casanova MJ, Chaparro M, Domènech E, et al. Safety of thiopurines and anti-TNF-α drugs during pregnancy in patients with inflammatory bowel disease. *Am J Gastroenterol*. 2013;108(3):433-440.

56. de Meij TG, Jharap B, Kneepkens CM et al. Long-term follow-up of children exposed intrauterine to maternal thiopurine therapy during pregnancy in females with inflammatory bowel disease. *Aliment Pharm Ther*. 2013;38:38-43.

57. Jharap B, Boer NKH de, Stokkers P, et al. Intrauterine exposure and pharmacology of conventional thiopurine therapy in pregnant patients with inflammatory bowel disease. *Gut*. 2014;63(3):451-457.

58. Mahadevan U, McConnell RA, Chambers CD. Drug safety and risk of adverse outcomes for pregnant patients with inflammatory bowel disease. *Gastroenterology*. 2017;152(2):451-462.e2.

59. Weisshof R, Ollech JE, El Jurdi K, et al. Ciclosporin therapy after infliximab failure in hospitalized patients with severe acute colitis is effective and safe. *J Crohns Colitis*. 2019;13(9):1105-1110.

60. Bar Oz B, Hackman R, Einarson T, Koren G. Pregnancy outcome after cyclosporine therapy during pregnancy: a meta-analysis. *Transplantation*. 2001;71(8):1051-1055.

61. Reddy D, Murphy SJ, Kane SV, et al. Relapses of inflammatory bowel disease during pregnancy: in-hospital management and birth outcomes. *Am J Gastroenterol*. 2008;103(5):1203-1209.

62. Branche J, Cortot A, Bourreille A, et al. Cyclosporine treatment of steroid-refractory ulcerative colitis during pregnancy. *Inflamm Bowel Dis*. 2009;15(7):1044-1048.

63. Kainz A, Harabacz I, Cowlrick IS, et al. Analysis of 100 pregnancy outcomes in women treated systemically with tacrolimus. *Transpl Int*. 2000;13(1):S299-S300.

64. Baumgart DC, Sturm A, Wiedenmann B, Dignass AU. Uneventful pregnancy and neonatal outcome with tacrolimus in refractory ulcerative colitis. *Gut*. 2005;54(12):1822-1823.

65. Shibuya T, Haga K, Kamei M, et al. Successful remission of ulcerative colitis flare-up during pregnancy with adsorptive granulomonocytapheresis plus tacrolimus. *Intest Res*. 2018;16(3):484-488.

66. Mahadevan U, Dubinsky MC, Su C, et al. Outcomes of pregnancies with maternal/paternal exposure in the tofacitinib safety databases for ulcerative colitis. *Inflamm Bowel Dis*. 2018;24(12):2494-2500.

67. Clowse MEB, Feldman SR, Isaacs JD, et al. Pregnancy outcomes in the tofacitinib safety databases for rheumatoid arthritis and psoriasis. *Drug Saf*. 2016;39(8):755-762.

68. Gisbert JP, Chaparro M. Safety of anti-TNF agents during pregnancy and breastfeeding in women with inflammatory bowel disease. *Am J Gastroenterol*. 2013;108(9):1426-1438.

69. Mahadevan U, Wolf DC, Dubinsky M, et al. Placental transfer of anti–tumor necrosis factor agents in pregnant patients with inflammatory bowel disease. *Clin Gastroenterol Hepatol*. 2013;11(3):286-292.

70. U. S. Food and Drug Administration. Biosimilar and Interchangeable Products, content current as of 10/23/2017. Available at https://www.fda.gov/drugs/biosimilars/biosimilar-and-interchangeable-products#biological.

71. Chaparro M, Verreth A, Lobaton T, et al. Long-term safety of in utero exposure to anti-TNFα drugs for the treatment of inflammatory bowel disease: results from the multicenter European TEDDY study. *Am J Gastroenterol*. 2018;113(3):396-403.

72. Luu M, Benzenine E, Doret M, et al. Continuous anti-TNFα use throughout pregnancy: possible complications for the mother but not for the fetus. A retrospective cohort on the French National Health Insurance Database (EVASION). *Am J Gastroenterol*. 2018;113(11):1669-1677.

73. Mahadevan U, Martin CF, Sandler RS, et al. PIANO: a 1000 patient prospective registry of pregnancy outcomes in women with IBD exposed to immunomodulators and biologic therapy. *Gastroenterology*. 2012;142(5 Suppl 1):S-149.

74. Mahadevan U, Martin CF, Dubinsky M, et al. Exposure to anti-TNFα therapy in the third trimester of pregnancy is not associated with increased adverse outcomes: results from the PIANO Registry. *Gastroenterology*. 2014;146(5 Suppl 1):S-170.

75. Shihab Z, Yeomans ND, De Cruz P. Anti-tumour necrosis factor α therapies and inflammatory bowel disease pregnancy outcomes: a meta-analysis. *J Crohns Colitis*. 2016;10(8):979-988.

76.  Chambers CD, Johnson DL, Xu R, et al. Birth outcomes in women who have taken adalimumab in pregnancy: a prospective cohort study. *PLoS One.* 2019;14(10).

77.  Clowse MEB, Scheuerle AE, Chambers C, et al. Pregnancy outcomes after exposure to certolizumab pegol. *Arthritis Rheum.* 2018;70(9):1399-1407.

78.  Eworuke E, Panucci G, Goulding M, Neuner R, Toh S. Use of tumor necrosis factor-alpha inhibitors during pregnancy among women who delivered live born infants. *Pharmacoepidemiol Drug Saf.* 2019;28(3):296-304.

79.  Duricova D, Dvorakova E, Hradsky O, et al. Safety of anti-TNF-alpha therapy during pregnancy on long-term outcome of exposed children: a controlled, multicenter observation. *Inflamm Bowel Dis.* 2019;25(4):789-796.

80.  Nielsen OH, Loftus Jr EV, Jess T. Safety of TNF-α inhibitors during IBD pregnancy: a systematic review. *BMC Med.* 2013;11:174.

81.  Kolar M, Bortlik M, Duricova D, et al. Pregnancy outcomes in women with IBD treated with biosimilar infliximab. *Gastroent Hepatol.* 2018;72(1):20-26.

82.  Mahadevan U, Martin CF, Chambers C, et al. Achievement of developmental milestones among offspring of women with inflammatory bowel disease: the PIANO Registry. *Gastroenterology.* 2014;146(5 Suppl 1):S-1.

83.  Cheent K, Nolan J, Shariq S, et al. Case report: fatal case of disseminated BCG infection in an infant born to a mother taking infliximab for Crohn's disease. *J Crohns Colitis.* 2010;4(5):603-605.

84.  Beaulieu DB, Ananthakrishnan AN, Martin C, Cohen RD, Kane SV, Mahadevan U. Use of biologic therapy by pregnant women with inflammatory bowel disease does not affect infant response to vaccines. *Clin Gastroenterol Hepatol.* 2018;16(1):99-105.

85.  McConnell RA, Mahadevan U. Use of immunomodulators and biologics before, during and after pregnancy. *Inflamm Bowel Dis.* 2016;22(1):213-223.

86.  Deepak P, Stobaugh DJ. Maternal and foetal adverse events with tumour necrosis factor-alpha inhibitors in inflammatory bowel disease. *Aliment Pharm Ther.* 2014;40:1035-1043.

87.  Julsgaard M, Christensen LA, Gibson PR, et al. Concentrations of adalimumab and infliximab in mothers and newborns, and effects on infection. *Gastroenterology.* 2016;151(1):110-119.

88.  Vande Casteele N, Herfarth H, Katz J. et al. American Gastroenterological Association Institute Technical Review on the role of therapeutic drug monitoring in the management of inflammatory bowel diseases. *Gastroenterology.* 2017;153:835-857.

89.  Seow CH, Leung Y, Casteele NV, et al. The effects of pregnancy on the pharmacokinetics of infliximab and adalimumab in inflammatory bowel disease. *Aliment Pharm Ther.* 2017;45(10):1329-1338.

90.  Grisic A-M, Rasmussen M, Ungar B, et al. Infliximab clearance is decreased during 2nd and 3rd trimesters of pregnancy in inflammatory bowel disease. *Gastroenterology.* 2019;156(6 Suppl 1):S-18.

91.  Bar-Gil Shitrit A, Grisaru-Granovsky S, Ben Ya'acov A, Goldin E. Management of inflammatory bowel disease during pregnancy. *Dig Dis Sci.* 2016;61(8):2194-2204.

92.  Picardo S, Seow CH. A pharmacological approach to managing inflammatory bowel disease during conception, pregnancy and breastfeeding: biologic and oral small molecule therapy. *Drugs.* 2019;79(10):1053-1063.

93.  Park SC, Jeen YT. Anti-integrin therapy for inflammatory bowel disease. *World J Gastroenterol.* 2018;24(17):1868-1880.

94.  Portaccio E, Moiola L, Martinelli V, et al. Pregnancy decision-making in women with multiple sclerosis treated with natalizumab: II: maternal risks. *Neurology.* 2018;90(10):e832-e839.

95.  Wehner NG, Shopp G, Oneda S, Clarke J. Embryo/fetal development in cynomolgus monkeys exposed to natalizumab, an α4 inhibitor. *Birth Defects Res (Part B).* 86:117-130.

96.  Haghikia A, Langer-Gould A, Rellensmann G, et al. Natalizumab use during the third trimester of pregnancy. *JAMA Neurol.* 2014;71(7):891-895.

97.  Ebrahimi N, Herbstritt S, Gold R, et al. Pregnancy and fetal outcomes following natalizumab exposure in pregnancy. A prospective, controlled observational study. *Mult Scler.* 2015;21:198-205.

98.  Mahadevan U, Vermeire S, Lasch K, et al. Vedolizumab exposure in pregnancy: outcomes from clinical studies in inflammatory bowel disease. *Aliment Pharm Ther.* 2017;45(7):941-950.

99.  Moens A, Woude CJ van der, Julsgaard M, et al. Pregnancy outcomes in inflammatory bowel disease patients treated with vedolizumab, anti-TNF or conventional therapy: results of the European CONCEIVE study. *Aliment Pharm Ther.* 2020;51(1):129-138.

100. Chambers CD, Adams J, Xu R, Johnson D, Luo Y, Jones KL. Results from the vedolizumab pregnancy exposure registry: an OTIS pregnancy study. *Am J Gastroenterol.* 2018;113:S416.

101. Mahadevan U, Martin C, Kane SV, Dubinsky M, Sands BE, Sandborn W. 437 Do infant serum levels of biologic agents at birth correlate with risk of adverse outcomes? Results from the PIANO registry. *Gastroenterol.* 2016;150(4):S91–S92.

102. Martin PL, Sachs C, Imai N, et al. Development in the cynomolgus macaque following administration of ustekinumab, a human anti-il-12/23p40 monoclonal antibody, during pregnancy and lactation. *Birth Defects Research Part B: Developmental and Reproductive Toxicology.* 2010;89(5):351-363.

103. Mahadevan U, Naureckas S, Sharma B, et al. Su1799 - Pregnancy outcomes in women exposed to ustekinumab. *Gastroenterology.* 2018;154(6 Suppl 1):S-588.

104. Scherl E, Jacobstein D, Murphy C, et al. Pregnancy outcomes in women exposed to ustekinumab in the Crohn's disease clinical development program. *J Can Assoc Gastroenterol.* 2018;1(Suppl 2):166-166.

105. Klenske E, Osaba L, Nagore D, et al. Drug levels in the maternal serum, cord blood and breast milk of a ustekinumab-treated patient with Crohn's disease. *J Crohns Colitis.* 2019;13(2):267-269.

106. Rowan CR, Cullen G, Mulcahy HE, et al. Ustekinumab drug levels in maternal and cord blood in a woman with Crohn's disease treated until 33 weeks of gestation. *J Crohns Colitis.* 2018;12(3):376-378.

107. Farraye FA, Melmed GY, Lichtenstein GR, and Kane SV. ACG clinical guideline: preventive care in inflammatory bowel disease. *Am J Gastroenterol.* 2017;112(2):241-258.

108. Patlas N, Golomb G, Yaffe P, et al. Transplacental effects of bisphosphonates on fetal skeletal ossification and mineralization in rats. *Teratology.* 1999;60(2):68-73.

109. Green SB, Pappas AL. Effects of maternal bisphosphonate use on fetal and neonatal outcomes. *Am J Health Syst Pharm.* 2014;71(23):2029-2036.

110. Machairiotis N, Ntali G, Kouroutou P, Michala L. Clinical evidence of the effect of bisphosphonates on pregnancy and the infant. *Horm Mol Biol Clin Investig.* 2019;40(2):21.

111. Quigley EMM. Overlapping irritable bowel syndrome and inflammatory bowel disease: less to this than meets the eye? *Therap Adv Gastroenterol.* 2016;9(2):199-212.

112. Einarson A, Mastroiacovo P, Arnon J, et al. Prospective, controlled, multicentre study of loperamide in pregnancy. *Can J Gastroenterol.* 2000;14(3):185-187.

113. Källén B, Nilsson E, Otterblad Olausson P. Maternal use of loperamide in early pregnancy and delivery outcome. *Acta Paediatr.* 2008;97(5):541-545.

114. Lomotil, Drugs.com (available at https://www.drugs.com/pro/lomotil.html).

115. Riis L, Vind I, Politi P, et al. Does pregnancy change the disease course? A study in a European cohort of patients with inflammatory bowel disease. *Am J Gastroenterol.* 2006;101(7):1539-1545.

116. Lever G, Glanville T, Selinger C. PTH-120 Maternal obstetric outcomes in women with IBD compared to the general population. *Gut.* 2019;68(Suppl 2):A94-A94.

117. Afzali A. Inflammatory bowel disease during pregnancy: management of a disease flare or remission. *Curr Opin Gastro.* 2019;35(4):281-287.

118. Sharaf AA, Nguyen GC. Predictors of cesarean delivery in pregnant women with inflammatory bowel disease. *J Can Assoc Gastroenterol.* 2018;1(2):76-81.

119. Steinhart AH, Panaccione R, Targownik L, et al. Clinical practice guideline for the medical management of perianal fistulizing Crohn's disease: the Toronto Consensus. *Inflamm Bowel Dis.* 2019;25(1):1-13.

120. Foulon A, Dupas JL, Sabbagh C, et al. Defining the most appropriate delivery mode in women with inflammatory bowel disease: a systematic review. *Inflamm Bowel Dis.* 2017;23:712-720.

121. Hatch Q, Champagne BJ, Maykel JA, et al. Crohn's disease and pregnancy: the impact of perianal disease on delivery methods and complications. *Dis Colon Rectum.* 2014;57(2):174-178.

122. Rajaratnam SG, Eglinton TW, Hider P, Fearnhead NS. Impact of ileal pouch-anal anastomosis on female fertility: meta-analysis and systematic review. *Int J Colrectal Dis.* 2011;26(11):1365-1374.

123. Hahnloser D, Pemberton JH, Wolff BG, et al. Pregnancy and delivery before and after ileal pouch-anal anastomosis for inflammatory bowel disease: immediate and long-term consequences and outcomes. *Dis Colon Rectum.* 2004;47(7):1127-1135.

124. Juhasz ES, Fozard B, Dozois RR, et al. Ileal pouch-anal anastomosis function following childbirth. An extended evaluation. *Dis Colon Rectum.* 1995;38(2):159-165.

125. Remzi FH, Gorgun E, Bast J, et al. Vaginal delivery after ileal pouch-anal anastomosis: a word of caution. *Dis Colon Rectum.* 2005;48(9):1691-1699.

126. Ravid A, Richard CS, Spencer LM, et al. Pregnancy, delivery, and pouch function after ileal pouch-anal anastomosis for ulcerative colitis. *Dis Colon Rectum.* 2002;45(10):1283-1288.

127. Sultan AH, Kamm MA, Hudson CN, Thomas JM, Bartram CI. Anal-sphincter disruption during vaginal delivery. *N Engl J Med.* 1993;329(26):1905-1911.

128. Moss AC, Wolf JL. Adverse influences of pregnancy on IBD. In: Advanced Therapy in Inflammatory Bowel Disease. Vol 1: IBD and Ulcerative Colitis. *PMPH USA;* 2011:267-270.

129. McConnell RA, Mahadevan U. Pregnancy and the patient with inflammatory bowel disease: fertility, treatment, delivery, and complications. *Gastro Clin N Am.* 2016;45(2):285-301.

130. Rubin DT, Anathakrishnan AN, Seigel CA, et al. ACG clinical guideline ulcerative colitis in adults. *Am J Gastroenterol.* 2019;114(3):384-413.

131. De Lima A, Galjart B, Wisse PH, et al. Does lower gastrointestinal endoscopy during pregnancy pose a risk for mother and child? – a systematic review. *BMC Gastroenterol.* 2015;15-25.

132. Cappell MS, Colon VJ, Sidhom OA. A study at 10 medical centers of the safety and efficacy of 48 flexible sigmoid-oscopies and 8 colonoscopies during pregnancy with follow-up of fetal outcome and with comparison to control groups. *Dig Dis Sci.* 1996;41(12):2353-2361.

133. Shergill AK, Ben-Menachem T, Chandrasekhara V, et al. Guidelines for endoscopy in pregnant and lactating women. *Gastrointest Endosc.* 2012;76(1):18-24.

134. Visser BC, Glasgow RE, Mulvihill KK, et al. Safety and timing of non-obstetric abdominal surgery in pregnancy. *Dis Surg.* 2001;18:409-417.

135. Lambers DS, Clark KE. The maternal and fetal physiologic effects of nicotine. *Semin Perinatol.* 1996;20(2):115-126.

136. Kane S, Lemieux N. The role of breastfeeding in postpartum disease activity in women with inflammatory bowel disease. *Am J Gastroenterol.* 2005;100(1):102-105.

137. Lakatos PL, Szamosi T, Lakatos L. Smoking in inflammatory bowel diseases: good, bad or ugly? *World J Gastroenterol.* 2007;13(46):6134-6139.

138. Mullin GE. Micronutrients and inflammatory bowel disease. *Nutr Clin Pract.* 2012;27(1):136-137.

139. Van Assche G, Dignass A, Reinisch W, et al. The second European evidence-based consensus on the diagnosis and management of Crohn's disease: special situations. *J Crohns Colitis.* 2010;4(1):63-101.

140. Bengtson M-B, Aamodt G, Mahadevan U, Vatn MH. Inadequate gestational weight gain, the hidden link between maternal IBD and adverse pregnancy outcomes: results from the Norwegian mother and child cohort study. *Inflamm Bowel Dis.* 2017;23(7):1225-1233.

141. Bengtson M-B, Solberg IC, Aamodt G, et al. Relationships between inflammatory bowel disease and perinatal factors: both maternal and paternal disease are related to preterm birth of offspring. *Inflamm Bowel Dis.* 2010;16(5):847-855.

142. Selinger CP, Eaden J, Selby W, et al. Inflammatory bowel disease and pregnancy: lack of knowledge is associated with negative views. *J Crohns Colitis.* 2013;7(6):e206-e213.

143. Bixenstine PJ, Cheng TL, Cheng D, Connor KA, Mistry KB. Association between preconception counseling and folic acid supplementation before pregnancy and reasons for non-use. *Matern Child Health J.* 2015;19(9):1974-1984.

144. de Lima A, Zelinkova Z, Mulders AGMGJ, van der Woude CJ. Preconception care reduces relapse of inflammatory bowel disease during pregnancy. *Clin Gastroenterol Hepatol.* 2016;14(9):1285-1292.e1.

145. Williams L, Zapata LB, D'Angelo DV, et al. Associations between preconception counseling and maternal behaviors before and during pregnancy. *Matern Child Health J.* 2012;16(9):1854-1861.

146. Puchner A, Gröchenig HP, Sautner J, et al. Immunosuppressives and biologics during pregnancy and lactation. *Wien Klin Wochenschr.* 2019;131(1):29-44.

147. Johns DG, Rutherford LD, Leighton PC, Vogel CL. Secretion of methotrexate into human milk. *Am J Obstet Gynecol.* 1972;112(7):978-980.

# 9

# Breastfeeding in the Postpartum Woman With IBD

Rebecca Matro, MD | Anil Sharma, MD

## Introduction

Most organizations and guidelines, including the American Academy of Pediatrics (AAP), World Health Organization (WHO), and Centers for Disease Control and Prevention recommend breastfeeding and the exclusive use of human milk for about 6 months for all infants if possible.[1-3] Breastfeeding should continue for 1 year or longer if it is felt to be mutually beneficial for mother and child.[1,2] These recommendations are both national and international and apply to infants born to mothers with or without inflammatory bowel disease (IBD). Breast milk provides all the nutrients an infant needs in the first few months of life. According to the WHO, breast milk is the ideal food for infants—it is safe, clean, and provides antibodies that help protect infants from many childhood illnesses. This chapter will review the nutritional recommendations for postpartum women with IBD who are breastfeeding, the known benefits and risks of breastfeeding, as well as the compatibility of medications used to treat IBD and breastfeeding.

## Nutrition

In general, no specific diet has been found to be superior or recommended in the setting of breastfeeding, and women are encouraged to eat a healthy diet. Breastfeeding mothers with IBD should follow all standard nutritional recommendations. This includes increasing their caloric intake by 450 to 500 kcal/day.[1] The number of additional calories required will also vary depending on a breastfeeding woman's age, body mass index, and physical activity level. There are also

Abraham BP, Kane SV, Glassner KL, eds.
*Women's Health in IBD: The Spectrum of Care
From Birth to Adulthood* (pp 177-189).
© 2022 Taylor & Francis Group.

increased requirements for vitamins A, C, $B_1$ (thiamine), $B_2$ (riboflavin), $B_3$ (niacin), $B_6$ (pyridoxine), $B_{12}$, and E, along with iodine, selenium, and zinc for women who are breastfeeding. As such, ensuring a well-balanced diet with a moderate increase in daily calorie intake is recommended for all nursing mothers. In addition, certain long-chain polyunsaturated fatty acids, such as docosahexaenoic acid (DHA), have been noted to play an important role in infant neurobehavioral development with regards to formation of the phospholipid membrane in the brain and retina.[4] Nursing mothers are recommended to consume 200 to 300 mg/day of omega-3 fatty acids. This amounts to one to 2 servings of fish per week (specifically, fish lower in mercury content such as salmon, pollock, catfish, and canned light tuna).

Iodine is an important component of thyroid hormones thyroxine (T4) and triiodothyronine (T3). Maternal thyroid hormone levels affect fetal growth and neurological development during pregnancy and after birth. The recommended daily allowance of iodine for lactating women is 290 µg. Women who do not consume dairy are at risk for iodine deficiency. The AAP recommends that lactating women take an iodine supplement containing 150 µg of iodine daily, such as a prenatal vitamin.[5]

Vitamin $B_{12}$ is important for brain development and healthy red blood cell production in the infant. Vitamin $B_{12}$ is found in food from animals, including meat, fish, milk, and eggs. Women who follow a vegetarian or vegan diet, and those with a history of small bowel surgery and/or ileal inflammation from Crohn's disease (CD) are at risk of deficiency and may require supplementation.

Vitamin D plays an important role in the absorption and regulation of calcium and phosphate, enabling normal bone growth and remodeling. In addition to its role in bone health, vitamin D has been increasingly recognized for its effects on the immune system, including expression of tight junctions in the intestinal epithelial barrier, promotion of anti-inflammatory cytokines, and regulation of the gut microbiome.[6] It has been established that vitamin D deficiency is quite prevalent in the IBD population and that patients with IBD are at increased risk of deficiency as compared to those without IBD (odds ratio [OR], 1.64, 95% confidence interval, 1.30 to 2.08, $P < .0001$).[7] Furthermore, osteopenia and osteoporosis are recognized as complications of IBD with the incidence of fractures in the IBD population found to be 40% higher than in the general population.[8] More recently, studies have noted an association between vitamin D deficiency and disease activity, including increased risk of flares and need for surgeries in patients with IBD.[9,10] As such, women with IBD should be screened for vitamin D deficiency to determine any supplementation needs. Due to the fact that only a small percentage of maternal serum vitamin D is transmitted into breast milk, the AAP emphasizes the importance of vitamin D supplementation to infants of cholecalciferol (D3) 400 IU daily to prevent vitamin D deficiency and rickets.[11,12] Prior studies assessing supplementation of 1000 to 2000 IU daily in breastfeeding mothers did not demonstrate significant effect on infant stores of vitamin D.[13] Studies assessing higher doses of maternal vitamin D supplementation suggest vitamin D concentrations can be increased in breast milk[14,15]; however, given concerns with regards to safety and the risk of vitamin D toxicity, the AAP does not recommend universal supplementation to breastfeeding mothers.[11] Women who avoid dairy products may also need to consider calcium and vitamin D supplementation.

Patients with IBD may have iron deficiency due to chronic gastrointestinal blood loss or malabsorption and may require supplementation. While iron deficiency is often a concern in patients with IBD, due to amenorrhea associated with lactation, the nutritional requirements for iron are lower when lactating. As such, there are no specific universal recommendations for iron supplementation in the setting of breastfeeding.

Women with IBD may have unique nutritional considerations. Patients with an ostomy or active disease may have difficulty staying hydrated and well-nourished. In these situations, mothers should be referred for nutritional counseling.[16] IBD patients may also follow specific or restricted diets to control their disease or gastrointestinal symptoms. Commonly reported diets include a gluten-free diet; dairy-free diet; the Specific Carbohydrate Diet; low fermented oligosaccharides, disaccharides, monosaccharides, and polyols (FODMAP) diet; and anti-inflammatory diet.[17] These diets may increase the risk of certain nutritional deficiencies that should be addressed during breastfeeding. In particular, with diets that involve carbohydrate restriction, such as the Specific Carbohydrate Diet and low FODMAP diet, there are risks of deficiencies in folate, thiamine, and vitamin $B_6$ (from restricting cereals and breads), as well as potassium and vitamins A and C (from restricting certain fruits and vegetables).[18] Those adhering to a gluten-free diet are similarly at risk of deficiencies of folate, thiamine, and vitamin $B_6$; however, with incorporation of gluten-free alternatives to traditional cereals and breads, these deficiencies can be avoided. Additionally, individuals are at risk for insufficient caloric intake and weight loss with these diets that involve significant restrictions.

Finally, fenugreek is a dietary supplement commonly used to increase milk supply among lactating women. Women with IBD who perceive their milk supply to be low should avoid fenugreek, as diarrhea is a common side effect and bleeding has been reported.[11,19]

# Benefits

Numerous benefits are attributed to breastfeeding with regard to both maternal and infant outcomes, and are derived from various prospective observational cohort studies, systematic reviews, and meta-analyses. Infant outcomes include reduced risk of otitis media, upper respiratory tract infection, lower respiratory tract infection, asthma, atopic dermatitis, and celiac disease.[1] Maternal benefits of breastfeeding include reduction in postpartum blood loss with accelerated return of the uterus to its pre-partum size, delay in return of ovulation, and improved maternal-infant bonding. While breastfeeding may delay the return of ovulation, it should not be considered an adequate form of contraception. Prospective cohort studies also suggest that mothers who breastfeed are at reduced risk of postpartum depression. Cumulative lactation experience is also associated with a reduced risk of breast and ovarian cancer.[1]

Benefits are also seen specifically with regard to IBD. Several studies have looked at the role of breastfeeding and the development of pediatric IBD. One systematic review looking at 1632 cases of pediatric IBD found that breast milk exposure had a significant protective benefit against the development of early onset IBD (OR, 0.69; 95% confidence interval, 0.51 to 0.94; $P = .02$).[20] This protective effect may be due to an immunomodulating effect from human milk. In addition, type of infant feeding is an important determinant of infant microbiome composition, and thus may play a role in the development of IBD.[21] Additional case-control and cohort studies have reinforced this protective effect, suggesting that breastfeeding may decrease the risk of development of IBD.[22-24] However, these data are limited by small sample size and quality of the included studies. More recently, a population-based study assessing more than 2 million births in Scotland between 1981 and 2017 found no association between type of feeding and risk of developing pediatric IBD.[25]

Studies also suggest that breastfeeding may be beneficial for IBD activity. One population-based study of women with IBD showed that breastfeeding was not associated with an increased risk of disease flare and may have a protective effect against disease flare in the first year postpartum.[26] However, women who discontinue their IBD medications to breastfeed are at increased risk of flare in the postpartum period.

# Risks

The benefits of breastfeeding are numerous for both women and infants. However, breastfeeding can take time to master and can be painful. Infants may have trouble latching and may have inadequate milk intake leading to weight loss and dehydration. Insufficient milk intake is the leading cause of early termination of breastfeeding. Mothers are also at risk of nipple or breast pain, commonly caused by nipple injury, vasoconstriction, engorgement, plugged ducts, or infections. Nipple and breast pain are also common causes of premature discontinuation of breastfeeding.[27]

As mentioned earlier, breastfeeding may have a protective effect against disease flare. However, older studies previously suggested an increased risk of disease flare in the postpartum period and a possible association between disease activity and breastfeeding. A closer look at the data shows that the primary factor driving the increase in disease activity while breastfeeding is non-adherence and cessation of medical therapy.[28] Specifically, in a study of 122 women with IBD who gave birth in the preceding 5 years, 44% of the women had breastfed their infant and 43% of these women experienced a flare of disease postpartum (OR 2.2). After accounting for cessation of IBD medication, there was no longer an association between breastfeeding and disease activity.[29]

For mothers on medications, the benefits of breastfeeding for both mother and infant must be weighed against potential risks of drug exposure to the infant. While most medications are compatible with breastfeeding, many mothers are inappropriately advised to discontinue breastfeeding or avoid taking essential medications because of fears of adverse effects on their infants.[30]

In the United States, women with IBD breastfeed at a slightly lower rate than the national rate.[31] The Pregnancy in Inflammatory Bowel Disease and Neonatal Outcomes (PIANO) registry is a multicenter national prospective study of pregnancy and neonatal outcomes in women with IBD and their offspring. The registry aims to determine the effect of medication use and disease activity on pregnancy and infant outcomes among women with IBD and their offspring up to 4 years from birth. More than 1000 women with IBD have been enrolled and provided data regarding breastfeeding practices as well as medication use and infant outcomes.

Among women with IBD participating in the PIANO registry, the overall rate of breastfeeding was 75%, compared to 83.2%, the national average rate in the United States.[3,31] For PIANO, 824 women answered questions regarding their breastfeeding practices. Women who were not exposed to biologics and immunomodulators were significantly more likely to breastfeed (85%) compared with women on immunomodulators (65%), biologics (75%), or combination therapy (67%, $P <$ .0001). The most commonly cited reason for not breastfeeding was concern about exposing the infant to IBD medications. Additional factors affecting the decision to not breastfeed include personal preference, patients reporting being too ill from IBD, and clinician recommendation, similar to prior studies assessing barriers to breastfeeding in the IBD population. Other reasons for not breastfeeding included difficulty with latching or milk production and work schedules. Finally, women with increased disease activity were also less likely to breastfeed.

The PIANO registry also compared infants who were breastfed with those who were not breastfed. There was no difference in development, milestone achievement, or rates of infection to 12 months of age in infants who were breastfed compared to those who were not breastfed.

In the absence of notable risks concerning lactation in the setting of IBD, the decision to breastfeed should be made between a woman and her physicians (gastroenterologist, obstetrician, and pediatrician), with counseling focused on the benefits of breastfeeding, a treatment plan with appropriate medications, medication compliance, and risk of flare if medications are discontinued.

# Medications

The safety of medications while breastfeeding can garner concern among both women with IBD and their physicians. As described, women are often inappropriately advised to discontinue medications for breastfeeding, and women who stop their IBD medications are more likely to suffer disease flare, which may subsequently affect the ability to care for their newborn infant. The main concern is whether medications taken by the mother can be transferred to the infant via breast milk and what effects that might have on the infant. LactMed is a free database produced by the National Library of Medicine that is a reliable reference for lactation compatibility for prescription and over-the-counter drugs. It provides data on drug levels in human milk and infant serum, potential adverse effects on breastfeeding infants and lactation, and suggested therapeutic alternative medications. It is revised and updated frequently and can serve as a useful resource for patients and physicians. This next section will focus on medications used to treat IBD and their compatibility with breastfeeding (Table 9-1).

# Aminosalicylates

The 5-aminosalicylic acids (5-ASA) include sulfasalazine, mesalamine, olsalazine, and balsalazide. Balsalazide, and olsalazine are metabolized to the active drug mesalamine. Mesalamine is poorly excreted in breast milk but the mesalamine metabolite N-acetyl-5-ASA does appear in breast milk. In one study that reported mesalamine and N-acetyl-5-ASA concentration in breast milk of a woman with ulcerative colitis (UC), the authors estimated that a fully fed breastfed infant whose mother was taking mesalamine 1.5 g daily would receive 0.015 mg/kg of mesalamine and 2.3 mg/kg of N-acetyl-5-ASA daily.[32] In another study of 12 women taking mesalamine, mesalamine was detected in 3 out of 12 women with levels ranging from 20 to 81 μg/L. N-acetyl-5-ASA was also detected in milk samples, and the authors estimated that a fully breastfed infant would receive the equivalent of 1% of the usual daily mesalamine dose.[33] Several other case reports confirm that mesalamine is excreted into breast milk at exceedingly low levels.[34,35]

Sulfasalazine consists of 5-ASA linked to sulfapyridine and is metabolized to mesalamine and sulfapyridine, which is associated with the majority of adverse effects of this medication, including nausea and vomiting. Studies have demonstrated that both sulfasalazine and the sulfapyridine moiety are excreted into breast milk at levels 30% to 50% lower than their serum concentrations,[36] but sulfapyridine is excreted at higher concentrations and has hemolytic and antimicrobial properties.[16,37] Sulfasalazine and sulfapyridine have also been detected in serum of infants being breastfed by mothers on sulfasalazine. Based on this, experts prefer mesalamine, balsalazide, and olsalazine over sulfasalazine while breastfeeding. If a breastfeeding woman requires sulfasalazine, she should receive folic acid supplementation of 1 to 2 mg daily.

There are rare reports of diarrhea in infants exposed to mesalamine when mothers were taking these agents while breastfeeding.[38] The diarrhea resolved with cessation of mesalamine. Otherwise, there have been no significant adverse effects from mesalamine exposure on breastfed infants. Although women should be aware of the complication of diarrhea in the infant, they may breastfeed unless the infant develops diarrhea. Based on the available literature and extensive experience with these older medications, the various formulations of 5-ASA, including topical forms of the drug, are considered low risk and compatible with breastfeeding.

# Immunomodulators

Thiopurines (azathioprine[AZA], 6-mercaptopurine[6-MP]) work as antimetabolites, targeting DNA synthesis and have been used to treat IBD for decades. 6-MP is the active metabolite of AZA, and it is further broken down to the active metabolites 6-thioguanine (6-TGN) and 6-methylmercaptopurine (6-MMPN). The enzyme thiopurine methyltransferase (TPMT) is responsible for metabolism of 6-TGN, and deficiencies in this enzyme can lead to toxicity.

Prior studies have demonstrated that 6-TGN and 6-MMPN are undetectable in breast milk and in infants of breastfeeding mothers with wild-type genotypes of thiopurine methyltransferase.[39-41] Another study of 8 lactating women taking AZA 75 to 200 mg daily demonstrated variability in bioavailability of the drug based on a wide range of peak maternal serum drug levels within 3 hours of drug administration. There were correlating but lower and clinically insignificant levels of the drug in breast milk, with a peak seen within 4 hours of drug dosing.[42] Several studies have also

## Table 9-1. IBD Medications and Breastfeeding

| MEDICATION | COMPATIBILITY IN BREASTFEEDING | KEY CONSIDERATIONS |
|---|---|---|
| *AMINOSALICYLATES* | | |
| Sulfasalazine | Compatible | Monitor for infant diarrhea; ensure maternal folic acid supplementation |
| Mesalamine (including olsalazine and balsalazide) | Compatible | Monitor for infant diarrhea; preferred over sulfasalazine |
| *IMMUNOMODULATORS* | | |
| Thiopurines (AZA, 6-MP) | Compatible | Higher levels in breastmilk if reduced maternal TPMT activity but no reports of harm from breastfeeding |
| Methotrexate | Use not advised | Limited human data but known teratogen |
| CSA | Compatible | No reports of adverse effects |
| *BIOLOGIC AGENTS* | | |
| IFX | Compatible | |
| ADA | Compatible | |
| CZP | Compatible | |
| GOL | Compatible | Limited data |
| NAT | Compatible | |
| VDZ | Compatible | |
| UST | Compatible | |
| *SMALL MOLECULE THERAPIES* | | |
| Tofacitinib | Use not advised | No human data |
| *CORTICOSTEROIDS* | | |
| Systemic | Compatible | Dose-dependent effect on levels in breast milk; delaying breastfeeding for 4 hours after dosing can minimize exposure but not advised |
| Budesonide | Compatible | Extrapolated from data on inhaled budesonide and systemic corticosteroids |
| *ANTIBIOTICS* | | |
| Amoxicillin-clavulanic acid | Compatible | Report of restlessness, rash, and change in bowel habits |
| Ciprofloxacin | Compatible | Preferred over metronidazole in lactation |
| Metronidazole | Compatible | Report of *Candida* infection and diarrhea |

evaluated serum 6-TGN and 6-MMPN levels in infants breastfed during maternal use of AZA and found undetectable metabolites in the infants.[40,43]

Effects in breastfed infants are also largely reassuring. One study followed breastfeeding mothers on AZA (with a median dose of 150 mg daily) during pregnancy and in the postpartum period for up to 3 to 4 years. Compared to the infants of women who did not breastfeed, infants exposed to AZA had no increased risk of infection or delayed mental or physical development.[44] In the prospective cohort study PIANO, the use of a thiopurine alone was not associated with any infant complication, infection, or effect on growth and development to 12 months of age.[45] Mothers with decreased TPMT enzyme activity may transmit higher levels of drug to their infants in breast milk, and cases of mild, asymptomatic neutropenia and anemia have been reported after in utero exposure.[46] Nevertheless, experts do not currently recommend routine lab monitoring for breastfeeding infants if azathioprine is used during lactation. Additionally, while avoiding breastfeeding for 4 hours after dosing may decrease the dose received by nursing infants in breast milk, we do not recommend this practice and consider thiopurines compatible with lactation.

Methotrexate is a known teratogen and contraindicated in pregnancy. Methotrexate is excreted in breast milk, raising concern for accumulation in the tissue of infants. While breast milk concentrations after anti-inflammatory dosing appear to be clinically insignificant, data are extremely limited.[47] It is currently contraindicated while breastfeeding.[16,48]

Cyclosporine (CSA) is detected in breast milk of nursing mothers, but most studies show undetectable levels in breastfed infants.[49] Only 2 infants have had measurable CSA serum levels while breastfeeding. Nevertheless, there have been no reports of adverse effects on infant growth, development, or overall health after breastfeeding. We consider CSA compatible with breastfeeding.[16]

# Biologic Agents

Biologic agents are monoclonal antibodies and large molecules that target various receptors. The most commonly used and well-studied are the anti–tumor necrosis factor alpha (TNF-α) agents, which include infliximab (IFX), adalimumab (ADA), certolizumab pegol (CZP), and golimumab (GOL).

IFX is a chimeric monoclonal IgG1 antibody that targets TNF-α and is indicated to treat CD and UC. ADA, which is indicated to treat CD and UC, and GOL, which is indicated to treat UC, are humanized monoclonal IgG1 antibodies against TNF-α. Fc receptors in the lining of the gastrointestinal tract of the infant bind maternal antibodies to transport them across the mucosa, thereby conferring immunity to the infant. These receptors in particular have high affinity for IgG1 and thus there is risk of exposure of IFX, ADA, and GOL to the infant. CZP is a pegylated Fab fragment of humanized antibody to TNF-α and is indicated to treat CD. Given the lack of an Fc receptor, transfer to the infant should be minimal. Among the anti-TNF-α agents used to treat IBD, the most well studied are IFX, ADA, and CZP.

Much of the data evaluating the concentrations of IFX, ADA, and CZP in breast milk has come from case reports and case series. The PIANO registry has provided the largest prospective series of breast milk analysis among women on biologics. Seventy-two women on biologic agents submitted breast milk samples at 1, 12, 24, and 48 hours after dosing. Additional samples were taken at 72, 96, 120, and 168 hours in some women.

In 1 case report of 3 women with IBD on IFX who submitted breast milk samples, the level of IFX peaked at 0.101 µg/mL within 2 to 3 days of infusion.[50] This level was 1/200th of the corresponding IFX level in the maternal blood. Similar low breast milk levels were measured in 2 women on IFX while breastfeeding.[51] In PIANO, 29 women on IFX submitted samples and 19 (66%) women had detectable drug levels in breast milk. The peak IFX level was 0.74 µg/mL and occurred 24 to 48 hours after infusion.[31]

For ADA, in 1 nursing mother who provided breast milk and serum samples while on the medication, the peak breast milk level was 0.031 µg/mL at day 6 after injection, 1/100th of the corresponding level in serum.[52] Another case series reported levels of 0.483 µg/mL and 0.488 µg/mL in 2 women who submitted breast milk samples 7 and 9 days after ADA injection, respectively.[51] Twenty-one women on ADA submitted breast milk samples in PIANO and drug was detected in breast milk of 2 (9.5%) women, including one on an immunomodulator. The maximum concentration was 0.71 µg/mL and was seen 12 to 24 hours after injection. Seven women also provided breast milk samples out to 168 hours (7 days) after injection, and ADA was undetectable at all time points.[31]

The prospective CRADLE study evaluated the breast milk levels of CZP in lactating women. Seventeen women submitted breast milk samples and 77 of 137 (56%) samples had no measurable CZP. For 4 of 17 women, all breast milk samples were below the lower limit of quantification (LLOQ). Thirteen women had measurable CZP during at least one time point, with a maximum CZP concentration of 0.076 µg/mL, which was less than 3 times the LLOQ (0.032 µg/mL) or less than 1% of the expected serum concentration.[53] Thirteen women on CZP in the PIANO registry submitted breast milk samples and 3 (23%) had detectable levels in breast milk between 12 and 48 hours after injection. The peak level was 0.29 µg/mL. Two women submitted samples out to 7 days, and CZP was undetectable at every time point.

Very limited data are available regarding GOL and lactation. Only one woman from the PIANO registry was on GOL and had undetectable drug levels in breast milk for up to 7 days after injection.[31]

After the anti-TNF-α agents, the anti-integrin antibodies were the next class of drugs used to treat IBD and include natalizumab (NAT) and vedolizumab (VDZ). NAT is a chimeric recombinant human monoclonal antibody (IgG4) that targets the α4 subunit of α4β1 and α4β7 integrins and VDZ is a humanized monoclonal antibody (IgG1) that targets the α4β7 integrin. Much less lactation data are available for these drugs.

Two women on NAT submitted breast milk samples in the PIANO registry, and no women were on VDZ. Low but detectable drug levels were seen in the breast milk of one of the 2 women on NAT, with a peak level of 0.46 µg/mL at 24 hours.[31] Several other case reports show detectable NAT in breast milk of nursing mothers with multiple sclerosis and suggest that peak levels can be seen weeks after infusion and may increase with subsequent doses.[54]

One study evaluated breast milk samples provided by 5 women on VDZ. VDZ was detectable in all samples collected from 30 minutes to 14 days after infusion, with a peak concentration of 0.318 µg/mL, which is less than 1% of the serum-equivalent concentration.[55] Another study measured breast milk levels in 5 women lactating on VDZ. Peak milk concentrations occurred from day 2 to 4 after infusion and ranged from 0.108 to 0.478 µg/mL, 1/100th of the comparable serum levels.[56] Exposed infants had normal development to 10 months and no increase in general or gastrointestinal infections.

Finally, ustekinumab (UST) is a human antibody (IgG1) against the p40 subunit of both IL-12 IL-23 and is indicated to treat CD and UC. Of 6 women on UST in the PIANO registry who submitted breast milk samples, low but detectable drug levels were seen in the breast milk of 4 (67%) women. The peak concentrations ranged from 0.72 to 1.57 µg/mL and were seen 12 and 72 hours after injection.[31]

There has not been any significant adverse effect on infant outcomes among infants exposed to biologic agents through breast milk. The PIANO registry compared breastfed infants based on type of drug exposure from the nursing mother (immunomodulators, biologics, combination of the 2, or neither [unexposed]). Among infants who are breastfed by mothers on these biologic medications, there was no difference in milestone achievement, development, or rates of infection in the first 12 months of life, compared to infants who were not breastfed or were breastfed by mothers on immunomodulators, combination therapy, or no medications.

As illustrated, a majority of women breastfeeding while on biologic medications have undetectable or very low drug concentrations in their breast milk. The levels are less than 1% of corresponding serum concentration and result in no negative impact of breastfeeding on infant health outcomes. While a small amount of drug may be ingested by the infant and it is hypothesized that these large protein molecules are likely broken down and inactivated via digestive enzymes making it clinically unlikely to have intestinal absorption of these drugs, further study is needed. At this time, there is no indication of harm from breastfeeding while on biologic medications and they are considered compatible with breastfeeding.

# Small Molecule Therapies

As the newest class of medications to treat IBD, small molecule therapies are typically taken orally and target a number of inflammatory pathways. At this time, the only small molecule therapy approved for the treatment of IBD (specifically UC) is tofacitinib (Xeljanz), a Janus kinase (JAK) inhibitor. Animal studies have demonstrated detectable drug levels in milk during lactation. There are no human studies assessing excretion of tofacitinib in breast milk. The manufacturer recommends that breastfeeding be discontinued for 18 hours after the last dose of Xeljanz or 36 hours after the last dose of Xeljanz XR.[57] Experts recommend against breastfeeding while on this medication.[16]

# Corticosteroids

Corticosteroids (prednisone, prednisolone, budesonide) can be used to treat flares of IBD and are not recommended for maintenance therapy, including while breastfeeding. No adverse effects have been reported in infants being breastfed by mothers on any corticosteroid. Amounts of prednisone in breast milk are low, and human studies of prednisolone have suggested breast milk concentrations of less than 0.05% of the ingested dose.[58] Peak milk steroid levels occur about 2 hours after a dose. An older study suggested a degree of dose-dependence with regards to breast milk levels.[59] Based on this, maternal prednisolone doses of 20 mg once or twice daily or lower provide minimal drug levels to the infant. At a daily maternal dose of 80 mg, the breastfed infant would ingest less than 0.1% of the dose. In 2 women taking oral prednisone, one 2 mg every 12 hours and one 15 mg daily, drug concentrations in breast milk were undetectable after 12 hours for prednisone and 6 hours for prednisolone.[60] Using prednisolone instead of prednisone and avoiding breastfeeding for 1 to 4 hours after dosing can minimize infant exposure, but this practice is not recommended.[16,61] While the bulk of the data assessing use of budesonide in the setting of lactation comes from the asthma literature with inhaled budesonide, given its low oral bioavailability, budesonide and budesonide MMX are similarly felt to be safe to use during lactation.[62] Both corticosteroids and budesonide are compatible with breastfeeding.

# Antibiotics

Antibiotics in IBD are used for perianal disease, intra-abdominal abscesses, or pouchitis and are not recommended for maintenance therapy. The most commonly used antibiotics are amoxicillin/clavulanic acid, ciprofloxacin, and metronidazole. Amoxicillin without clavulanic acid is detected in low concentrations in breast milk.[63] In a prospective, controlled study of mothers who called an information service about adverse reactions experienced by their breastfed infants, adverse reactions reported among those exposed to amoxicillin-clavulanic acid included restlessness, diarrhea, rash, and constipation. Nevertheless, amoxicillin-clavulanic acid is considered low risk and compatible with breast feeding. Similarly, ciprofloxacin is detectable in breast milk at low levels.[64] A single case of pseudomembranous colitis was reported in a 2-month-old infant with a history of necrotizing enterocolitis being breastfed by a mother taking ciprofloxacin.[65] However, a systematic review of the use of ciprofloxacin in infants suggests breastfeeding is low risk.[66] Metronidazole is also detected in breast milk and in low levels in the serum of infants breastfed by mothers on the medication. While data on the effects of metronidazole exposure among breastfed infants are limited, cases of *Candida* infection and diarrhea have been reported.[67] Ciprofloxacin is preferred over metronidazole if needed during lactation.[16]

# Conclusion

The universal recommendations that support breastfeeding and the exclusive use of human milk for at least 6 months if possible also apply to women with IBD. There are a number of benefits associated with breastfeeding for both infant and mother. These include reduced risk of infections, atopy, and inflammatory conditions in the infant, along with increased maternal-infant bonding and reduced risk of postpartum depression. There are few, if any, risks of breastfeeding specific to IBD, and breastfeeding is not associated with flare of disease. For those on medical therapy, the benefits of breastfeeding must be weighed against potential risks of drug exposure to the infant; however, the majority of medications are compatible with breastfeeding based on data to support undetectable to low drug levels in breast milk and no adverse effects on infant outcomes.

---

## KEY POINTS

1. Mothers with IBD should be encouraged to attempt breastfeeding as per guidance by the AAP and other organizations. Women should continue their current medications while breastfeeding with the exception of methotrexate or tofacitinib for which use is not advised while breastfeeding.

2. No specific diet has been demonstrated to be superior in the setting of breastfeeding with IBD; however, those women who are breastfeeding should increase their caloric intake by 450 to 500 kcal/day and aim for 200 to 300 mg/day of omega-3 fatty acids. Additional considerations and guidance on nutrition may be required for those mothers with an ostomy and/or active disease.

3. To date, the available studies have demonstrated either undetectable or very low concentrations of aminosalicylates, thiopurines, and biologic agents in the breastmilk of mothers with IBD on these therapies. Infants who were breastfed and exposed to these medications have similar health and development outcomes as compared to infants who were not breastfed or not exposed.

---

# References

1. Johnston M, Landers S, Noble L, Szucs K, Viehmann L. Breastfeeding and the use of human milk. *Pediatrics.* 2012;129(3):e827-e841.

2. Bagci Bosi AT, Eriksen KG, Sobko T, Wijnhoven TM, Breda J. Breastfeeding practices and policies in WHO european region member states. *Public Health Nutr.* 2016;19(4):753-764.

3. Breastfeeding Report Card. Centers for Disease Control and Prevention. https://www.cdc.gov/breastfeeding/data/reportcard.htm. Published 2018. Accessed January 12, 2020.

4.  Carlson SE. Docosahexaenoic acid supplementation in pregnancy and lactation. *Am J Clin Nutr.* 2009;89(2):678S-684S.

5.  Rogan WJ, Paulson JA, Baum C, et al. Iodine deficiency, pollutant chemicals, and the thyroid: new information on an old problem. *Pediatrics.* 133(6):1163-1166.

6.  Gubatan J, Moss AC. Vitamin D in inflammatory bowel disease: more than just a supplement. *Curr Opin Gastroenterol.* 2018;34(4):217-225.

7.  Del Pinto R, Pietropaoli D, Chandar AK, Ferri C, Cominelli F. Association between inflammatory bowel disease and vitamin D deficiency: a systematic review and meta-analysis. *Inflamm Bowel Dis.* 2015;21(11):2708-2717.

8.  Bernstein CN, Blanchard JF, Leslie W, Wajda A, Yu BN. The incidence of fracture among patients with inflammatory bowel disease: a population-based cohort study. *Ann Intern Med.* 2000;133(10):795-799.

9.  Nielsen OH, Rejnmark L, Moss AC. Role of vitamin D in the natural history of inflammatory bowel disease. *J Crohns Colitis.* 2018;12(6):742-752.

10. Ham NS, Hwang SW, Oh EH, et al. Influence of severe vitamin D deficiency on the clinical course of inflammatory bowel disease. *Dig Dis Sci.* 2021;66(2):587-596.

11. Wagner CL, Greer FR. Prevention of rickets and vitamin D deficiency in infants, children, and adolescents. *Pediatrics.* 2008;122(5):1142-1152.

12. Pilz S, Zittermann A, Obeid R, et al. The role of vitamin D in fertility and during pregnancy and lactation: a review of clinical data. *Int J Environ Res Public Health.* 2018;15(10):2241.

13. Ala-Houhala M. 25(OH)D levels during breast-feeding with or without maternal or infantile supplementation of vitamin D. *J Pediatr Gastroenterol Nutr.* 1985;4(2):220-226.

14. Hollis BW, Wagner CL. Vitamin D requirements during lactation: high-dose maternal supplementation as therapy to prevent hypovitaminosis D in both mother and nursing infant. *Am J Clin Nutr.* 2004;80:1752S-1758S.

15. Wagner CL, Hulsey TC, Fanning D, Ebeling M, Hollis BW. High dose vitamin D3 supplementation in a cohort of breastfeeding mothers and their infants: a six-month follow-up pilot study. *Breastfeed Med.* 2006;1(2):59-70.

16. Mahadevan U, Robinson C, Bernasko N, et al. Inflammatory bowel disease in pregnancy clinical care pathway: a report from the american gastroenterological association IBD parenthood project working group. *Gastroenterology.* 2019;156(5):1508-1524.

17. Knight-Sepulveda K, Kais S, Santaolalla R, Abreu MT. Diet and inflammatory bowel disease. *Gastroenterol Hepatol.* 2015;11(8):511-520.

18. Hwang C, Ross V, Mahadevan U. Popular exclusionary diets for inflammatory bowel disease: the search for a dietary culprit. *Inflamm Bowel Dis.* 2014;20(4):732-741.

19. Brodribb W. ABM clinical protocol #9: use of galactogogues in initiating or augmenting maternal milk production, second revision 2018. *Breastfeed Med.* 2018;13(5):307-314.

20. Barclay AR, Russell RK, Wilson ML, Gilmour WH, Satsangi J, Wilson DC. Systematic review: the role of breastfeeding in the development of pediatric inflammatory bowel disease. *J Pediatr.* 2009;155(3):421-426.

21. Penders J, Thijs C, Vink C, et al. Factors influencing the composition of the intestinal microbiota in early Iifancy. *Pediatrics.* 2006;118(2):511-521.

22. Gearry RB, Richardson AK, Frampton CM, Dodgshun AJ, Barclay ML. Population-based cases control study of inflammatory bowel disease risk factors. *J Gastroenterol Hepatol.* 2010;25(2):325-333.

23. Hansen TS, Jess T, Vind I, et al. Environmental factors in inflammatory bowel disease: a case-control study based on a Danish inception cohort. *J Crohns Colitis.* 2011;5(6):577-584.

24. Ng SC, Tang W, Leong RW, et al. Environmental risk factors in inflammatory bowel disease: a population-based case-control study in Asia-Pacific. *Gut.* 2015;64(7):1063-1071.

25. Burgess C, Schnier C, Chalmers I, et al. OP19 Perinatal factors do not affect paediatric inflammatory bowel disease risk: a Scottish nationwide cohort study using administrative health data 1981–2017. *J Crohns Colitis.* 2020;14(Suppl 1):S016-S016.

26. Moffatt D, Ilnyckyj A, Bernstein C. A population-based study of breastfeeding in inflammatory bowel disease: initiation, duration, and effect on disease in the postpartum period. *Am J Gastroenterol.* 2009;104(10):2517-2523.

27. Spencer J. Common problems of breastfeeding and weaning. In: Post T, ed. *UpToDate.* www.uptodate.com. Published 2020.

28. Mogadam M, Korelitz BI, Ahmed SW, Dobbins WO, Baiocco PJ. The course of inflammatory bowel disease during pregnancy and postpartum. *Am J Gastroenterol.* 1981;75(4):265-269.

29. Kane S, Lemieux N. The role of breastfeeding in postpartum disease activity in women with inflammatory bowel disease. *Am J Gastroenterol.* 2005;100(1):102-105.

30. Sachs HC. The transfer of drugs and therapeutics into human breast milk: an update on selected topics. *Pediatrics.* 2013;132(3):e796-809.

31. Matro R, Martin CF, Wolf D, Shah SA, Mahadevan U. Exposure concentrations of infants breastfed by women receiving biologic therapies for inflammatory bowel diseases and effects of breastfeeding on infections and development. *Gastroenterology.* 2018;155(3):696-704.

32.  Klotz U, Harings-Kaim A. Negligible excretion of 5-aminosalicylic acid in breast milk. *Lancet*. 1993;342(8871):618-619.

33.  Christensen LA, Rasmussen SN, Hansen SH. Disposition of 5-aminosalicylic acid and N-acetyl-5-aminosalicylic acid in fetal and maternal body fluids during treatment with different 5-aminosalicylic acid preparations. *Acta Obstet Gynecol Scand*. 1994;73:399-402.

34.  Miller LG, Hopkinson JM, Motil KJ, Corboy JE, Andersson S. Disposition of olsalazine and metabolites in breast milk. *J Clin Pharmacol*. 1993;33(8):703-706.

35.  Datta P, Rewers-Felkins K, Kallem RR, T. B, Hale TW. Determination of mesalamine levels in human milk as a function of dose. *Breastfeed Med*. 2019;14(2):98-101.

36.  Khan AK, Truelove SC. Placental and mammary transfer of sulphasalazine. *Br Med J*. 1979;2(6204):1553.

37.  Esbjorner E, Jarnerot G, Wranne L. Sulphasalazine and sulphapyridine serum levels in children to mothers treated with sulphasalazine during pregnancy and lactation. *Acta Paediatr Scand*. 1987;76:137-142.

38.  Nelis GF. Diarrhoea due to 5-aminosalicylic acid in breast milk. *Lancet*. 1989;1(8634):383.

39.  Kane SV, Present DH. Metabolites to immunomodulators are not detected in breast milk. *Am J Gastroenterol*. 2004;99(10):S246-247.

40.  Gardiner SJ, Gearry RB, Roberts RL, Zhang M, Barclay ML, Begg EJ. Exposure to thiopurine drugs through breast milk is low based on metabolite concentrations in mother-infant pairs. *Br J Clin Pharmacol*. 2006;62(4):453-456.

41.  Ter Horst P, Smolders EJ, den Besten-Bertholee D. Mercaptopurine and metabolites in breast milk. *Breastfeed Med*. 2019;15(4):277-279.

42.  Christensen LA, Dahlerup JF, Nielsen MJ, Fallingborg JF, Schmiegelow K. Azathioprine treatment during lactation. *Aliment Pharmacol Ther*. 2008;28(10):1209-1213.

43.  Sau A, Clarke S, Bass J, Kaiser A, Marinaki A, Nelson-Piercy C. Azathioprine and breastfeeding: is it safe? *BJOG*. 2007;114:498-501.

44.  Angelberger S, Reinisch W, Messerschmidt A, et al. Long-term follow-up of babies exposed to azathioprine in utero and via breastfeeding. *J Crohns Colitis*. 2011;5(2):95-100.

45.  Mahadevan U, Martin CF, Sandler RS, et al. PIANO: a 1000 patient prospective registry of pregnancy outcomes in women with IBD exposed to immunomodulators and biologic therapy. *Gastroenterology*. 2012;142(5):S149.

46.  Jharap B, de Boer NK, Stokkers P, et al. Intrauterine exposure and pharmacology of conventional thiopurine therapy in pregnant patients with inflammatory bowel disease. *Gut*. 2014;63(3):451-457.

47.  Delaney S, Colantonio D, Ito S. Methotrexate in breast milk. *Birth Defects Res*. 2017;109:711.

48.  Nguyen GC, Seow CH, Maxwell C, et al. The Toronto consensus statements for the management of inflammatory bowel disease in pregnancy. *Gastroenterology*. 2016;150(3):734-757.e731.

49.  Drugs and Lactation Database (LactMed) [Internet]. Bethesda (MD): National Library of Medicine (US); 2006-. Cyclosporine. [Updated 2018 Oct 31]. Available from: https://www.ncbi.nlm.nih.gov/books/NBK501683/.

50.  Ben-Horin S, Yavzori M, Kopylov U, et al. Detection of infliximab in breast milk of nursing mothers with inflammatory bowel disease. *J Crohns Colitis*. 2011;5(6):555-558.

51.  Fritzsche J, Pilch A, Mury D, Schaefer C, Weber-Schoendorfer C. Infliximab and adalimumab use during breastfeeding. *J Clin Gastroenterol*. 2012;46(8):718-719.

52.  Ben-Horin S, Yavzori M, Katz L, et al. Adalimumab level in breast milk of a nursing mother. *Clin Gastroenterol Hepatol*. 2010;8(5):475-476.

53.  Clowse ME, Förger F, Hwang C, et al. Minimal to no transfer of certolizumab pegol into breast milk: results from CRADLE, a prospective, postmarketing, multicentre, pharmacokinetic study. *Ann Rheum Dis*. 2017;76(11):1890-1896.

54.  Baker TE, Cooper SD, Kessler L, Hale TW. Transfer of natalizumab into breast milk in a mother with multiple sclerosis. *J Hum Lact*. 2015;31:233-236.

55.  Julsgaard M, Kjeldsen J, Bibby BM, Brock B, Baumgart DC. Vedolizumab concentrations in the breast milk of nursing mothers with inflammatory bowel disease. *Gastroenterology*. 2018;154(3):752-754.e751.

56.  Lahat A, Shitrit AB, Naftali T, et al. Vedolizumab levels in breast milk of nursing mothers with inflammatory bowel disease. *J Crohns Colitis*. 2018;12(1):120-123.

57.  Highlights of prescribing information: tofacitinib. Federal Drug Administration. https://www.accessdata.fda.gov/drugsatfda_docs/label/2019/208246s009lbl.pdf. Published 2019.

58.  Greenberger PA, Y.K. O, Frederiksen MC, Atkinson A. Pharmacokinetics of prednisolone transfer to breast milk. *Clin Pharmacol Ther*. 1993;53(3):324-328.

59.  Ost L, Wettrell G, Björkhem I, Rane A. Prednisolone excretion in human milk. *J Pediatr*. 1985;106(6):1008-1011.

60.  Ryu RJ, Easterling TR, Caritis SN, et al. Prednisone pharmacokinetics during pregnancy and lactation. *J Clin Pharmacol*. 2018;58:1223-1232.

61.  Drugs and Lactation Database (LactMed) [Internet]. Bethesda (MD): National Library of Medicine (US); 2006-. Prednisolone. [Updated 2018 Oct 31]. Available from: https://www.ncbi.nlm.nih.gov/books/NBK501076/.

62. Drugs and Lactation Database (LactMed) [Internet]. Bethesda (MD): National Library of Medicine (US); 2006-. Budesonide. [Updated 2018 Oct 31]. Available from: https://www.ncbi.nlm.nih.gov/books/NBK501215/.

63. Kafetzis DA, Siafas CA, Georgakopoulos PA, Papadatos CJ. Passage of cephalosporins and amoxicillin into the breast milk. *Acta Paediatr Scand*. 1981;70:285-288.

64. Giamarellou H, Kolokythas E, Petrikkos G, Gazis J, Aravantinos D, Sfikakis P. Pharmacokinetics of three newer quinolones in pregnant and lactating women. *Am J Med*. 1989;87:49S-51S.

65. Harmon T, Burkhart G, Applebaum H. Perforated pseudomembranous colitis in the breast-fed infant. *J Pediatr Surg*. 1992;27:744-746.

66. Kaguelidou F, Turner MA, Choonara I, Jacqz-Aigrain E. Ciprofloxacin use in neonates: a systematic review of the literature. *Pediatr Infect Dis J*. 2011;30:e29-37.

67. Drugs and Lactation Database (LactMed) [Internet]. Bethesda (MD): National Library of Medicine (US); 2006-. Metronidazole. [Updated 2018 Oct 31]. Available from: https://www.ncbi.nlm.nih.gov/books/NBK501315/.

# 10

# IBD in Menopause

Sunanda V. Kane, MD, MSPH | Daniela Guerrero Vinsard, MD

## Introduction

Menopause is the cessation of menstrual periods in women who have naturally experienced 12 months of amenorrhea. The median age of occurrence is 51.4 years.[1,2] While the majority of women spontaneously experience menopause between age 45 and 55 years, around 5% will experience early menopause between 40 and 45 years[3] and 1% will experience premature menopause before 40 years.[4,5]

Surgical menopause after bilateral salpingo-oophorectomy occurs in women with conditions such as endometriosis, ovarian tumors, ovarian torsion, or prophylactic removal of the ovaries for prevention of breast and ovarian cancer. Bilateral salpingo-oophorectomy that occurs before the natural onset of menopause has been associated with increased overall mortality, coronary heart disease, dementia, parkinsonism, osteoporosis, mood disorders, and sexual dysfunction.[6,7] But little is known about inflammatory bowel disease (IBD) in the post-menopause stage. Although the majority of patients are diagnosed with IBD between ages 15 and 30 years,[8,9] women can be diagnosed with IBD after menopause, with scant literature pertaining to the hormonal impact on the disease course.

A 2018 pooled analysis of sex-age based differences in the incidence of IBD found that female patients had a lower risk of Crohn's disease (CD) until the age of 10 to 14 years, but they had a higher risk of CD thereafter, which was statistically significant for women older than 35 years.[10] Importantly, this shift begins after puberty, suggesting that hormones play an important role. The

Abraham BP, Kane SV, Glassner KL, eds.
*Women's Health in IBD: The Spectrum of Care
From Birth to Adulthood* (pp 191-194).
© 2022 Taylor & Francis Group.

incidence of ulcerative colitis (UC) did not differ significantly for female vs male patients until age 45 years; thereafter, men had a significantly higher incidence of UC than women, suggesting that hormones may also be implicated on the type of IBD affecting a patient.[11]

# Menopause Onset

The existing evidence of menopause onset in women with IBD is conflicting. A 2008 retrospective study reported that the median age for menopause in women with IBD was similar to historical controls.[12] Conversely, another retrospective study reported that women with CD had menopause at 47.6 years compared with 49.6 years in a group of healthy women from the same region and with the same smoking habits, concluding that CD may be associated with premature onset of menopause. In this same study, the mean age at menopause for women with CD was similar in people who do and do not smoke and in those diagnosed with CD before and after menopause.[13] A more recent 2018 study included 1202 women with IBD from which 454 women experienced menopause at a mean age of 46.4 years old.[14] From the reported ages of menopause onset in available studies, it appears that women with IBD experience menopause within the standard timeframe (45 to 55 years old) of the natural onset of menopause in the average woman.

# Effects of Menopause in IBD Symptomatology

Several studies propose estrogen as a hormone capable of exacerbating gastrointestinal symptoms and pain perception due to an inhibitory effect on smooth muscle contractility, increase in gastrointestinal permeability, and a pronociceptive effect.[15] Furthermore, it has been well established by both experimental and human observations that women are more likely to report abdominal pain and discomfort to colorectal distension and pain-related irritable bowel syndrome (IBS) symptoms than men do.[16] Therefore, the quiescent estrogen milieu after menopause has been associated with a positive impact in patient's symptomatology in IBD and in other gastrointestinal-related issues, such as IBS, in several studies.[17-20]

CD and UC follow different cytokine pathways, with inflammation in CD mostly mediated by T helper (Th) 1-related cytokines and UC mediated by Th2-related cytokines.[21]

High estrogen environments, such as pregnancy, stimulate Th lymphocytes to secrete type 2 cytokines and have been implicated in the pathogenesis and progression of Th2-mediated diseases, such as primary biliary cirrhosis and systemic lupus erythematous. Conversely, androgens create a shift toward type 1 cytokine excretion stimulating T CD8 and reducing Th2 response, potentially improving Th2-mediated diseases but worsening Th1-mediated diseases.[22] A decrease in estrogens, such as in the postpartum period or menopause, has been associated with improvement of Th2-mediated autoimmunity, expecting menopause to be protective at least against UC, which is a Th2-mediated disease.[21]

In a recent prospective study by Rolston et al, women with IBD were asked to rate their symptoms during their menstrual cycle, pregnancy, postpartum, and after menopause. The authors hypothesize that times of hormonal surge, rather than hormonal depletion, are associated with an exacerbation of gastrointestinal symptoms. In this study, which included 454 postmenopausal women with IBD, about two-thirds reported no variation in IBD symptoms due to menopause itself, while 16% reported improvement in symptoms during and after menopause.[14] Similarly, a study by Kane and Reddy demonstrated that the likelihood of having a flare before menopause is not different from having it after menopause.[12]

A 2018 study by Abdalla et al of 2252 postmenopausal women with IBD found that menopause was associated with increased disease activity in women age ≤ 45 years but not for women > 45 years. Similar to previous studies, neither the type of menopause (surgical or natural), nor the use of hormone replacement therapy (HRT), was a predictor for disease activity in postmenopausal women.[23] Another study on hormonal fluctuations in women with IBD demonstrated that among menopausal women, those who were diagnosed with IBD at an older age experienced worse symptoms (44 vs 32 years old).[19]

# Impact of Hormone Replacement Therapy in IBD

The use of HRT was not associated with changes in IBD symptoms in a recent study by Rolston et al in which 24% of postmenopausal women reported taking HRT and 8% reported taking supplements such as soy or black cohosh for control of menopausal symptoms.[14] Conversely, in the study by Kane and Reddy, HRT was thought to be protective of disease activity in postmenopausal women. The authors hypothesized that this observation results from the anti-inflammatory effect of estrogens, although this has yet to be proven in larger controlled studies.[12]

However, HRT in postmenopausal women is not free of risks. A 2002 randomized controlled trial from the women's health initiative, which compared HRT against placebo, demonstrated that overall health risks exceeded benefits from use of combined estrogen plus progestin, including increased risk for coronary artery disease, venous thromboembolism, and breast cancer.[24,25] Another large prospective study by Khalili et al showed that HRT was associated with an increased risk of UC but not CD and the risk was directly associated with the length of time use for HRT. The authors speculated that the effects of the estrogenic compound on gut permeability, contractility, pain perception, and type 2 cytokine stimulation was associated with this finding.[21]

# Future Perspectives

Clear evidence of hormones playing an important role in IBD pathogenesis throughout a woman's lifespan has been reported in several studies but there is scarce literature pertaining to the relationship between menopause, IBD, and mucosal inflammation. Some of the aspects that require further research efforts include the incidence of women diagnosed with IBD after menopause, with special attention to the natural history and disease phenotype in this subgroup of patients. Early, premature, and surgical menopause may affect the course and severity of the disease in different ways, and this should be further elucidated. Establishing differences between CD and UC in postmenopausal women is key as both diseases may entail a distinct hormonal and immunological pathway and respond differently to hormone replacement therapy. Physicians may need to have specific considerations when treating menopause-related symptoms in women with IBD. Randomized controlled trials assigning postmenopausal women (with CD vs UC) to placebo vs HRT may be the ideal study design to further describe the hormonal interactions between menopause and IBD.

## KEY POINTS

1. While menopause occurs either surgically or naturally in all women it is unclear what this does to the natural history of underlying IBD.
2. Menopause appears to occur earlier in women with IBD.
3. More study is needed in this area before definitive recommendations can be given.

# References

1.   Bonthala N, Kane S. Updates on women's health issues in patients with inflammatory bowel disease. *Curr Treat Options Gastroenterol.* 2018;16(1):86-100. doi:10.1007/s11938-018-0172-4

2.   Takahashi TA, Johnson KM. Menopause. *Med Clin North Am.* 2015;99(3):521-534. doi:10.1016/j.mcna.2015.01.006

3.   Miro F, Parker SW, Aspinall LJ, Coley J, Perry PW, Ellis JE. Sequential classification of endocrine stages during reproductive aging in women: the FREEDOM study. *Menopause.* 12(3):281-290. http://www.ncbi.nlm.nih.gov/pubmed/15879917. Accessed July 29, 2019.

4.   Faubion SS, Kuhle CL, Shuster LT, Rocca WA. Long-term health consequences of premature or early menopause and considerations for management. *Climacteric.* 2015;18(4):483-491. doi:10.3109/13697137.2015.1020484

5.   Cox L, Liu JH. Primary ovarian insufficiency: an update. *Int J Womens Health.* 2014;6:235-243. doi:10.2147/IJWH.S37636

6.   Shuster LT, Gostout BS, Grossardt BR, Rocca WA. Prophylactic oophorectomy in premenopausal women and long-term health. *Menopause Int.* 2008;14(3):111-116. doi:10.1258/mi.2008.008016

7.   Rocca WA, Ulrich LG. Oophorectomy for whom and at what age? Primum non nocere. *Maturitas.* 2012;71(1):1-2. doi:10.1016/j.maturitas.2011.10.006

8.   Johnston RD, Logan RFA. What is the peak age for onset of IBD? *Inflamm Bowel Dis.* 2008;14 Suppl 2:S4-5. doi:10.1002/ibd.20545

9.   Nee J, Feuerstein JD. Optimizing the care and health of women with inflammatory bowel disease. *Gastroenterol Res Pract.* 2015;2015:435820. doi:10.1155/2015/435820

10.  Shah SC, Khalili H, Gower-Rousseau C, et al. Sex-based differences in incidence of inflammatory bowel diseases—pooled analysis of population-based studies from Western countries. *Gastroenterology.* 2018;155(4):1079-1089.e3. doi:10.1053/j.gastro.2018.06.043

11.  Ruel J, Ruane D, Mehandru S, Gower-Rousseau C, Colombel JF. IBD across the age spectrum—is it the same disease? *Nat Rev Gastroenterol Hepatol.* 2014;11:88-98. doi:10.1038/nrgastro.2013.240

12.  Kane SV, Reddy D. Hormonal replacement therapy after menopause is protective of disease activity in women with inflammatory bowel disease. *Am J Gastroenterol.* 2008;103(5):1193-1196. doi:10.1111/j.1572-0241.2007.01700.x

13.  Lichtarowicz A, Norman C, Calcraft B, Morris JS, Rhodes J, Mayberry J. A study of the menopause, smoking, and contraception in women with crohn's disease. *Q J Med.* 1989;72(1):623-631. doi:10.1093/oxfordjournals.qjmed.a068355

14.  Rolston VS, Boroujerdi L, Long MD, et al. The influence of hormonal fluctuation on inflammatory bowel disease symptom severity—a cross-sectional cohort study. *Inflamm Bowel Dis.* 2018;24(2):387-393. doi:10.1093/ibd/izx004

15.  Meleine M, Matricon J. Gender-related differences in irritable bowel syndrome: potential mechanisms of sex hormones. *World J Gastroenterol.* 2014;20(22):6725-6743. doi:10.3748/wjg.v20.i22.6725

16.  Adeyemo MA, Spiegel BMR, Chang L. Meta-analysis: do irritable bowel syndrome symptoms vary between men and women? *Aliment Pharmacol Ther.* 2010;32(6):738-755. doi:10.1111/j.1365-2036.2010.04409.x

17.  Donaldson EK, Huang V, Ross S, Sydora BC. Experience of menopause in women with inflammatory bowel disease: pilot study. *Climacteric.* 2017;20(6):545-551. doi:10.1080/13697137.2017.1360861

18.  Bharadwaj S, Kulkarni G, Shen B. Menstrual cycle, sex hormones in female inflammatory bowel disease patients with and without surgery. *J Dig Dis.* 2015;16(5):245-255. doi:10.1111/1751-2980.12247

19.  Boroujerdi L, Long MD, McGovern DP, et al. Inflammatory bowel disease symptom severity is influenced by hormone fluctuations in many women with IBD. *Gastroenterology.* 2013;144(5):S-632. doi:10.1016/S0016-5085(13)62339-2

20.  Kane S. Gender issues in the management of inflammatory bowel disease and irritable bowel syndrome. *Int J Fertil Womens Med.* 2002;47(3):136-142. http://www.ncbi.nlm.nih.gov/pubmed/12081259. Accessed July 15, 2019.

21.  Khalili H, Higuchi LM, Ananthakrishnan AN, et al. Hormone therapy increases risk of ulcerative colitis but not Crohn's disease. *Gastroenterology.* 2012;143(5):1199-1206. doi:10.1053/j.gastro.2012.07.096

22.  González DA, Díaz BB, Rodríguez Pérez M del C, Hernández AG, Chico BND, de León AC. Sex hormones and autoimmunity. *Immunol Lett.* 2010;133(1):6-13. doi:10.1016/j.imlet.2010.07.001

23.  Abdalla M, Baird DD, Sandler RS, et al. Menopause and hormone replacement therapy in women with inflammatory bowel diseases in CCFA partners. https://cgibd.med.unc.edu/ccfapartners/docs/menopause abstract-DDW 2016.pdf. Accessed July 29, 2019.

24.  Rossouw JE, Anderson GL, Prentice R. Risks and benefits of estrogen plus progestin in healthy postmenopausal women: principal results from the women's health initiative randomized controlled trial. *JAMA J Am Med Assoc.* 2002;288(3):321-333. doi:10.1001/jama.288.3.321

25.  Manson JE, Hsia J, Johnson KC, et al. Estrogen plus progestin and the risk of coronary heart disease. *N Engl J Med.* 2003;349(6):523-534. doi:10.1056/nejmoa030808

# 11

# Irritable Bowel Syndrome in Women With IBD

Bincy P. Abraham, MD, MS | Kerri L. Glassner, DO | Eamonn M. M. Quigley, MD

## Introduction

Irritable bowel syndrome (IBS) is a functional gastrointestinal disorder characterized by recurrent abdominal pain and altered bowel habits. In order to fulfill Rome IV diagnostic criteria, abdominal pain must occur at least 1 day/week within the prior 3 months, be related to defecation, and associated with a change in stool frequency or form.[1] Many factors are considered to contribute to the pathogenesis of symptoms that characterize IBS: dysmotility, visceral hypersensitivity, disordered central sensing of intestinal activity, low-grade intestinal inflammation, and an abnormal gut microbiota. Given the somewhat negative connotations attendant on the term "functional," IBS and related disorders are now referred to collectively as "disorders of gut-brain interaction." IBS affects up to 10% to 12% of the adult population in North America and is more common in younger adults and women.[2] IBS and inflammatory bowel disease (IBD) share many similarities including their cardinal symptoms: abdominal pain, bloating, diarrhea, and urgency. Furthermore, in IBD, clinical symptoms often do not correlate with the degree of intestinal inflammation,[3-5] rendering the clinical assessment of IBS symptoms in women with IBD especially challenging. However, correctly making this distinction is critical if one is to an avoid an inappropriate escalation of immunosuppressive therapy.

In patients with IBD in remission, the prevalence of IBS-type symptoms has been found to range from 19% to 45% depending upon disease subtype (Crohn's disease [CD] or ulcerative colitis [UC]) and the criteria used to define remission.[6-12] IBS-type symptoms have been found to occur more frequently in patients with CD than in those with UC (46% vs 36%, odds ratio 1.62, 95% confidence interval [CI] 1.21 to 2.18) according to data from a meta-analysis.[13] Symptoms of IBS in

Abraham BP, Kane SV, Glassner KL, eds.
*Women's Health in IBD: The Spectrum of Care
From Birth to Adulthood* (pp 195-212).
© 2022 Taylor & Francis Group.

patients with IBD have been shown to have a negative effect on psychological well-being and quality of life (QOL) that equals that of patients with active IBD.[6,10] IBS-type symptoms in IBD have also been associated with increased health care utilization, fatigue, sleep disturbance, and narcotic use.[6,14]

The difficulty in diagnosing and managing IBS-type symptoms in women with IBD lies in determining whether IBS-like symptoms fall into one of the following categories: subclinical IBD, complications of IBD, or "true" IBS superimposed on IBD. In those with subclinical IBD, there may be ongoing histologic evidence of inflammation or small bowel disease missed with ileo-colonoscopy. Alternative etiologies for IBS-like symptoms such as small intestinal bacterial overgrowth (SIBO), bile acid diarrhea (BAD), and complications of IBD such as structural damage from chronic inflammation leading to fibrosis should be considered and evaluated for. A diagnosis of "true" IBS in IBD should only be made once the previously mentioned etiologies have been excluded.

# Similarities Between IBS and IBD

Not only do IBS and IBD share similar symptoms, they are also both thought to have a genetic basis that involves alterations in immune response, gut microbiota, and microbiota-host interactions (Table 11-1). Although a genetic basis has been well established for IBD and involves a number of microbiota-host interactions and inflammatory pathways, genetic polymorphisms in tumor necrosis factor (TNF) genes have also been associated with susceptibility to IBS and drug efficacy for IBS in children.[15] One such gene, the CD risk allele rs4263839 G in the TNF super family (TNFSF) 15 gene has been shown to be significantly associated with an increased risk of IBS.[16] Individuals who carry this gene are thought to have increased expression of the TL1A protein in immune cells, which leads to T-cell activation and an inflammatory response in the gastrointestinal mucosa.[16] While such shared genetic loci are persuasive that IBS and IBD may involve a similar predisposition, more than 200 risk loci have been identified for IBD, compared to significantly fewer for IBS.[17]

There is also evidence to suggest that low-grade inflammation and immune activation may play a role in the pathophysiology of IBS, especially in certain subgroups. Several studies have found increased numbers of inflammatory cells in the colon of individuals with IBS compared to healthy controls. In particular, IBS has been associated with increased colonic mucosal macrophages, mast cells, and CD3+ T cells.[18,19] Other immunological phenomena described in IBS include increases in circulating B7+ T cells and activated B cells.[19] Further studies have identified upregulation of Toll-like receptors (TLRs) and mediated cytokines in IBS. Patients with IBS were found to have higher levels of both TLR-4 and TLR-5, as well as increased expression of the pro-inflammatory cytokine interleukin (IL) 6, the chemokine CXCL-11 and its receptor CXCR-3 together with decreased expression of the anti-inflammatory cytokine IL-10.[20] Women with IBS have been found to have much higher expression of TLR-4 and TLR-5 compared to controls.[21] It is possible that these immune-mediated mechanisms could contribute to the apparent increased prevalence of IBS seen in individuals with IBD.

Similar to IBD, studies have shown that gut microbiota in IBS are different to that of healthy controls. A recent systematic review identified increases in *Lactobacillaceae*, *Bacteroides*, and *Enterobacteriaceae*, and decreases in *Bifidobacterium* and *Faecalibacterium* in IBS compared to controls.[22] The *Enterobacteriaceae* family contains several pathogenic bacteria responsible for common enteric infections including *Escherichia*, *Shigella*, *Campylobacter*, and *Salmonella*. Post-infectious IBS is thought to occur in as many as 30% of patients after an episode of gastroenteritis; therefore, increases in *Enterobacteriaceae* may correlate with this.[23] As in IBD, diversity of the stool microbiota in IBS is decreased. In IBD, *Proteobacteria*, *Pasturellaceae*, *Veillonellaceae*, *Fusobacterium* species, and *Ruminoccocus gnavus* species are increased while *Bacteroides*, *Bifidobacterium*, *Clostridium* XIVa and IV, *Faecalibacterium prausnitzii*, *Roseburia*, and *Suterella* are decreased (24). Common to both IBD and IBS are decreases in *Bifidobacterium* and *Faecalibacterium* and increases in

## Table 11-1. Similarities Between IBS and IBD

| | IBS | IBD |
|---|---|---|
| *GENETICS* | TNF gene polymorphisms | More than 200 risk loci identified |
| *IMMUNE RESPONSE* | Increased colonic mucosal macrophages, mast cells, and CD3+ T cells<br><br>Increased circulating B7+ T cells and activated B cells<br><br>Upregulation of toll-like receptors and mediated cytokines | Increased mucosal neutrophils, macrophages, dendritic cells, natural killer T cells, B cells, and T cells<br><br>Increased cytokines including tumor necrosis factor (TNF-α), IL-1β, IL-6, IL-12, IL-23, interferon-γ, and chemokines |
| *GUT MICROBIOTA* | Increased:<br>• Lactobacillaceae<br>• Bacteroides<br>• Enterobacteriaceae<br>Decreased:<br>• Bifidobacterium<br>• Faecalibacterium | Increased:<br>• Proteobacteria<br>• Pasturellaceae<br>• Veillonellaceae<br>• Fusobacterium species<br>• Ruminoccocus gnavus<br>Decreased:<br>• Bacteroides<br>• Bifidobacterium<br>• Clostridium XIVa and IV<br>• Faecalibacterium prausnitzii<br>• Roseburia<br>• Suterella |

*Proteobacteria.* Although similarities do exist, the role of the microbiome in IBD has more consistent and supporting data than that of the microbiome in IBS.

# Diagnosing IBS in IBD

## History and Physical Examination

The first step in evaluating persistent symptoms in women with IBD should be a careful history and physical exam. Clinicians should begin by asking about the location, duration, and severity of symptoms. Questions about weight loss, frequency of bowel movements, nocturnal symptoms, hematochezia, and fever should be elicited; these alarm symptoms necessitate further workup for inflammatory activity. Medication compliance should be assessed; poor compliance should prompt assessment of disease activity and medication optimization. The history should also evaluate for episodes of incontinence, use of narcotics or antibiotics and symptoms that may point toward various organic etiologies.

The importance of a meticulous physical examination should not be overlooked. The detection of tachycardia or hypotension would certainly indicate an organic basis for symptoms and should prompt urgent assessment immediately and even hospital admission. The abdominal exam should include evaluation for important findings such as distension, masses, guarding, or rebound. A rectal exam should be performed with inspection for perianal disease such as an abscess or fistula. The digital rectal examination may also reveal signs of a defecatory disorder, such as dyssynergia.

## Assessment of Inflammation

Information gathered from a thorough history and physical examination will help to guide the next steps in evaluation (Figure 11-1). Patients with history or physical exam findings concerning for active disease should undergo assessment for inflammation. Laboratory markers such as erythrocyte sedimentation rate (ESR) and C-reactive protein (CRP) have not been found to be as useful because of poor sensitivity compared to fecal calprotectin.[25] Furthermore, up to 20% of people do not express CRP in inflammatory conditions; this is genetically determined.[26] In some patients, starting with a non-invasive test such as fecal calprotectin or lactoferrin may be appropriate. Many studies have examined the utility of fecal calprotectin as a non-invasive marker in the assessment of inflammation. Some suggested a cutoff of ≤ 250 µg/g as indicative of endoscopic remission,[27,28] whereas others have shown that using a cutoff of ≤ 60 µg/g accurately predicted both remission and histologic healing.[29] In patients without a known diagnosis of IBD presenting for evaluation of symptoms consistent with IBS, a meta-analysis found there was a ≤ 1% probability of having active IBD when the fecal calprotectin level was ≤ 40 µg/g.[30] Fecal calprotectin values ≤ 40 µg/g are reassuring; however, those in between 40 and 250 µg/g are more difficult to assess and may require further evaluation with endoscopy or imaging. As previously mentioned, the prevalence of IBS in IBD has ranged from 19% to 45% depending upon the fecal calprotectin cutoff used to define remission.[6-12] The use of higher fecal calprotectin values may mis-diagnose some patients who have persistent inflammatory activity as having IBS. In addition, enteric infections can cause elevations in fecal calprotectin.[31] Patients with diarrhea who have risk factors for an infectious etiology should have stool testing to exclude *Clostridioides difficile* and other gastrointestinal pathogens.

Symptomatic patients who have not recently had an endoscopic evaluation or those with an elevated fecal marker (calprotectin, lactoferrin) should have endoscopy performed to evaluate for disease activity. Women with IBD who have a history of upper gastrointestinal tract involvement should have both upper and lower endoscopic evaluation. Biopsies should be obtained even when there appears to be mucosal healing visually. Histologic disease activity with normal-appearing mucosa on endoscopic evaluation should prompt consideration for optimization of medical therapy. How aggressively histologic remission should be targeted continues to be debated and has not yet been established as a treatment endpoint.[32]

In CD, small bowel inflammation, strictures, or fistulizing disease can lead to symptoms that may be missed on ileo-colonoscopy and can mistakenly be labeled as IBS. As part of disease activity assessment, patients should undergo imaging (ie, magnetic resonance [MR] enterography, computed tomography [CT] enterography) or endoscopic assessment (ie, capsule endoscopy, balloon enteroscopy) of the small bowel, as appropriate. Although there has been some concern that fecal calprotectin may not correlate with small bowel disease activity, recent studies have not found this to be the case; fecal calprotectin has in fact correlated with video capsule, radiologic, and endoscopic findings in patients with small bowel CD.[33-35] Therefore, patients with CD who have an elevated fecal calprotectin warrant investigation for small bowel, as well as colonic, inflammation.

## Exclusion of Alternative Etiologies

Once active disease and/or infectious etiologies have been excluded, alternative diagnoses such as medication side effects, SIBO, carbohydrate malabsorption, BAD, pancreatic exocrine insufficiency (PEI), and pelvic floor dysfunction should be considered. Medications are often overlooked

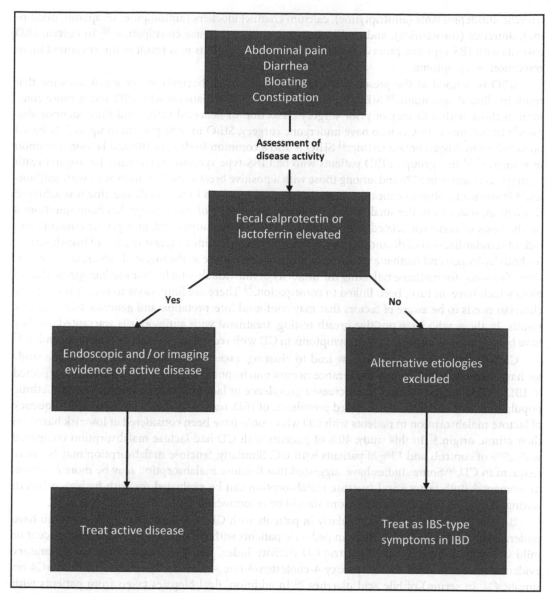

**Figure 11-1.** Diagnostic algorithm to distinguish IBD from IBS.

and can be associated with symptoms of diarrhea or constipation. Pharmacologic agents can contribute to diarrhea through effects on motility, by causing malabsorption or through osmotic and secretory mechanisms.[36] Macrolide antibiotics (erythromycin, metoclopramide) and stimulant laxatives (bisacodyl, senna) can produce diarrhea by increasing gastrointestinal motility. Acarbose, an alpha-glucosidase inhibitor, causes carbohydrate malabsorption, and orlistat used for weight loss, inhibits gastric and pancreatic lipases leading to fat malabsorption.[37] Malabsorption can also be induced by aminoglycoside antibiotics and thyroid supplements. Secretory diarrhea can occur with the use of antiarrhythmics (quinine), antibiotics (amoxicillin/clavulanate), colchicine, prostaglandins (misoprostol), cardiac glycosides (digitalis), calcitonin, and biguanides (metformin). Sugar alcohols (mannitol, sorbitol, xylitol) and magnesium-containing medications can cause osmotic diarrhea. Conversely, many commonly used medications including opiates, anticholinergics (scopolamine, oxybutynin, hyoscyamine, dicyclomine, promethazine), antihistamines (diphenhydramine), tricyclic antidepressants (amitriptyline), calcium channel blockers (amlodipine, verapamil, nifedipine), diuretics (furosemide), and oral iron supplements can cause constipation.[38] In certain IBD patients with IBS-type symptoms, eliminating culprit medications may result in improvement in, or resolution of, symptoms.

SIBO is defined as the presence of excessive numbers of bacteria in the small intestine that result in clinical symptoms.[39] SIBO is present in up to 22% of patients with IBD and is more common in those with a history of prior surgery (resection of ileocecal valve) and fibro-stenotic disease.[40] In patients with CD who have undergone surgery, SIBO may be present in up to 30% based on lactulose hydrogen breath testing.[41] SIBO is also a common finding in IBS and is more common in women.[42,43] In a group of IBD patients who had IBS-type symptoms, lactulose hydrogen breath testing was positive in 57% and among those with a positive breath test 57% improved with antibiotics.[44] Historically, objective measurements of bacterial numbers in the small intestine was achieved through aspirates from the small bowel. However, the validity of this strategy has been questioned on the basis of concerns related to contamination with oral, esophageal, and gastric contents and lack of standardization of diagnostic thresholds. Current guidelines suggest the use of breath testing for both hydrogen and methane using either glucose or lactulose as the ingested substrate; the inclusion of an assay for methane reflecting the minority of individuals who harbor methanogenic microbiota which have, in turn, been linked to constipation.[39] There are limitations to breath testing; the clinician needs to be aware of factors that may confound interpretation and generate false-positive results. In those who have positive breath testing, treatment with antibiotics is warranted, as they have been shown to improve clinical symptoms in CD with reductions in Harvey-Bradshaw Index.[45]

Carbohydrate malabsorption may lead to bloating, excessive flatus, and diarrhea. Some studies have suggested that lactose intolerance occurs much more frequently than would be expected in IBD.[46] Taking into account the increased prevalence of lactose malabsorption in certain ethnic populations that also have an increased prevalence of IBD, one study found an increased frequency of lactose malabsorption in patients with CD who would have been considered at low risk based on their ethnic origin.[47] In this study, 40% of patients with CD had lactose malabsorption compared with 29% of controls and 13% of patients with UC. Similarly, fructose malabsorption may be more frequent in CD.[46] Some studies have suggested that fructose malabsorption may be more common in women.[48] Both lactose and fructose malabsorption can be evaluated for with hydrogen breath testing. If positive, dietary modifications should be recommended.

BAD is common in IBD, particularly in patients with CD who have ileal disease or who have undergone ileal resection.[49] A study in pediatric patients with persistent diarrhea with quiescent or mild CD activity based on the Pediatric CD Activity Index, found that up to 86% had laboratory evidence (elevated levels of 7α-hydroxy-4-cholesten-3-one – commonly referred to as 7 αC4 or, simply, C4, in serum) of bile acid diarrhea.[50] In addition, ileal biopsies taken from patients with CD without inflammation were found to have decreased expression of the apical sodium bile acid co-transporting polypeptide that participates in ileal bile acid absorption.[51] In another study of patients with CD with persistent diarrhea unresponsive to conventional treatment, 90% of those who had undergone prior bowel resections had an abnormal selenium homotaurocholic acid seven-day retention test (SeHCAT), and 28% of those who had not undergone resection had an abnormal SeHCAT.[52] The various diagnostic tests for BAD, SeHCAT, plasma FGF19, fecal measurements of bile acids, or serum C4 levels[53] are not widely available, and patients can be empirically treated with bile acid chelators such as cholestyramine, colestipol, or colesevelam.

Some authors have suggested that PEI may be an extraintestinal manifestation of IBD which can account for symptoms of diarrhea, particularly steatorrhea. A study of 100 patients with CD, 100 with UC, and 100 controls found PEI in 22% of patients with UC and 14% of patients with CD by fecal elastase testing.[54] The odds ratio for PEI in patients with IBD was 10.5 (95% CI 2.5 to 44.8) compared to controls. However, PEI may be transient as elastase values became normal in 24 of the patients with IBD at a 6-month follow-up. Another study of 237 patients with IBD found that 21% had PEI demonstrated by 4-para-aminobenzoic acid test, and 19% had abnormally low bicarbonate secretion in response to a secretin test.[55] A major limitation of fecal elastase testing is that it has poor diagnostic accuracy in patients with diarrhea (may be falsely low); thus, other etiologies of diarrhea must be excluded.

Finally, women with quiescent IBD complaining of constipation or diarrhea should be evaluated for fecal incontinence, overflow diarrhea, or a defecatory disorder. A clinical suspicion of this warrants a rectal examination, anorectal manometry, and balloon expulsion testing. There is a 2-fold increased risk of fecal incontinence in women who have had vaginal deliveries complicated by third- or fourth-degree lacerations resulting in injury to the anal sphincter.[56,57] The risk of fecal incontinence is highest in deliveries that required forceps or vacuum extraction.[58] Surgery for anorectal conditions including fistula, fissures, hemorrhoids, or anorectal carcinoma can also damage the anal sphincter and lead to incontinence.[59] Functional defecation disorders, which include dyssynergic defecation and inadequate defecatory propulsion, are up to 3 times more prevalent in women than in men.[60,61] In women, functional defecation disorders are associated with a history of sexual abuse.[60] A recent meta-analysis concluded that, in patients with IBD who had ongoing symptoms suggestive of defecatory dysfunction, the rate of dyssynergic defecation ranged from 45% to 97% in patients without an ileal pouch-anal anastomosis (IPAA) and 25% to 75% in those with an IPAA.[62] Another study of 30 patients with IBD in remission found that 97% fulfilled anorectal manometric criteria for dyssynergia.[63] If testing confirms dyssynergia, patients should be referred for biofeedback therapy, as response rates have been shown to be up to 70% in IBD patients without an IPAA and 86% in those with an IPAA.[62]

## Structural Complications of IBD

Chronic intestinal inflammation can lead to fibrosis in both CD and UC. Fibrotic changes lead to changes in motility of the colon, small bowel, and anorectal function. As previously discussed, in women with CD it is important to exclude fibro-stenotic disease with imaging studies such as MR or CT enterography. While, in general, the severity of fibrosis in UC has been linked to longer disease duration,[64,65] some recent studies have suggested that even those with a disease duration of less than 1 year may develop fibrosis.[66] Unfortunately, no antifibrotic therapies have been approved for IBD, although several agents have shown encouraging results in preclinical studies.[67]

# Hormonal Effects on IBS

In women with IBD, hormones may play a role in the development of IBS-like symptoms, similar to what is seen in women without IBD. IBS is more common in women, with a female to male sex ratio ranging from 2:1 to 4:1.[68] Variants on chromosome 9q31.2 in a region previously linked to age at menarche and 13 additional loci were found to affect the risk of IBS in women, and were associated with constipation predominant IBS.[69] The hormones estrogen and progesterone are known to inhibit smooth muscle contraction. Progesterone also modulates the colonic 5-hydroxytryptamine (5-HT) system, which is involved in the control of peristalsis.[70] Mucosal 5-HT release has been shown to be significantly higher in IBS than in healthy controls and correlates with the severity of abdominal pain.[71] Women have been shown to have slower colonic and gastric emptying, which may explain, in part, the increased prevalence rates for constipation and gastroparesis that have been documented among females.[72,73] Women with slow transit constipation exhibit progesterone receptor overexpression in colon muscle that impairs contractility.[70] Not surprisingly, therefore, the subtype of IBS with constipation is significantly more common in women than men.[74,75] Estrogen is involved in the hormonal regulation of pain through the function of the nervous, immune, skeletal, and cardiovascular systems.[76] Along these lines, pain is reported more commonly in women with IBS, as well as in chronic pain disorders such as fibromyalgia, chronic fatigue syndrome, chronic pelvic pain, and migraine headache—disorders that commonly overlap with IBS.[77-81] In addition,

IBS symptoms are increased in frequency and severity during menstruation, further evidence for a hormonal effect on gut motility.[81]

Studies have shown that there are gender-based differences in response to certain medications used to treat IBS. One such example is the 5-HT3 receptor antagonist alosetron, which was shown to significantly improve the symptoms of women, but not men, with IBS.[82] Another 5-HT3 receptor antagonist cilansetron and a 5-HT4 receptor agonist tegaserod have also shown greater efficacy in women.[83-85] Lubiprostone, an orally active prostone that stimulates chloride secretion through the activation of type-2 chloride channels in the gastrointestinal tract is approved by the US Food and Drug Administration (FDA) for use in women with IBS-C.[86] Lubiprostone may also have greater efficacy in women; however, the clinical trials included fewer men than women limiting the ability to draw any firm conclusions.

# Management

Effective therapy for IBS-like symptoms in IBD is imperative due to the significant impact on psychological well-being and QOL, as well as increased health care utilization and costs. Unfortunately, there have been few trials that specifically addressed the impact of different treatment options on IBS-like symptoms in IBD. However, in clinical practice, therapies with efficacy in IBS are often used in patients with IBD. Strategies employed include pharmacologic, dietary, psychological, and microbiota-based methods (Table 11-2). Treatments targeting IBS-like symptoms are almost always used concomitantly with standard IBD-directed medical therapy for inflammation.

# Pharmacologic Treatment

## Fiber Supplements

In IBS, soluble fiber such as psyllium is recommended for overall symptom improvement.[2] The use of fiber to treat IBS-like symptoms in IBD has been shown to be beneficial in some patients, while it may be contraindicated in others with luminal narrowing or fibro-stenotic disease. Intake of dietary fiber, in a large study of patients with IBD in remission, was associated with a decreased risk of disease flare at 6-month follow-up.[87] In a small placebo-controlled trial of patients with UC with IBS-like symptoms in endoscopic remission, ispaghula husk, a soluble fiber, was found to improve symptoms of pain, diarrhea, urgency, constipation, and bloating compared to placebo.[88] Certain fibers, especially insoluble fiber, can contribute to worsening symptoms and should be avoided.[89]

## Antispasmodics

Antispasmodics, although not specifically studied in patients with quiescent IBD, may help with abdominal cramping and diarrhea as their use in IBS has been shown to significantly improve symptoms.[2] In IBD patients with IBS-like symptoms related to hypermotility, antispasmodics may be particularly helpful. Active disease and strictures should be evaluated for and excluded prior to the use of antispasmodics to avoid the risk of adverse outcomes such as toxic megacolon from anticholinergic side effects.[90]

## Table 11-2. Treatment Options for IBS–Like Symptoms in IBD

### TREATMENT OPTIONS

| |
|---|
| *PHARMACOLOGIC* |
| Fiber |
| • Soluble fiber |
| Antispasmodics |
| • Dicyclomine, hyoscyamine |
| Antidiarrheals |
| • Loperamide, eluxadoline, alosetron |
| Constipation-directed therapy |
| • Linaclotide, plecanatide, lubiprostone, polyethylene glycol, naloxegol, methylnaltrexone |
| Antibiotics |
| • Rifaximin |
| Probiotics |
| • Various strains |
| Neuromodulators |
| • TCA, SSRI |
| 5-aminosalicylates |
| • Further studies needed |
| Narcotics |
| • Avoid or discontinue |
| Nonsteroidal anti-inflammatories |
| • Avoid if possible, consider cyclooxygenase-2 inhibitors |
| *DIETARY* |
| Food diary |
| Low FODMAP diet |
| *PSYCHOLOGIC* |
| Medications: TCA, SSRI |
| Cognitive behavioral therapy |
| Relaxation therapy |
| Hypnotherapy |
| Sleep optimization |
| *MICROBIOTA* |
| FMT: clinical trials needed |

# Antidiarrheals

Although there are no studies evaluating the efficacy of loperamide or other antidiarrheals for IBS-like symptoms in IBD, current guidelines recommend against the use of loperamide for IBS.[2] Previous randomized controlled trials of loperamide compared to placebo in patients with IBS did not show any significant symptom improvement.[91,92] In CD, in general, loperamide use for chronic diarrhea has been shown to improve abdominal pain and diarrhea.[93] Eluxadoline, a μ-opioid and κ-opioid receptor agonist and α-opioid receptor antagonist is FDA-approved for IBS with diarrhea (IBS-D), and improves symptoms and stool consistency.[94] Eluxadoline must be avoided in patients who have undergone cholecystectomy or who have a history of sphincter of Oddi dysfunction, pancreatitis, alcohol abuse, or severe liver problems due to the risk of pancreatitis. The serotonergic agent alosetron has been shown to improve symptoms in women with IBS-D.[95] There have been reports of severe constipation and ischemic colitis with alosetron, and the current recommended dose is lower than used in the original clinical trials.[96] Eluxadoline and alosetron have not been studied in women with IBD and should be used with caution.

# Constipation-Directed Therapy

In constipation-predominant IBS (IBS-C), the prosecretory agents linaclotide, plecanatide, and lubiprostone all improve symptoms compared to placebo.[2] These medications have not been studied in IBD and caution must be taken to avoid the major side effect of diarrhea. Most stool softeners are safe to use in IBD, and polyethylene glycol, an osmotic laxative, is often recommended for constipation due to its safety with low side effect profile. However, in IBS trials, polyethylene glycol has not been shown to improve pain symptoms.[97,98] Women with IBD on opioid medications should be weaned off opioids and can be treated with the peripheral opioid antagonists naloxegol and methylnaltrexone which have been shown to improve the frequency of spontaneous bowel movements and pain symptoms.[99-102]

# Antibiotics

Rifaximin has been approved for treatment of IBS-D and improves global IBS symptoms, as well as bloating.[103,104] In IBD, rifaximin has shown efficacy in the induction and maintenance of remission in adults with moderate CD activity.[105,106] The use of rifaximin leads to minor, though detectable, changes in the fecal microbiome.[107,108] As the microbiome is thought to be a contributing factor to the development of and symptoms in both IBD and IBS-D, it may be an ideal option for IBS-like symptoms in IBD. However, clinical trials are needed to evaluate efficacy in this population.

# Probiotics

In IBS, probiotics, as a group, improve global symptoms, bloating, and flatulence.[2] Probiotics have shown benefit in the induction and maintenance of remission in mild UC.[109] In IBD patients with pouchitis, there is evidence of efficacy with the use of probiotics for the primary prevention and maintenance of remission of pouchitis.[110] Based on the evidence of efficacy in both IBS and IBD, probiotic use seems to be an attractive option for treating IBS-like symptoms in IBD. However, further studies are needed to specifically address its use in IBD patients with IBS-like symptoms and to determine appropriate strains and duration of use.

# Neuromodulators

Tricyclic antidepressants (TCAs) and selective serotonin reuptake inhibitors (SSRIs) have been shown to improve IBS symptoms in clinical trials.[111-114] These agents work as central neuromodulators targeting pain and psychological disorders such as anxiety, depression, and somatization. TCAs also improve diarrhea due to effects on gastrointestinal motility, while SSRIs are beneficial for constipation. In a retrospective cohort study of IBD patients with concomitant IBS-type symptoms, low-dose TCAs led to moderate improvement of gastrointestinal symptoms in 59.3% of patients.[115] Another study evaluating the effects of antidepressant use in IBD found that when used to treat concomitant mood disorders, antidepressants reduced relapse rates, use of steroids, and endoscopies in the year after their introduction.[116]

# 5-Aminosalicylates

Immune activation and low-grade inflammation have been suggested to play a role in the pathophysiology of IBS, and anti-inflammatory medications such as 5-aminosalicylates (5-ASAs) have been evaluated in IBS. The use of 5-ASAs overall has not been shown to be beneficial for IBS in randomized controlled trials.[117,118] However, one of the studies did show that a secondary endpoint, overall symptom improvement, yielded a positive outcome in the 5-ASA group compared to placebo.[117] Pooled data from a recent IBS monograph showed a significant effect of mesalamine on symptom reduction, although the result depended upon the endpoint used and the conclusion drawn was that 5-ASAs are not recommended for use in IBS.[2] There have not been any trials performed in IBD patients with IBS-type symptoms and this is an area that could be further explored in the future.

# Narcotics

Narcotics are not beneficial in the treatment of IBS and should be avoided in patients with IBD. Studies have shown that narcotic use in patients with CD leads to an increased risk of mortality and infection.[119] Opiate use in IBD patients has also been associated with a higher risk of emergency department visits and increased health care costs.[120] Opiate use can lead to narcotic bowel syndrome resulting in a paradoxical increase in abdominal pain.[121] Alternative treatment strategies should be used in women with IBD who have IBS-like symptoms, and those who are already on chronic narcotic medications should undergo gradual discontinuation.

# Nonsteroidal Anti-Inflammatories

Nonsteroidal anti-inflammatory medications are not used for IBS, and, in general, are avoided in IBD. Nonsteroidal anti-inflammatory medications are associated with risk of disease relapse in IBD and gastrointestinal mucosal injury.[122-124] The use of cyclooxygenase-2 inhibitors in IBD was shown in a small study to be safe[125]; their use, however, has not been evaluated in the context of IBS-like symptoms.

# Dietary Strategies

## Food Diary

Keeping a food diary may benefit certain patients with IBD and concomitant IBS-type symptoms by helping them avoid "trigger" foods that contribute to their symptoms.[126] Lactose malabsorption is common in IBD and avoiding lactose-containing products may improve IBS-like symptoms in women with IBD.[46,47] Other foods that have been implicated in IBS-like symptoms in IBD patients include caffeine-containing products, alcoholic beverages, diet foods and beverages, fatty and fried foods, and processed foods such as cookies, cakes, crackers, and pretzels.[126] Foods that have been shown to ameliorate IBS-symptoms in patients with IBD include water, plain pasta, rice, eggs, baked potatoes, plain fish, chicken, and turkey.

## Low FODMAP Diet

A low fermentable oligosaccharides, disaccharides, monosaccharides, and polyols (FODMAP) diet has shown efficacy in both IBS[127] and in IBD patients who have IBS-type symptoms.[128] In a randomized trial of 52 patients with quiescent IBD, symptoms of bloating and flatulence improved the most with the low FODMAP diet while abdominal pain did not improve.[128] Patients on the low FODMAP diet experienced a decline in *Bifidobacteria* and *Faecalibacterium prausnitzii* abundance but no adverse effects were seen on disease activity. The authors concluded that a 4-week low FODMAP diet is safe and effective in managing persistent symptoms in quiescent IBD.

# Psychologic Interventions

IBS-like symptoms in IBD are associated with anxiety, depression, and decreased QOL.[6,7] Psychological distress in both IBS and IBD was found to have a stronger direct effect on health-related QOL than gastrointestinal symptoms.[129] In addition to the use of antidepressant medications such as TCAs and SSRIs, other psychiatric interventions such as mindfulness therapy may be of benefit in IBD patients with IBS-type symptoms or high perceived stress levels.[130] The use of cognitive behavioral therapy has been associated with mixed results in IBD, and while it has generally not been shown to improve physical symptoms or disease status in adult patients, it may improve QOL and coping skills.[131-133] In IBS, cognitive behavioral therapy, relaxation therapy, and hypnotherapy have been shown to improve symptoms[2]; however, there are limited data in women with IBD who have IBS-like symptoms. IBD patients with IBS-type symptoms have poor sleep quality.[134] Sleep disturbances contribute to pain, mood disturbances, and decreased QOL; optimizing sleep hygiene may be of benefit in these patients.

# Fecal Microbiota Transplantation

To date no studies have been conducted on the use of fecal microbiota transplantation (FMT) in women with IBD who have IBS-type symptoms. IBS-type symptoms in patients with quiescent IBD were not associated with specific changes of the fecal microbiome in a study of 270 patients; however, there was concern that unmeasured confounding factors may have impacted the significance of the findings.[12] A recent randomized controlled trial of FMT in IBS showed improved QOL and decreased fatigue in patients who received FMT compared to placebo.[135] In the patients who received FMT, there were changes in the intestinal bacterial composition. FMT was administered by esophagogastroduodenoscopy to the duodenum and a single super donor was used. Another randomized controlled trial of FMT in IBS administered by colonoscopy into the cecum led to significant improvement in the IBS severity scoring system.[136] FMT in IBD has limited supporting evidence. There have been no published randomized controlled trials of FMT in CD. In UC some studies have suggested efficacy,[137-139] although specific donors were found to produce the majority of the treatment benefit.[140]

# Future Perspectives

Although recognized more frequently, IBS-like symptoms in IBD remain challenging to diagnose and manage. Establishing whether certain biomarkers, genetic testing, or microbial signatures could assist in the diagnosis of, or risk for, "IBS in IBD" could potentially decrease the costs and risks associated with repeated invasive evaluations. Despite IBS-like symptoms in women with IBD being quite common, evidenced-based therapy for this group of patients is lacking. Future trials investigating the use of therapies that have been effective for IBS are urgently needed in patients with quiescent IBD who have symptoms of IBS. Clinical trials addressing gender-based outcomes are important because of the frequency of IBS-like symptoms in women with IBD. Studies targeting the use of probiotics, antibiotics, dietary modifications, and other microbiota-directed therapies will help guide management strategies in this group of patients.

---

## KEY POINTS

1. Gastrointestinal symptoms such as pain, bloating, and altered bowel habit are common among patients with IBD who are in apparent remission.

2. Care must be taken to exclude IBD activity before attaching a label of IBS—fecal levels of calprotectin or lactoferrin may prove helpful in this regard though endoscopic studies may be necessary for confirmation.

3. Once active disease has been excluded, alternative diagnoses such as medication side effects, SIBO, carbohydrate malabsorption, BAD, PEI, and pelvic floor dysfunction should be considered.

4. If it is concluded that IBS is the cause of persistent symptoms, therapy should follow principles developed for the management of IBS, in general, though one should remain mindful of any impacts on IBD complications, such as stenosis.

5. There are very little evidence-based data to guide the use of IBS therapies in IBS; though there are data to support the use of the low-FODMAP diet.

---

# References

1. Drossman DA, Hasler WL. Rome IV-functional GI disorders: disorders of gut-brain interaction. *Gastroenterology.* 2016;150(6):1257-1261.

2. Ford AC, Moayyedi P, Chey WD, et al. American College of Gastroenterology monograph on management of irritable bowel syndrome. *Am J Gastroenterol.* 2018;113(Suppl 2):1-18.

3. Baars JE, Nuij VJ, Oldenburg B, Kuipers EJ, van der Woude CJ. Majority of patients with inflammatory bowel disease in clinical remission have mucosal inflammation. *Inflamm Bowel Dis.* 2012;18(9):1634-1640.

4. Gracie DJ, Williams CJ, Sood R, et al. Poor correlation between clinical disease activity and mucosal inflammation, and the role of psychological comorbidity, in inflammatory bowel disease. *Am J Gastroenterol.* 2016;111(4):541-551.

5.  Colombel JF, Keir ME, Scherl A, et al. Discrepancies between patient-reported outcomes, and endoscopic and histological appearance in UC. *Gut.* 2017;66(12):2063-2068.

6.  Gracie DJ, Hamlin JP, Ford AC. Longitudinal impact of IBS-type symptoms on disease activity, healthcare utilization, psychological health, and quality of life in inflammatory bowel disease. *Am J Gastroenterol.* 2018;113(5):702-712.

7.  Gracie DJ, Williams CJ, Sood R, et al. Negative effects on psychological health and quality of life of genuine irritable bowel syndrome-type symptoms in patients with inflammatory bowel disease. *Clin Gastroenterol Hepatol.* 2017;15(3):376-384 e5.

8.  Henriksen M, Hoivik ML, Jelsness-Jorgensen LP, Moum B, Group IS. Irritable bowel-like symptoms in ulcerative colitis are as common in patients in deep remission as in inflammation: results from a population-based study [the IBSEN study]. *J Crohns Colitis.* 2018;12(4):389-393.

9.  Hoekman DR, Zeevenhooven J, D'Haens GR, Benninga MA. The prevalence of irritable bowel syndrome-type symptoms in inflammatory bowel disease patients in remission. *Eur J Gastroenterol Hepatol.* 2017;29(9):1086-1090.

10. Jonefjall B, Ohman L, Simren M, Strid H. IBS-like symptoms in patients with ulcerative colitis in deep remission are associated with increased levels of serum cytokines and poor psychological well-being. *Inflamm Bowel Dis.* 2016;22(11):2630-2640.

11. Jonefjall B, Strid H, Ohman L, Svedlund J, Bergstedt A, Simren M. Characterization of IBS-like symptoms in patients with ulcerative colitis in clinical remission. *Neurogastroenterol Motil.* 2013;25(9):756-e578.

12. Shutkever O, Gracie DJ, Young C, Wood HM, Taylor M, John Hamlin P, et al. No significant association between the fecal microbiome and the presence of irritable bowel syndrome-type symptoms in patients with quiescent inflammatory bowel disease. *Inflamm Bowel Dis.* 2018;24(7):1597-1605.

13. Halpin SJ, Ford AC. Prevalence of symptoms meeting criteria for irritable bowel syndrome in inflammatory bowel disease: systematic review and meta-analysis. *Am J Gastroenterol.* 2012;107(10):1474-1482.

14. Abdalla MI, Sandler RS, Kappelman MD, et al. Prevalence and impact of inflammatory bowel disease-irritable bowel syndrome on patient-reported outcomes in CCFA partners. *Inflamm Bowel Dis.* 2017;23(2):325-331.

15. Sun MH, Sun LQ, Guo GL, Zhang S. Tumour necrosis factor-alpha gene -308 G > A and -238 G > A polymorphisms are associated with susceptibility to irritable bowel syndrome and drug efficacy in children. *J Clin Pharm Ther.* 2019;44(2):180-187.

16. Zucchelli M, Camilleri M, Andreasson AN, et al. Association of TNFSF15 polymorphism with irritable bowel syndrome. *Gut.* 2011;60(12):1671-1677.

17. Momozawa Y, Dmitrieva J, Theatre E, et al. IBD risk loci are enriched in multigenic regulatory modules encompassing putative causative genes. *Nat Commun.* 2018;9(1):2427.

18. Bashashati M, Moossavi S, Cremon C, et al. Colonic immune cells in irritable bowel syndrome: a systematic review and meta-analysis. *Neurogastroenterol Motil.* 2018;30(1).

19. Burns G, Carroll G, Mathe A, et al. Evidence for local and systemic immune activation in functional dyspepsia and the irritable bowel syndrome: a systematic review. *Am J Gastroenterol.* 2019;114(3):429-436.

20. Shukla R, Ghoshal U, Ranjan P, Ghoshal UC. Expression of toll-like receptors, pro-, and anti-inflammatory cytokines in relation to gut microbiota in irritable bowel syndrome: the evidence for its micro-organic basis. *J Neurogastroenterol Motil.* 2018;24(4):628-642.

21. Brint EK, MacSharry J, Fanning A, Shanahan F, Quigley EM. Differential expression of toll-like receptors in patients with irritable bowel syndrome. *Am J Gastroenterol.* 2011;106(2):329-336.

22. Pittayanon R, Lau JT, Yuan Y, et al. Gut microbiota in patients with irritable bowel syndrome-a systematic review. *Gastroenterology.* 2019;157(1):97-108.

23. Spiller R, Garsed K. Postinfectious irritable bowel syndrome. *Gastroenterology.* 2009;136(6):1979-1988.

24. Glassner KL, Abraham BP, Quigley EMM. The microbiome and inflammatory bowel disease. *J Allergy Clin Immunol.* 2020;145(1):16-27.

25. Mosli MH, Zou G, Garg SK, et al. C-reactive protein, fecal calprotectin, and stool lactoferrin for detection of endoscopic activity in symptomatic inflammatory bowel disease patients: a systematic review and meta-analysis. *Am J Gastroenterol.* 2015;110(6):802-819; quiz 20.

26. Panes J, Jairath V, Levesque BG. Advances in use of endoscopy, radiology, and biomarkers to monitor inflammatory bowel diseases. *Gastroenterology.* 2017;152(2):362-373 e3.

27. D'Haens G, Ferrante M, Vermeire S, et al. Fecal calprotectin is a surrogate marker for endoscopic lesions in inflammatory bowel disease. *Inflamm Bowel Dis.* 2012;18(12):2218-2224.

28. Kawashima K, Ishihara S, Yuki T, et al. Fecal calprotectin more accurately predicts endoscopic remission of Crohn's disease than serological biomarkers evaluated using balloon-assisted enteroscopy. *Inflamm Bowel Dis.* 2017;23(11):2027-2034.

29. Patel A, Panchal H, Dubinsky MC. Fecal calprotectin levels predict histological healing in ulcerative colitis. *Inflamm Bowel Dis.* 2017;23(9):1600-1604.

30.  Menees SB, Powell C, Kurlander J, Goel A, Chey WD. A meta-analysis of the utility of C-reactive protein, erythrocyte sedimentation rate, fecal calprotectin, and fecal lactoferrin to exclude inflammatory bowel disease in adults with IBS. *Am J Gastroenterol.* 2015;110(3):444-454.

31.  Chen CC, Huang JL, Chang CJ, Kong MS. Fecal calprotectin as a correlative marker in clinical severity of infectious diarrhea and usefulness in evaluating bacterial or viral pathogens in children. *J Pediatr Gastroenterol Nutr.* 2012;55(5):541-57.

32.  Chateau T, Feakins R, Marchal-Bressenot A, Magro F, Danese S, Peyrin-Biroulet L. Histological remission in ulcerative colitis: under the microscope is the cure. *Am J Gastroenterol.* 2020;115(2):179-189.

33.  Monteiro S, Barbosa M, Curdia Goncalves T, et al. Fecal calprotectin as a selection tool for small bowel capsule endoscopy in suspected Crohn's disease. *Inflamm Bowel Dis.* 2018;24(9):2033-2038.

34.  Stawczyk-Eder K, Eder P, Lykowska-Szuber L, et al. Is faecal calprotectin equally useful in all Crohn's disease locations? A prospective, comparative study. *Arch Med Sci.* 2015;11(2):353-361.

35.  Ye L, Cheng W, Chen BQ, et al. Levels of faecal calprotectin and magnetic resonance enterocolonography correlate with severity of small bowel Crohn's disease: a retrospective cohort study. *Sci Rep.* 2017;7(1):1970.

36.  Abraham B, Sellin JH. Drug-induced diarrhea. *Curr Gastroenterol Rep.* 2007;9(5):365-372.

37.  Juckett G, Trivedi R. Evaluation of chronic diarrhea. *Am Fam Physician.* 2011;84(10):1119-1126.

38.  Bharucha AE, Pemberton JH, Locke GR, 3rd. American Gastroenterological Association technical review on constipation. *Gastroenterology.* 2013;144(1):218-238.

39.  Pimentel M, Saad RJ, Long MD, Rao SSC. ACG clinical guideline: small intestinal bacterial overgrowth. *Am J Gastroenterol.* 2020;115(2):165-178.

40.  Shah A, Morrison M, Burger D, et al. Systematic review with meta-analysis: the prevalence of small intestinal bacterial overgrowth in inflammatory bowel disease. *Aliment Pharmacol Ther.* 2019;49(6):624-635.

41.  Castiglione F, Del Vecchio Blanco G, Rispo A, et al. Orocecal transit time and bacterial overgrowth in patients with Crohn's disease. *J Clin Gastroenterol.* 2000;31(1):63-66.

42.  Sachdeva S, Rawat AK, Reddy RS, Puri AS. Small intestinal bacterial overgrowth (SIBO) in irritable bowel syndrome: frequency and predictors. *J Gastroenterol Hepatol.* 2011;26 Suppl 3:135-138.

43.  Pimentel M, Chow EJ, Lin HC. Eradication of small intestinal bacterial overgrowth reduces symptoms of irritable bowel syndrome. *Am J Gastroenterol.* 2000;95(12):3503-3506.

44.  Gu P, Patel D, Lakhoo K, et al. Breath test gas patterns in inflammatory bowel disease with concomitant irritable bowel syndrome-like symptoms: a controlled large-scale database linkage analysis. *Dig Dis Sci.* 2020;65(8):2388-2396

45.  Cohen-Mekelburg S, Tafesh Z, Coburn E, et al. Testing and treating small intestinal bacterial overgrowth reduces symptoms in patients with inflammatory bowel disease. *Dig Dis Sci.* 2018;63(9):2439-2444.

46.  Barrett JS, Irving PM, Shepherd SJ, Muir JG, Gibson PR. Comparison of the prevalence of fructose and lactose malabsorption across chronic intestinal disorders. *Aliment Pharmacol Ther.* 2009;30(2):165-174.

47.  Mishkin B, Yalovsky M, Mishkin S. Increased prevalence of lactose malabsorption in Crohn's disease patients at low risk for lactose malabsorption based on ethnic origin. *Am J Gastroenterol.* 1997;92(7):1148-1153.

48.  Szilagyi A, Malolepszy P, Yesovitch S, et al. Fructose malabsorption may be gender dependent and fails to show compensation by colonic adaptation. *Dig Dis Sci.* 2007;52(11):2999-3004.

49.  Vitek L. Bile acid malabsorption in inflammatory bowel disease. *Inflamm Bowel Dis.* 2015;21(2):476-483.

50.  Gothe F, Beigel F, Rust C, Hajji M, Koletzko S, Freudenberg F. Bile acid malabsorption assessed by 7 alpha-hydroxy-4-cholesten-3-one in pediatric inflammatory bowel disease: correlation to clinical and laboratory findings. *J Crohns Colitis.* 2014;8(9):1072-1078.

51.  Jung D, Fantin AC, Scheurer U, Fried M, Kullak-Ublick GA. Human ileal bile acid transporter gene ASBT (SLC10A2) is transactivated by the glucocorticoid receptor. *Gut.* 2004;53(1):78-84.

52.  Nyhlin H, Merrick MV, Eastwood MA. Bile acid malabsorption in Crohn's disease and indications for its assessment using SeHCAT. *Gut.* 1994;35(1):90-93.

53.  Camilleri M. Bile Acid diarrhea: prevalence, pathogenesis, and therapy. *Gut Liver.* 2015;9(3):332-339.

54.  Maconi G, Dominici R, Molteni M, et al. Prevalence of pancreatic insufficiency in inflammatory bowel diseases. Assessment by fecal elastase-1. *Dig Dis Sci.* 2008;53(1):262-270.

55.  Heikius B, Niemela S, Lehtola J, Karttunen T, Lahde S. Pancreatic duct abnormalities and pancreatic function in patients with chronic inflammatory bowel disease. *Scand J Gastroenterol.* 1996;31(5):517-523.

56.  Borello-France D, Burgio KL, Richter HE, Zyczynski H, Fitzgerald MP, Whitehead W, et al. Fecal and urinary incontinence in primiparous women. *Obstet Gynecol.* 2006;108(4):863-872.

57.  Bols EM, Hendriks EJ, Berghmans BC, Baeten CG, Nijhuis JG, de Bie RA. A systematic review of etiological factors for postpartum fecal incontinence. *Acta Obstet Gynecol Scand.* 2010;89(3):302-314.

58.  Pretlove SJ, Thompson PJ, Toozs-Hobson PM, Radley S, Khan KS. Does the mode of delivery predispose women to anal incontinence in the first year postpartum? A comparative systematic review. *BJOG.* 2008;115(4):421-434.

59. Nyam DC, Pemberton JH. Long-term results of lateral internal sphincterotomy for chronic anal fissure with particular reference to incidence of fecal incontinence. *Dis Colon Rectum*. 1999;42(10):1306-1310.

60. Rao SS, Tuteja AK, Vellema T, Kempf J, Stessman M. Dyssynergic defecation: demographics, symptoms, stool patterns, and quality of life. *J Clin Gastroenterol*. 2004;38(8):680-685.

61. Rao SS, Bharucha AE, Chiarioni G, et al. Functional Anorectal Disorders. *Gastroenterology*. 2016;150(6):1430-1442.

62. Rezaie A, Gu P, Kaplan GG, Pimentel M, Al-Darmaki AK. Dyssynergic defecation in inflammatory bowel disease: a systematic review and meta-analysis. *Inflamm Bowel Dis*. 2018;24(5):1065-1073.

63. Perera LP, Ananthakrishnan AN, Guilday C, et al. Dyssynergic defecation: a treatable cause of persistent symptoms when inflammatory bowel disease is in remission. *Dig Dis Sci*. 2013;58(12):3600-3605.

64. Mitomi H, Okayasu I, Bronner MP, et al. Comparative histologic assessment of proctocolectomy specimens from Japanese and American patients with ulcerative colitis with or without dysplasia. *Int J Surg Pathol*. 2005;13(3):259-265.

65. Yamagata M, Mikami T, Tsuruta T, et al. Submucosal fibrosis and basic-fibroblast growth factor-positive neutrophils correlate with colonic stenosis in cases of ulcerative colitis. *Digestion*. 2011;84(1):12-21.

66. de Bruyn JR, Meijer SL, Wildenberg ME, Bemelman WA, van den Brink GR, D'Haens GR. Development of fibrosis in acute and longstanding ulcerative colitis. *J Crohns Colitis*. 2015;9(11):966-972.

67. D'Haens G, Rieder F, Feagan BG, et al. Challenges in the pathophysiology, diagnosis and management of intestinal fibrosis in inflammatory bowel disease. *Gastroenterology*. 2019;S0016-5085(19)41035-4.

68. Chial HJ, Camilleri M. Gender differences in irritable bowel syndrome. *J Gend Specif Med*. 2002;5(3):37-45.

69. Bonfiglio F, Zheng T, Garcia-Etxebarria K, et al. Female-specific association between variants on chromosome 9 and self-reported diagnosis of irritable bowel syndrome. *Gastroenterology*. 2018;155(1):168-179.

70. Guarino M, Cheng L, Cicala M, Ripetti V, Biancani P, Behar J. Progesterone receptors and serotonin levels in colon epithelial cells from females with slow transit constipation. *Neurogastroenterol Motil*. 2011;23(6):575-e210.

71. Cremon C, Carini G, Wang B, et al. Intestinal serotonin release, sensory neuron activation, and abdominal pain in irritable bowel syndrome. *Am J Gastroenterol*. 2011;106(7):1290-1298.

72. Hutson WR, Roehrkasse RL, Wald A. Influence of gender and menopause on gastric emptying and motility. *Gastroenterology*. 1989;96(1):11-17.

73. Meier R, Beglinger C, Dederding JP, et al. Influence of age, gender, hormonal status and smoking habits on colonic transit time. *Neurogastroenterol Motil*. 1995;7(4):235-238.

74. Adeyemo MA, Spiegel BM, Chang L. Meta-analysis: do irritable bowel syndrome symptoms vary between men and women? *Aliment Pharmacol Ther*. 2010;32(6):738-755.

75. Lovell RM, Ford AC. Effect of gender on prevalence of irritable bowel syndrome in the community: systematic review and meta-analysis. *Am J Gastroenterol*. 2012;107(7):991-1000.

76. Craft RM. Modulation of pain by estrogens. *Pain*. 2007;132 Suppl 1:S3-12.

77. Kim YS, Kim N. Sex-gender differences in irritable bowel syndrome. *J Neurogastroenterol Motil*. 2018;24(4):544-558.

78. Chang L, Toner BB, Fukudo S, et al. Gender, age, society, culture, and the patient's perspective in the functional gastrointestinal disorders. *Gastroenterology*. 2006;130(5):1435-1446.

79. Georgescu D, Reisz D, Gurban CV, et al. Migraine in young females with irritable bowel syndrome: still a challenge. *Neuropsychiatr Dis Treat*. 2018;14:21-28.

80. Heitkemper MM, Chang L. Do fluctuations in ovarian hormones affect gastrointestinal symptoms in women with irritable bowel syndrome? *Gend Med*. 2009;6 Suppl 2:152-167.

81. Mulak A, Tache Y. Sex difference in irritable bowel syndrome: do gonadal hormones play a role? *Gastroenterol Pol*. 2010;17(2):89-97.

82. Camilleri M, Mayer EA, Drossman DA, et al. Improvement in pain and bowel function in female irritable bowel patients with alosetron, a 5-HT3 receptor antagonist. *Aliment Pharmacol Ther*. 1999;13(9):1149-1159.

83. Ford AC, Brandt LJ, Young C, Chey WD, Foxx-Orenstein AE, Moayyedi P. Efficacy of 5-HT3 antagonists and 5-HT4 agonists in irritable bowel syndrome: systematic review and meta-analysis. *Am J Gastroenterol*. 2009;104(7):1831-1843; quiz 44.

84. Scott LJ, Perry CM. Tegaserod. *Drugs*. 1999;58(3):491-496; discussion 7-8.

85. Zheng Y, Yu T, Tang Y, et al. Efficacy and safety of 5-hydroxytryptamine 3 receptor antagonists in irritable bowel syndrome: a systematic review and meta-analysis of randomized controlled trials. *PLoS One*. 2017;12(3):e0172846.

86. Drossman DA, Chey WD, Johanson JF, et al. Clinical trial: lubiprostone in patients with constipation-associated irritable bowel syndrome—results of two randomized, placebo-controlled studies. *Aliment Pharmacol Ther*. 2009;29(3):329-341.

87. Brotherton CS, Martin CA, Long MD, Kappelman MD, Sandler RS. Avoidance of fiber is associated with greater risk of Crohn's disease flare in a 6-month period. *Clin Gastroenterol Hepatol*. 2016;14(8):1130-1136.

88. Hallert C, Kaldma M, Petersson BG. Ispaghula husk may relieve gastrointestinal symptoms in ulcerative colitis in remission. *Scand J Gastroenterol*. 1991;26(7):747-750.

89. Bijkerk CJ, Muris JW, Knottnerus JA, Hoes AW, de Wit NJ. Systematic review: the role of different types of fibre in the treatment of irritable bowel syndrome. *Aliment Pharmacol Ther*. 2004;19(3):245-251.

90. Rubin DT, Ananthakrishnan AN, Siegel CA, Sauer BG, Long MD. ACG clinical guideline: ulcerative colitis in adults. *Am J Gastroenterol*. 2019;114(3):384-413.

91. Hovdenak N. Loperamide treatment of the irritable bowel syndrome. *Scand J Gastroenterol Suppl*. 1987;130:81-84.

92. Lavo B, Stenstam M, Nielsen AL. Loperamide in treatment of irritable bowel syndrome--a double-blind placebo controlled study. *Scand J Gastroenterol Suppl*. 1987;130:77-80.

93. van Outryve M, Toussaint J. Loperamide oxide for the treatment of chronic diarrhoea in Crohn's disease. *J Int Med Res*. 1995;23(5):335-341.

94. Lembo AJ, Lacy BE, Zuckerman MJ, et al. Eluxadoline for irritable bowel syndrome with diarrhea. *N Engl J Med*. 2016;374(3):242-253.

95. Krause R, Ameen V, Gordon SH, et al. A randomized, double-blind, placebo-controlled study to assess efficacy and safety of 0.5 mg and 1 mg alosetron in women with severe diarrhea-predominant IBS. *Am J Gastroenterol*. 2007;102(8):1709-1719.

96. Miller DP, Alfredson T, Cook SF, Sands BE, Walker AM. Incidence of colonic ischemia, hospitalized complications of constipation, and bowel surgery in relation to use of alosetron hydrochloride. *Am J Gastroenterol*. 2003;98(5):1117-1122.

97. Awad RA, Camacho S. A randomized, double-blind, placebo-controlled trial of polyethylene glycol effects on fasting and postprandial rectal sensitivity and symptoms in hypersensitive constipation-predominant irritable bowel syndrome. *Colorectal Dis*. 2010;12(11):1131-1138.

98. Chapman RW, Stanghellini V, Geraint M, Halphen M. Randomized clinical trial: macrogol/PEG 3350 plus electrolytes for treatment of patients with constipation associated with irritable bowel syndrome. *Am J Gastroenterol*. 2013;108(9):1508-1515.

99. Chey WD, Webster L, Sostek M, Lappalainen J, Barker PN, Tack J. Naloxegol for opioid-induced constipation in patients with noncancer pain. *N Engl J Med*. 2014;370(25):2387-2396.

100. Michna E, Blonsky ER, Schulman S, et al. Subcutaneous methylnaltrexone for treatment of opioid-induced constipation in patients with chronic, nonmalignant pain: a randomized controlled study. *J Pain*. 2011;12(5):554-562.

101. Webster L, Chey WD, Tack J, Lappalainen J, Diva U, Sostek M. Randomised clinical trial: the long-term safety and tolerability of naloxegol in patients with pain and opioid-induced constipation. *Aliment Pharmacol Ther*. 2014;40(7):771-779.

102. Webster L, Dhar S, Eldon M, Masuoka L, Lappalainen J, Sostek M. A phase 2, double-blind, randomized, placebo-controlled, dose-escalation study to evaluate the efficacy, safety, and tolerability of naloxegol in patients with opioid-induced constipation. *Pain*. 2013;154(9):1542-1550.

103. Pimentel M, Park S, Mirocha J, Kane SV, Kong Y. The effect of a nonabsorbed oral antibiotic (rifaximin) on the symptoms of the irritable bowel syndrome: a randomized trial. *Ann Intern Med*. 2006;145(8):557-563.

104. Sharara AI, Aoun E, Abdul-Baki H, Mounzer R, Sidani S, Elhajj I. A randomized double-blind placebo-controlled trial of rifaximin in patients with abdominal bloating and flatulence. *Am J Gastroenterol*. 2006;101(2):326-333.

105. Jigaranu AO, Nedelciuc O, Blaj A, et al. Is rifaximin effective in maintaining remission in Crohn's disease? *Dig Dis*. 2014;32(4):378-383.

106. Prantera C, Lochs H, Grimaldi M, et al. Rifaximin-extended intestinal release induces remission in patients with moderately active Crohn's disease. *Gastroenterology*. 2012;142(3):473-481 e4.

107. Acosta A, Camilleri M, Shin A, et al. Effects of Rifaximin on transit, permeability, fecal microbiome, and organic acid excretion in irritable bowel syndrome. *Clin Transl Gastroenterol*. 2016;7:e173.

108. Soldi S, Vasileiadis S, Uggeri F, et al. Modulation of the gut microbiota composition by rifaximin in non-constipated irritable bowel syndrome patients: a molecular approach. *Clin Exp Gastroenterol*. 2015;8:309-325.

109. Whelan K, Quigley EM. Probiotics in the management of irritable bowel syndrome and inflammatory bowel disease. *Curr Opin Gastroenterol*. 2013;29(2):184-189.

110. Abraham BP, Quigley EMM. Probiotics in inflammatory bowel disease. *Gastroenterol Clin North Am*. 2017;46(4):769-782.

111. Agger JL, Schroder A, Gormsen LK, Jensen JS, Jensen TS, Fink PK. Imipramine versus placebo for multiple functional somatic syndromes (STreSS-3): a double-blind, randomised study. *Lancet Psychiatry*. 2017;4(5):378-388.

112. Drossman DA, Toner BB, Whitehead WE, et al. Cognitive-behavioral therapy versus education and desipramine versus placebo for moderate to severe functional bowel disorders. *Gastroenterology*. 2003;125(1):19-31.

113. Tabas G, Beaves M, Wang J, Friday P, Mardini H, Arnold G. Paroxetine to treat irritable bowel syndrome not responding to high-fiber diet: a double-blind, placebo-controlled trial. *Am J Gastroenterol*. 2004;99(5):914-920.

114. Vahedi H, Merat S, Momtahen S, et al. Clinical trial: the effect of amitriptyline in patients with diarrhoea-predominant irritable bowel syndrome. *Aliment Pharmacol Ther*. 2008;27(8):678-684.

115. Iskandar HN, Cassell B, Kanuri N, et al. Tricyclic antidepressants for management of residual symptoms in inflammatory bowel disease. *J Clin Gastroenterol*. 2014;48(5):423-429.

116. Goodhand JR, Greig FI, Koodun Y, et al. Do antidepressants influence the disease course in inflammatory bowel disease? A retrospective case-matched observational study. *Inflamm Bowel Dis.* 2012;18(7):1232-1239.

117. Barbara G, Cremon C, Annese V, et al. Randomised controlled trial of mesalazine in IBS. *Gut.* 2016;65(1):82-90.

118. Lam C, Tan W, Leighton M, et al. A mechanistic multicentre, parallel group, randomised placebo-controlled trial of mesalazine for the treatment of IBS with diarrhoea (IBS-D). *Gut.* 2016;65(1):91-99.

119. Lichtenstein GR, Feagan BG, Cohen RD, et al. Serious infection and mortality in patients with Crohn's disease: more than 5 years of follow-up in the TREAT registry. *Am J Gastroenterol.* 2012;107(9):1409-1422.

120. Alley K, Singla A, Afzali A. Opioid use is associated with higher health care costs and emergency encounters in inflammatory bowel disease. *Inflamm Bowel Dis.* 2019;25(12):1990-1995.

121. Drossman D, Szigethy E. The narcotic bowel syndrome: a recent update. *Am J Gastroenterol Suppl.* 2014;2(1):22-30.

122. Singh S, Graff LA, Bernstein CN. Do NSAIDs, antibiotics, infections, or stress trigger flares in IBD? *Am J Gastroenterol.* 2009;104(5):1298-1313; quiz 314.

123. Takeuchi K, Smale S, Premchand P, et al. Prevalence and mechanism of nonsteroidal anti-inflammatory drug-induced clinical relapse in patients with inflammatory bowel disease. *Clin Gastroenterol Hepatol.* 2006;4(2):196-202.

124. Wolfe MM, Lichtenstein DR, Singh G. Gastrointestinal toxicity of nonsteroidal antiinflammatory drugs. *N Engl J Med.* 1999;340(24):1888-1899.

125. Mahadevan U, Loftus EV, Jr., Tremaine WJ, Sandborn WJ. Safety of selective cyclooxygenase-2 inhibitors in inflammatory bowel disease. *Am J Gastroenterol.* 2002;97(4):910-914.

126. MacDermott RP. Treatment of irritable bowel syndrome in outpatients with inflammatory bowel disease using a food and beverage intolerance, food and beverage avoidance diet. *Inflamm Bowel Dis.* 2007;13(1):91-96.

127. Halmos EP, Power VA, Shepherd SJ, Gibson PR, Muir JG. A diet low in FODMAPs reduces symptoms of irritable bowel syndrome. *Gastroenterology.* 2014;146(1):67-75 e5.

128. Cox SR, Lindsay JO, Fromentin S, et al. Effects of low FODMAP diet on symptoms, fecal microbiome, and markers of inflammation in patients with quiescent inflammatory bowel disease in a randomized trial. *Gastroenterology.* 2020;158(1):176-188 e7.

129. Naliboff BD, Kim SE, Bolus R, Bernstein CN, Mayer EA, Chang L. Gastrointestinal and psychological mediators of health-related quality of life in IBS and IBD: a structural equation modeling analysis. *Am J Gastroenterol.* 2012;107(3):451-459.

130. Berrill JW, Sadlier M, Hood K, Green JT. Mindfulness-based therapy for inflammatory bowel disease patients with functional abdominal symptoms or high perceived stress levels. *J Crohns Colitis.* 2014;8(9):945-955.

131. Ballou S, Keefer L. Psychological interventions for irritable bowel syndrome and inflammatory bowel diseases. *Clin Transl Gastroenterol.* 2017;8(1):e214.

132. Knowles SR, Monshat K, Castle DJ. The efficacy and methodological challenges of psychotherapy for adults with inflammatory bowel disease: a review. *Inflamm Bowel Dis.* 2013;19(12):2704-2715.

133. von Wietersheim J, Kessler H. Psychotherapy with chronic inflammatory bowel disease patients: a review. *Inflamm Bowel Dis.* 2006;12(12):1175-1184.

134. Zargar A, Gooraji SA, Keshavarzi B, Haji Aghamohammadi AA. Effect of irritable bowel syndrome on sleep quality and quality of life of inflammatory bowel disease in clinical remission. *Int J Prev Med.* 2019;10:10.

135. El-Salhy M, Hatlebakk JG, Gilja OH, Brathen Kristoffersen A, Hausken T. Efficacy of faecal microbiota transplantation for patients with irritable bowel syndrome in a randomised, double-blind, placebo-controlled study. *Gut.* 2020;69(5):859-867.

136. Johnsen PH, Hilpusch F, Cavanagh JP, et al. Faecal microbiota transplantation versus placebo for moderate-to-severe irritable bowel syndrome: a double-blind, randomised, placebo-controlled, parallel-group, single-centre trial. *Lancet Gastroenterol Hepatol.* 2018;3(1):17-24.

137. Costello SP, Hughes PA, Waters O, et al. Effect of fecal microbiota transplantation on 8-week remission in patients with ulcerative colitis: a randomized clinical trial. *JAMA.* 2019;321(2):156-164.

138. Moayyedi P, Surette MG, Kim PT, et al. Fecal microbiota transplantation induces remission in patients with active ulcerative colitis in a randomized controlled trial. *Gastroenterology.* 2015;149(1):102-109 e6.

139. Paramsothy S, Kamm MA, Kaakoush NO, et al. Multidonor intensive faecal microbiota transplantation for active ulcerative colitis: a randomised placebo-controlled trial. *Lancet.* 2017;389(10075):1218-1228.

140. Paramsothy S, Paramsothy R, Rubin DT, et al. Faecal microbiota transplantation for inflammatory bowel disease: a systematic review and meta-analysis. *J Crohns Colitis.* 2017;11(10):1180-1199.

# Financial Disclosures

*Dr. Bincy P. Abraham* has no financial or proprietary interest in the materials presented herein.

*Dr. Anita Afzali* has financial interest in AbbVie, Celgene, Janssen, Pfizer, Takeda, and UCB.

*Jessica Barry* has no financial or proprietary interest in the materials presented herein.

*Dr. Nirupama Bonthala* has no financial or proprietary interest in the materials presented herein.

*Dr. Madalina Butnariu* has no financial or proprietary interest in the materials presented herein.

*Dr. Kindra Clark-Snustad* is a consultant for Takeda Pharmaceutical Company.

*Dr. Jordyn Feingold* has no financial or proprietary interest in the materials presented herein.

*Dr. Sonia Friedman* has no financial or proprietary interest in the materials presented herein.

*Dr. Jill K. J. Gaidos* has no financial or proprietary interest in the materials presented herein.

*Dr. Kerri L. Glassner* has no financial or proprietary interest in the materials presented herein.

*Kelly Issokson* has no financial or proprietary interest in the materials presented herein.

*Dr. Shelly Joseph* has no financial or proprietary interest in the materials presented herein.

*Dr. Sunanda V. Kane* has no financial or proprietary interest in the materials presented herein.

*Dr. Laurie Keefer* is a consultant to Abbvie, Eli Lilly, and Trellus Health and an equity owner in Trellus Health.

*Dr. Emilie S. Kim* has no financial or proprietary interest in the materials presented herein.

*Dr. Dana J. Lukin* is a consultant to Abbvie, Boehringer Ingelheim, Eli Lilly, Janssen, Palatin Technologies, and Pfizer; on the scientific advisory board for PSI; on the data and safety monitoring board for WuXi Apptec; and has received grants from Abbvie, Janssen, and Takeda.

*Dr. Rebecca Matro* was on the advisory board for Pfizer.

*Dr. Katrina H. Naik* has no financial or proprietary interest in the materials presented herein.

*Dr. Maria Oliva-Hemker* has no financial or proprietary interest in the materials presented herein.

*Dr. Jessica Philpott* has no financial or proprietary interest in the materials presented herein.

*Dr. Eamonn M. M. Quigley* has no financial or proprietary interest in the materials presented herein.

*Dr. Akriti P. Saxena* has no financial or proprietary interest in the materials presented herein.

*Dr. Ellen J. Scherl* has no financial or proprietary interest in the materials presented herein.

*Dr. Anil Sharma* has no financial or proprietary interest in the materials presented herein.

*Dr. Daniela Guerrero Vinsard* has no financial or proprietary interest in the materials presented herein.

*Ryan Warren* has no financial or proprietary interest in the materials presented herein.

*Dr. Sharmeel K. Wasan* has no financial or proprietary interest in the materials presented herein.

# Index

Printed in the United States
by Baker & Taylor Publisher Services